The Law of Deviation of Homeostasis and

Diseases of Aging

Vladimir M. Dilman, MD

Chief, Laboratory of Endocrinology
The Petrov Research Institute of Oncology
Leningrad, USSR

Edited by

Herman T. Blumenthal, PhD, MD

Research Professor of Gerontology
Department of Psychology
Washington University
St. Louis, Missouri

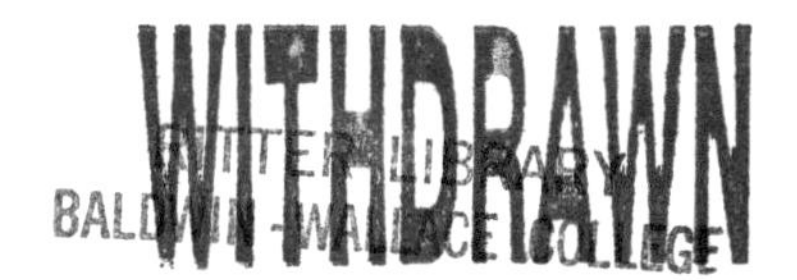

John Wright · PSG Inc
Boston · Bristol · London

Library of Congress Cataloging in Publication Data

Dil'man, Vladimir Mikhaĭlovich.
The law of deviation of homeostasis and diseases of aging.

Bibliography: p.
Includes index.
1. Age factors in disease. 2. Homeostasis. 3. Geriatrics. I. Title.
RB210.D54 618.9'7 79-21456
ISBN 0-88416-250-8

Printed in the United States of America.

International Standard Book Number: 0-88416-250-8

Library of Congress Catalog Card Number: 79-21456

To the memory of my daughter
Svetlana Blagosklonnaya

ABOUT THE AUTHOR

Vladimir M. Dilman was born in 1925 in Dnepropetrovsk, USSR. He graduated from the Medical Institute in Leningrad in 1947, and then studied internal medicine under Prof V.F. Lang, and later studied endocrinology under Prof V.G. Baranov. His work as a researcher at the Institute of Physiology of the USSR Academy of Sciences led to his PhD there in 1956. He has worked at the Petrov Research Institute of Oncology since 1958, and received a medical degree in 1964. Dr Dilman is the author of six books and over 260 contributions to scientific journals on the problems of endocrinology, gerontology, physiology, and oncology. He is a member of the board of the All-Union Society of Gerontologists, vice-president of the All-Union Problem Council for Combined Cancer Treatment, and is a member of the editorial boards of two journals, *Voprosy Onkologii* (Problems of Oncology) and *Fiziologiia Cheloveka* (Human Physiology). Dr Dilman's main scientific views in the field of research are represented in this monograph.

PERSONAL SKETCH ABOUT THE EDITOR

Herman T. Blumenthal was born in New York City in 1913. His graduate degrees include an MS in cellular physiology from the University of Pennsylvania (1936), a PhD in experimental pathology (1938) and an MD (1942) from Washington University in St. Louis. After completion of a residency in pathology he served in the US Army for three years during World War II, attaining the rank of Major, and the assignment as Commanding Officer of the 29th Medical Laboratory in the China-Burma-India Theater. Subsequent positions include those of Director of Laboratories of several hospitals, and of Associate Professor in the Department of Pathology of St. Louis University School of Medicine. Currently he is Research Professor of Gerontology in the Aging and Development Program of the department of Psychology at Washington University, Adjunct Professor in the Department of Community Medicine at St. Louis University School of Medicine, and Director-Pathologist of Medwest Medical Laboratory.

Dr. Blumenthal's interest in aging derives from research on his Master's program under Professor Louis V. Heilbrun and from studies on his PhD program under Professor Leo Loeb. His research includes some 160 papers on aging, endocrinology, cancer, transplantation, diabetes, and autoimmunity. He is co-author or editor of three books and editor of the first eight volumes of *Interdisciplinary Topics in Gerontology*. Dr. Blumenthal has also written articles for popular publications and is presently Book Editor of the Journal of Gerontology. He is a member of ten national and international scientific organizations and has served as an officer in three.

CONTENTS

FOREWORD

For many decades conventional thinking has held that normal aging is genetically programmed while aging-associated diseases are not so programmed, and therefore somehow separate. For some years I have taken issue with such a concept, and to emphasize the nature of the problem, I have even resorted to the eye-catching expression "Aging and Disease – A Casual or Causal Connection?" to the consternation of some proofreaders. It was therefore with great initial interest and subsequent enthusiasm that I first encountered Professor Dilman's 1971 *Lancet* article entitled "Age-Associated Elevation of Hypothalamic Threshold to Feedback Control and Its Role in Development, Aging, and Disease (Dilman 1971).

During the past decade several investigators have been converging, from somewhat different perspectives, on the concept that aging and aging-associated disease are linked in some direct fashion. In Great Britain P.R.J. Burch (1969) has provided mathematical formulations based on vital statistics which implicate somatic mutations and the immune system in both normal aging phenomena and aging-related disease. In Australia Burnet (1974), while proposing a similar mechanism, has suggested that the link between aging and associated diseases ultimately derives from the genetic programming of DNA polymerases and their ultimate loss of ability to repair DNA damage. In his view failure of this mechanism leads to the accumulation of mutated cells that affect all organs including the immune system, and to failure of the latter to censor deviant cells. And in the United States, Walford (1969) has approached the problem primarily from the standpoint of identifying mechanisms which express failure of the immune system, while this writer (Blumenthal 1968) has dealt with the identification of parameters in precise mechanism. Some physiological studies are currently in progress, particularly by Finch (1976), but there have been remarkably few morphologic studies dealing directly with aging changes in hypothalamic neurons, and virtually no investigations dealing with possible immunopathologic phenomena. In a recent volume edited by A.V. Everitt and J.S. Burgess, titled *Hypothalamus, Pituitary, and Aging* (1976), Aschheim (1976) notes that there is little certainty as to the diminution in the number of hypothalamic neurons with age. He cites Andrew (1956) as noting an absence of evidence of neuronal destruction in the senile hypothalamus; and Bottlar-Brentano (1954) as describing an increase in neuronal cellular volume leading to giant neurons up to ten times the adult size, and cells containing two to three nuclei showing increased basophilia, sometimes with two to six nucleoli. Andrew interprets these changes as "reactive" or "defensive." In this same volume, Frolkis (1976) reports on a study in rats from which he concludes that in old animals there is no evidence of a decrease in the production of neurosecretory granules, but rather retarded secretion. He also shows a failure (or diminution) of secretory activity following appropriate electrical stimulation of neurons.

These observations provide some support for Dilman's central thesis documented in this volume: namely, a loss of sensitivity of hypothalamic neurons to feedback signals, neural or endocrine, and indications of an elevation in hypothalamic set-point. But the mechanism(s) responsible for this phenomenon remains to be elucidated. My own hypothesis in this regard is that there may be aging-dependent changes in cell surface receptors and/or in hormonal feedback signals. Dilman's observations on non-phenolic steroids presented in this volume suggest the possibility of a more general aging-dependent mis-specification of hormones, particularly those of polypeptide character.

The foregoing remarks are intended solely to indicate some future lines of research deriving from the fundamental Dilman concept. His work would merit a comprehensive publication under any circumstances, but when one realizes that many of us in the Western world obtain much of our information through delayed abstracts and a limited number of selected translations, a comprehensive publication in English becomes imperative. Professor Dilman, with Mr. Arkhipov's assistance has now completed this difficult task. It is revealing, on the other hand, that the extensive bibliography accompanying this volume reflects his comprehension of investigations published in English.

Aside from the great intrinsic value of this volume, I would hope that it would also serve to broaden the bridge between Eastern and Western gerontology.

Herman T. Blumenthal, PhD, MD

SELECTED READINGS

Andrew, W. Structural alterations with aging in the nervous system. *J Chronic Dis.* 3:575, 1956.

Aschheim, P. Aging in the hypothalamic-hypophyseal ovarian axis in the rat. Edited by A.V. Everitt and J.A. Burgess. In *Hypothalamus, Pituitary, and Aging*. Springfield, Ill.: Charles C Thomas, Publisher, 1976, pp. 376–418.

Blumenthal, H.T., and Probstein, J.G. The pathogenesis of diseases of senescence. Edited by J.H. Powers. In *Surgery of the Aged and Debilitated Patient*. Philadelphia: W.B. Saunders Co., 1968, pp. 44–81.

Bottlar-Brentano, K. Zur Lebensgeschichte des Nucleus basalis, tuberomammilaris, supraopticus and paraventrincularis unter normalen und pathogenen Bedingungen. *J Hirnforschung*. 1:337, 1954.

Burch, P.R.J. *An Inquiry Concerning Growth, Disease, and Aging*. Toronto: University of Toronto Press, 1969.

Burnet, F.M. *Intrinsic Mutagenesis: A Genetic Approach of Aging*. New York: John Wiley and Sons, 1974.

Dilman, V. Age-associated elevation of hypothalamic threshold to feedback control, and its role in development, aging, and disease. *Lancet* 1:1211, 1971.

Everitt, A.V., and Burgess, J.A., Editors. *Hypothalamus, Pituitary, and Aging*. Springfield, Ill.: Charles C Thomas, Publisher, 1976.

Finch, C.E. Cell differentiation, extrinsic factors and aging. Edited by R.G. Cutler. In *Cellular Aging: General Concepts and Mechanism. Part I. Fidelity of Information Flow*. Basel: S. Karger, 1976, pp. 8–15.

Frolkis, V.V. The hypothalamic mechanisms of aging. Edited by A.V. Everitt, and J.A. Burgess. In *Hypothalamus, Pituitary and Aging*. Springfield, Ill.: Charles C Thomas, Publisher, 1976, pp. 614–633.

Walford, R.L. *The Immunologic Theory of Aging*. Baltimore: The Williams and Wilkins Co., 1969.

PART I
The Law of Deviation of Homeostasis and the Organism's Development

If the stability of internal environment of the organism provides the body with a certain degree of functional freedom from the variability of external and internal environmental factors, the programmed deviation of homeostasis is an essential condition of development of an organism. Therefore, along with the Law of Constancy of Internal Environment there exists the Law of Deviation of Homeostasis.

1 Introduction[1]

Природа—сфинкс. И тем она верней
Своим искусом губит человека,
Что, может статься, никакой от века
Загадки нет и не было у ней.[2]
ф.Тютчев (1869)

[1] In order to validate the basic theses of my concept, it is necessary that the reader familiarize himself with the numerous data presented in this book. However, it is possible to draw the same conclusions on the basis of purely logical reasoning. An attempt has been made to introduce the reader to the concept as a whole—by using mainly the generally known data and/or logical reasoning, which has resulted in this extensive "Introduction."

[2] Nature is a sphinx. And it ruling Man
In a surer way by challenging him to unravel
Its riddle which, perhaps, does not exist
And has never existed.

Let us consider a hypothetical situation that would seem both typical and somewhat unreal. A woman of 53 entered a consulting medical department divided into two sections, each with a doctor specializing in a particular branch of clinical medicine. Numerous tests were made on the patient. The results are shown in Table 1-1. Each doctor was supposed to determine whether the patient was suffering from any disease, and diagnose the disease, if any. The trouble was that each physician was very good in his field, but was not well versed in other specialties. (The situation would not seem improbable if one recalled that it took 54 highly qualified authors to compile one good book on diabetes mellitus [Williams 1960].)

Table 1-1
Endometrial Carcinoma – Illustration of Integrated Disease

Parameter (or disturbance)	Frequency of Disturbance
Diabetes mellitus (chemical, latent, or overt)	63%–73%
Obesity	21%–72%
Arterial hypertension	40%
Hypercholosterolemia (atherosclerosis)	64.1%
Climacteric bleeding and late menopause	27.7%–59%
Dexamethasone suppression test (dysadaptosis, latent cushingoid signs, psychic depression)	Resistance to inhibition in most patients
Metabolic immunodepression	In most patients
Antibodies to thyroglobulin	25%
Birth of large baby (acceleration of development)	42.6%
Glucose suppression test (aging-like symptom)	Resistance to inhibition or paradoxical reaction in most patients

Source: Dilman 1974a.

The patient consulted the first of the ten doctors, an endocrinologist, who promptly diagnosed diabetes mellitus on the strength of the blood and urine test results. He prescribed a course of treatment in the endocrinology department. The patient was then examined by the other doctors. Eventually she had ten prescriptions from different clinics. She was sent to an internal medicine clinic for treatment of high blood pressure, to a metabolic department for treatment of obesity, to a cardiology clinic for suspected ischemic heart disease because of high blood cholesterol and β-lipoprotein levels. The gynecologist diagnosed a late menopause and, at the same time, an early switching-on of the reproductive function. The patient was sent to a gynecology clinic to be treated for a uterine climacteric bleeding caused by adenomatous hyperplasia of the endometrium. The psychiatrist noticed an impaired sensitivity to dexamethasone suppression test (see Chapter 14), and had every reason to suppose an age-related depressive illness. Still another physician, taking part in this ideal round of medical examinations, was a specialist in clinical immunology; he determined two disorders: metabolic immunodepression (see Chapter 15) and autoimmune thyroiditis (see Chapter 16). The pediatric specialist was intrigued by the fact that the patient had had her baby 13 years before, and the baby had weighed more than 4 kg. Consequently the specialist was interested in both the patient and her daughter, because in his study of "accelerated development" he had often noticed a correlation between belated childbirth and a "large baby" (see Chapter 21). As a result, both the patient and her daughter were offered a thorough examination in a specialized pediatric clinic. The specialist in gerontology detected signs of early aging because the figures in nearly all tests were outside the upper limit allowed for her age (see Chapter 10). Finally the patient was taken into an oncology clinic with the diagnosis of endometrial carcinoma—her tenth disease diagnosed by the tenth specialist.

What could have caused all these diseases to develop in one person? Why those specific illnesses out of the vast spectrum of all possible diseases? Why does the frequency of a certain disease increase regularly with advancing age?

One could easily produce convincing arguments supporting not only the concept that the development of an organism is programmed, but also the concept that development of certain diseases is programmed, which eventually terminate in death, also a programmed phenomenon. Such an example is provided by the regulatory death of the spawning Pacific salmon (Robertson et al 1961a, 1961b). The direct cause of that regulatory death of the spawning Pacific salmon is the disturbance of metabolism (Wexler 1975). From the data given by Robertson et al (1961) for the period before spawning, when the salmon is still in the ocean, an intense accumulation of fat stores takes place in the liver and the muscles (formation of a hump). When the salmon is in the ocean during the spawning period the blood level of 11-hydroxysteroid is 11.8 mg%; when in the river, the concentration goes up to 105 mg%; glucose concentration is 99 mg% and 198 mg%, respectively. The blood cholesterol will rise to as much as 1000 mg% during spawning, leading to myocardial, cerebral, renal, and other infarction damage, and eventually programmed death (Wexler 1976). The concept of programmed disease and death seems even more likely when one compares the causes of natural death in such different species as the salmon, rat, and human (Table 1-2). Had we not been speaking of the mechanism of death, we ought to consider it a wonder of perfection, this similarity of natural causes of death in higher organisms.

Table 1-2
Age-Specific Pathology and Causes of Death in Pacific Salmon, Rats, and Humans

Pacific Salmon	Rat	Man
Hyperglycemia	Hyperglycemia	Hyperglycemia
Hyperlipidemia	Hyperinsulinemia	Hyperinsulinemia
	Hypertriglyceridemia	Hypertriglyceridemia
Hypercholesterolemia	Hypercholesterolemia	Hypercholesterolemia
Hyperplasia of adrenal cortex	Hyperplasia of adrenal cortex	Relative excess of glucocorticoids
Thymic involution	Thymic involution	Thymic involution
Obesity	Overweight	Overweight
Myocardial, cerebral, renal, and other infraction damage	Arterial hypertension, nephrosclerosis, arteriosclerosis, continuous estrus, myocardial infarction, adenoma of pituitary, tumors	Diseases of compensation: climacteric dysadaptosis, maturity-onset diabetes mellitus, metabolic immunodepression, autoimmune disorders, atherosclerosis, essential hypertension, psychic depression, cancer

Source: Wexler 1971.

Now, if we admit that some diseases and death are programmed, then we shall have to accept the unacceptable, ie, that Nature has a special purpose embodied in specially programmed mechanisms whose action provides for the death of every organism. On the other hand, if Nature had not set a purpose to discontinue every individual existence, why is that purpose achieved in similar ways?

If we consider the example of the "programmed death" of the Pacific salmon, the following answer to the above question seems probable. Although the direct cause of natural death of the Pacific salmon is the dramatic increase in blood levels of cholesterol, the high concentration of cholesterol is necessary for a high production of spawn in which cholesterol forms the structural basis of the cellular membrane. In turn, the higher cholesterol synthesis can only be provided by an increase of fat content that is accumulated in the liver and in the "reservoir" of the hump (see Chapter 6). Adiposity is caused by the overproduction of adrenal cortex hormones before spawning, which results in poor glucose utilization and speeds up the adiposity. An increased cholesterol synthesis is provided for by intensive utilization of free fatty acids (see Chapter 6). But simultaneously, the higher blood level of cholesterol causes atherosclerotic lesions of the heart, kidneys, brain, and lungs (Wexler 1971). Thus, the surplus of blood cholesterol level provides for the process of reproduction, while the death of the salmon is a by-product of the realization of the reproductive mechanism. Bearing this in mind, we can say that no special mechanism of death is programmed in the salmon, but at the same time the mechanism of death is realized with such regularity that one cannot help believing in the existence of such a mechanism. That is how Nature offers an optimal pathway to death for each organism of the species, based on regularities of the developmental program. Nature does not aim at discontinuing the individual existence of each organism, but only provides for the reproductive program.

But could this example be the particular case that Nature long ago rejected in the process of evolution? In order to be able to answer the question we should consider the particular and general aspects of this unique example.

Claude Bernard (1878) first stated that the composition of fluids bathing the cells of a multicellular organism has to be controlled, and that the stability of this internal environment provides the body with a degree of functional freedom from the variability of external and internal environmental factors.

From this fundamental statement, the natural death of the Pacific salmon is caused by violation of the Law of Constancy of Internal Environment. Strictly speaking, any permanent violation of the Law of Constancy of Internal Environment is a disease. Hence, it can be generally stated that the natural death of the salmon is a death caused by certain diseases which, in turn, are caused by disturbances in homeostasis.

We now face the question, what causes failure in homeostasis? In this particular case of regulatory death, it was discovered that in the Kokance salmon, prevention of spawning by castration prolonged the life span by several years (Robertson and Wexler 1962). That is why Wexler (1976) stresses the role of the "reproductive effort," which leads to activation of the hypothalamic-pituitary-adrenal axis and causes metabolic disturbances and death.

The particular meaning of the programmed death of the salmon is, therefore, defined by the disturbance of homeostasis promoted by the signals coming from the reproductive system, ie, the mechanism of death is switched on in strict accord with the demands of the reproductive mechanism. However, castration in mammals does not prolong the life span, as is the case with the salmon; actually, an early castration in women provokes an early development of atherosclerosis.

Thus, when considering the mechanism of natural death in the salmon, an impression may be formed that no similar mechanism exists in any other species, nor does it have an equivalent in Nature. The impression that this mechanism is an exclusive and special phenomenon will not hold if we stop looking for likeness and similarity, but try to discover the principle forming the basis for implementation of a developmental program in higher organisms.

As has been noted before, the metabolic shift toward an intense accumulation and utilization of fat is the key element in the mechanism providing for both reproduction and natural death of the Pacific salmon. A similar phenomenon takes place in higher organisms, too. This statement can be illustrated by the changes during pregnancy (see Chapter 21).

Fetal development requires certain metabolic conditions that provide for an intensive reproduction of the cellular mass of the fetus (similar to provisions for spawning in the salmon). In particular, cell division requires a lot of cholesterol which, as has been noted before, is an important element of the cellular membrane. Cholesterol synthesis requires both an accumulation and an intensive utilization of the fatty acids. How can this metabolic shift be achieved? It is known that carbohydrate tolerance decreases in pregnancy. In many cases, the development of the so-called diabetes of pregnancy may be observed. These two features, the decreased carbohydrate tolerance and the diabetes of pregnancy, are often considered to be nonphysiologic phenomena, so the following statement may seem a paradox. The so-called diabetes of pregnancy or, more precisely, the shift to predominant utilization of free fatty acids (FFA) for energy supply observed in the maternal organism, is the manifestation of a programmed deviation of homeostasis that ensures a rapid build-up of the cell mass of the fetus, and metabolic immunodepression that prevents the rejection of the fetus as a transplant (see Chapter 15). In other words, the normal course of pregnancy is ensured by a certain combination of diabetes-like changes in the maternal organism. Let us consider this paradox.

During pregnancy the secretion of chorionic somatomammatropin, which possesses the properties of growth hormone, and the increase in cortisol output, lower glucose utilization in the maternal organism. This shift leads to the development of compensatory hyperinsulinemia, which results in the accumulation of fat and, consequently, in an intensified lipolysis in the latter half of pregnancy. Since FFA fails to pass through the placenta (Felig 1977), cholesterol synthesis in the maternal organism is intensified (see Chapter 21). Cholesterol is transferred to the fetal-placental system where it is used for cell formation and synthesis of steroid hormones. Simultaneously, hypercholesterolemia inhibits the activity of cellular (transplantation) immunity, which counteracts the rejection of the fetus as a transplant. Hence, the reason that pregnancy is inconsistent with maintaining the constancy of internal environment is because the development and growth of an organism cannot be secured in a stable homeostasis. The necessary disturbance of homeostasis in pregnancy is actually a programmed disease. However, the mechanism that provides for the development of "the normal disease of a pregnant organism" is localized in the placenta; this is the reason why the disease ends after parturition.[1]

However, a programmed deviation of homeostasis is necessary to ensure the development and growth of the organism in the postnatal period. Then, the question naturally arises, how can the deviation of homeostasis be maintained in the postnatal period, thus providing the development and growth of an organism?

We know now that the stability of internal environment is attained by the functioning of complex homeostatic systems. The interrelation between them is most apparent in the hypothalamus, in which control, regulation, communication, and integration of all the main homeostatic systems take place. The most important general principle behind this stability is negative feedback control.

If the mechanism of homeostasis had always been functioning within the same range, then stability would have been permanently maintained, prohibiting an increase in the vigor of the system and, consequently, the very development of the organism.

Thus, the development of an organism is incompatible with the maintenance of constancy of the internal environment. According to this concept, the process of development and growth in higher organisms may be ensured only if the activity of homeostatic systems is increased in consonance with growth.

But in what manner can the vigor of the homeostatic system increase? Since the stability of homeostatic systems is maintained by negative feedback, it is easy to see that the homeostatic system potential may be increased, provided the threshold of sensitivity of the central element of the system to feedback control is elevated. Now, suppose that the system power is increased because of a primary intensification in the activity of the performer, ie, the peripheral part of homeostatic system. Then the enhanced signal of its activity would inhibit the regulator from functioning by negative feedback, which would make a further increase in homeostatic system vigor impossible. On the contrary, if the threshold of the regulator's sensitivity to homeostatic stimuli is elevated, the performer is stimulated and the overall potential of the homeostatic system is increased. I designate this feature of the homeostatic system functioning in higher organisms as the principle of self-development of homeostatic systems. This principle is fundamentally distinguished from classic

[1]The fetal requirements are met as a result of the growth of the placenta and gradual intensification of its hormonal activity uninhibited by negative feedback. However, the predetermined cessation of metabolic shifts after delivery seems to be accounted for by localization of an elevating mechanism of hormonal production in the placenta, which dies in accordance with its program of development. Of considerable interest is the hypothesis that the placental death is caused by autoimmune mechanisms (Burstein et al 1973).

cybernetic systems, since the latter are set to operate so that the parameters of homeostatic system functioning are maintained at the same level. For example, when an animal is born, the reproductive mechanism should be inhibited until the body development is completed. This occurs because the sensitivity of the hypothalamus (ie, the regulator of reproductive function) to inhibition by sex hormones is maximum in the early period of life. Therefore, even a low level of sex hormones produced in immature animals suppresses hypothalamic activity in accordance with the negative feedback mechanism. Under these conditions the hypothalamus does not stimulate production of gonadotropins, and the whole reproductive system is in a state nearing stability. Theoretically, such balance ought to be preserved for a long period, during the whole life span, if the sensitivity of the hypothalamus to sex hormones could be maintained at the same level.

In 1959, Donovan and Van der Werf ten Bosch postulated on the basis of the classical experiments of Hohlweg and Döhrn (1931) that the decrease in sensitivity of the sex center to inhibition by sex hormones constitutes a fundamental change that paves the way to sexual maturity. According to the genetic program of development the threshold of regulator sensitivity is elevated with aging; therefore, the suppression of hypothalamic activity by sex hormones will be gradually relieved. This situation results in enhanced activity of the hypothalamus, sex gland development, sexual maturity, and lastly, the switching-on of reproductive function. This is how the self-development of homeostatic systems ensures the development of the organism, and in this particular case, that of reproductive function.

Thus, the activity of any homeostatic system controlled by negative feedback may be increased only if the resistance to inhibition of the central regulator of the homeostatic system is also increased, in other words, if the hypothalamic threshold of sensitivity to homeostatic stimuli is elevated. The elevation of this hypothalamic set point will inevitably lead to a compensatory increase in the activity of the peripheral elements of the homeostatic system. The process of compensation contributes to the development of the overall potential of the system, thus securing the constantly increasing requirements of the growing organism.

Thus, the elevation of the hypothalamic threshold of sensitivity to feedback control is the only mechanism by which both feedback and deviation from constancy of internal environment can be simultaneously ensured in higher organisms. This mechanism makes sure that stability is maintained at a particular moment and is disturbed with time. There is a constant trend toward the development of the central type of homeostatic failure.[1]

---

[1]Theoretically, it is possible to distinguish three main mechanisms of homeostatic failure (see Chapter 2). The elevation of the threshold of sensitivity to regulatory signals is a feature of a central type of homeostatic failure. This type of disturbance is observed in Cushing's syndrome, with a failure of suppression by glucocorticoids.

In the first place, the mechanism of the age-associated switching-on of the reproductive cycle indicates that the development is realized through an increase in the vigor of the system, which in this case is the reproductive homeostat. In this respect, there is no difference between the processes taking place in higher organisms during pregnancy and during the postnatal period. Moreover, in higher organisms the requirements of development are met, in principle, in the same manner as in the spawning Pacific salmon. The only difference is in the mechanism providing for an elevation of potential of the homeostatic system in the spawning Pacific salmon, in pregnant organisms, and in the postnatal period.

Second, the increase of vigor is brought about by establishment of the central type of homeostatic failure. This proves that the mechanism of development cannot act without breaking the Law of Constancy of Internal Environment of the organism.

Therefore, while the stability of internal environment of an organism is a vital condition for its free existence, the programmed disturbance of stability is an essential condition for development. Consequently, I believe that in addition to the Law of Constancy of Internal Environment there exists the Law of Deviation of Homeostasis. It may be stressed once again that any chronic disturbance of constancy of internal environment is a disease. Therefore, strictly speaking, the mechanism of development is based upon the "programmed disease of homeostasis." This seemingly paradoxical statement reveals its true meaning when we take into account the later changes that take place in the reproductive homeostat after the age-associated switching-on of the reproductive function.

The hypothalamic factor which promotes the developmental program does not cease to act after the development and growth of the organism has been completed. If we restrict the consideration of the problem to an example related to the age-associated changes in reproductive homeostasis, then one more circumstance should be noted.

If the sex glands of an old animal in which the reproductive cycle has ceased functioning are transplanted into a young castrated animal, the activity of the sex glands will be restored. On the other hand, the sex glands of a young animal will not function properly in an old organism (Kushima et al 1961; Aschheim 1964–65). Therefore, it is clear from the consideration of such a purely age-connected process as the switching-off of reproductive function, that disturbances in regulation may be a key factor in aging.

I suggest that the age-associated switching-off of reproductive function is determined by the age-related increase in hypothalamic activity (Dilman 1958, unpublished data). Indeed, on completion of the growth and development of an organism, the same elevation of the hypothalamic threshold of sensitivity will inevitably lead to a failure in the feedback mechanism, and ultimately will switch off reproductive function.

This conclusion is based on results which indicate that gonadotropic secretion continues to increase after the switching-on of reproductive function (Dilman 1958, 1961). This process causes a still greater stimulation of ovarian activity. Such a compensatory intensificiation of hormonal activity maintains self-regulation of reproductive function as the hypothalamic threshold rises, and leads to an intensification of reproductive system function with age.

At the same time the increased activity of the reproductive system has a pathogenic stimulatory effect on target tissues, often causing uterine bleeding in the climacteric or menopausal hyperplasia of the endometrium that may progress in some menopausal patients to endomentrial carcinoma. In the end elevation of the hypothalamic threshold inevitably leads to a central type of homeostatic failure, which causes reproductive function in the female organism to be switched off at a certain age. The same phenomenon ensures that reproductive function is switched on and later switched off. However, such changes are not limited to reproductive function.

There are three indispensable attributes of any living organism: the ability to reproduce, the ability to adapt, and the ability to support the flow of energy. Therefore, it is natural that structural systems capable of self-development should correspond to these particular abilities. There are, accordingly, three main homeostats (I define "homeostat" as the system that controls homeostasis): reproductive, adaptive, and energy.

Yet we must ask why the formation of age-specific pathology is determined by changes in these particular systems? If the elevation of the hypothalamic set point is indispensable for the implementation of the neuroendocrine program for the development of the organism, it is clear that this phenomenon must occur in the systems that regulate the stream of energy and the ability for adaptation and reproduction, because these three functions are also indispensable.

Accordingly, the shift of homeostasis occurs in three main homeostats regulating reproduction, adaptation, and energy metabolism (see Chapters 3–6). At the same time, on completion of the growth and development of the organism, the same intensification of the activity of the main homeostatic system will inevitably result in a homeostatic failure, ie, in a number of disturbances and diseases and, eventually, in the regulatory death caused by this intrinsic factor of development. One of the specific features of this concept is, therefore, the idea that in addition to development and aging, some age-related diseases are considered part of the same mechanism. In view of this statement, age pathology formation is a by-product of the organism's developmental program.

This is why the climacteric is both a norm (because the menopause is a part of natural aging), and a disease (because the menopause is the product of a steady disturbance of homeostasis, which eventually results in a certain decline in the vital capacity of the organism. Thus there are diseases that can be called normal diseases because they develop regularly in the course of natural aging.

Now, if the climacteric is the normal disease of the reproductive homeostat, then in the other two main homeostatic systems, the adaptive and the energy homeostats (which are likely to increase their activity in order to provide for the development of the organism), the central type of homeostatic failure must also arise in ontogenesis, which, consequently, must bring about normal diseases connected with changes in those homeostatic systems. I shall refer to the normal disease arising in the adaptive homeostat as dysadaptosis (see Chapter 3). The typical clinical manifestations of dysadaptosis are the cushingoid features, such as a massive trunk and thin arms and legs, often observed in middle-aged and elderly persons. As the hypothalamic threshold for suppression is elevated, adaptational reactions become inadequate. Thus, as a result of normal age-associated changes in the adaptive homeostat, aging humans start living as if in a state of chronic stress, and, therefore, become more and more defenseless during actual stress. Aging is a natural stressor.

The normal disease that arises from regular changes in the energy homeostat is age-associated adiposity. During the course of aging, adiposity developes because of disturbances in the feeding and energy homeostats (see Chapters 5 and 6). Whatever its cause, adiposity begins to play a pathogenic role (see Chapters 6, 18, and 25), as it occurs in the Pacific salmon during spawning and in mammals during pregnancy. Obesity intensifies the development of nearly all specific diseases of aging (see Chapters 6 and 18).

Consequently, the fact that hypercholesterolemia is an attribute of age-associated pathology, in particular as a factor promoting the development of atherosclerosis (see Chapter 12), metabolic immunodepression (see Chapter 15), and cancer (see Chapter 17), results from the role of hypercholesterolemia in the development program.

Moreover, both in the dramatic mechanism of natural death of the Pacific salmon and in the mechanism of natural death of higher organisms (which is more prolonged in time but in many respects similar to the former mechanism), obesity plays a key role (see Chapters 18 and 25). Figuratively speaking, obesity forms the foundation of development and aging, and higher organisms are born and burned in the flames of fats. Therefore, overweight is not a problem of the lifetime of a generation; it is a problem of all times. Thus, both in the spawning Pacific salmon and in humans, the program of development of an organism transforms into the mechanism of the formation of specific diseases of aging and, eventually, natural death.

Natural death of higher organisms is a regulatory death. This concept eliminates the distinction between aging and certain diseases whose development is caused by programmed disturbances in homeostasis.

Consider Table 1-1 again. All those diseases that form an intricate pattern of syndromes in patients suffering from endometrial cancer can exist independently. However, out of the many hundred diseases known to modern medicine, only ten diseases arise regularly during natural aging; of these ten diseases, only seven or eight cause death in 85% of middle-aged and elderly patients. These diseases are obesity, dysadaptosis, climacteric, prediabetes and maturity-onset diabetes mellitus, atherosclerosis, metabolic immunodepression, autoimmune disorders, essential hypertension, psychic depression, and cancer (cancrophilia) (see Chapters 11–18).[1]

These diseases form a complex that is frequently revealed in cases of cancer of the uterus (see Table 1-1). All these diseases have some features in common (see Chapter 25). For example, obesity increases the probability of an early onset of maturity-onset diabetes mellitus, atherosclerosis, metabolic immunodepression, autoimmune disorders, and cancer. It is highly probable that such regularity is caused by some general factor in pathogenesis, and that the action of external or random factors cannot explain the regular age-associated increase in the frequency of occurrence of these diseases, individually or in combination.

I believe that this general factor is the hypothalamic mechanism which forms the basis for the development of a central type of homeostatic failure in the course of normal aging.[2]

Indeed, comparison of the data in Tables 1-1 and 1-2 shows that patients with endometrial carcinoma reveal signs of hypothalamic pathology (Dilman 1961; Dilman et al 1968), primarily those features of hypothalamic pathology that are characteristic of Cushing's syndrome and the syndrome causing the death of Pacific salmon after spawning (Wexler 1971; Dilman 1971).

Similarly, as the complex of main diseases of aging in a woman with endometrial carcinoma can be explained in terms of hypothalamic changes, so involvement of the hypothalamic mechanism can be traced in the formation of the main human diseases in the course of natural aging (see Chapters 18 and 25). Theoretically, even under ideal conditions,

---

[1] It may be mentioned that on this list of the main diseases of humans there are some terms which are not traditional, ie, dysadaptosis, metabolic immunodepression, and cancrophilia. The choice of these terms will be considered in the respective sections of this book.

[2] This statement is universal. Actually, the homeostatic failure in the spawning Pacific salmon, which is linked with the activation of the hypothalamus-pituitary–adrenal-gonadal axis (Wexler 1976), would have been theoretically impossible if the activation had not been combined with elevation of the sensitivity threshold in the homeostatic regulator to feedback inhibition by hormones and energy-producing substrates whose blood concentration must increase because of the activation of the homeostatic system. Consequently, even in this case, which has been discussed here as a particular case of implementation of developmental program, this program is carried out because of the development of a central type of homeostatic failure.

deviation of homeostasis takes place. Hence, the diseases of aging are a by-product of completion of an organism's development.[1]

However, analysis of causes that lead to age-associated pathology becomes more complicated because these same main diseases of the middle-aged and the elderly can develop at any age under the influence of external factors that are sufficiently well defined: stress, overeating, lowered physical activity, chemical carcinogens, etc. Though quite authentic, these data help create a false impression that the internal factors, ie, transformation of an organism's program of development into the mechanism of age-specific pathology, do not actually play the role suggested by the author.

In this connection it should be noted that the ability to promote the mechanism of age-specific pathology is not characteristic of just any external factors; it is a characteristic feature of those factors which can intensify the main elements involved in realizing the Law of Deviation of Homeostasis. This statement can be illustrated by the stress reaction (see Chapter 19). Adaptation to stress is effected through hormonal metabolic changes, eg, by an increase in blood levels of ACTH, cortisol, growth hormone, glucose, fatty acids, etc (see Chapter 19). Elevation of the levels of these substances would inhibit the activity of the hypothalamus-pituitary complex by negative feedback almost at once, thus making adaptation unavailable, unless the resistance of this complex to homeostatic suppression were increased simultaneously. Thus a sufficiently prolonged reaction to stress is a path to the formation of specific age pathology.

In general, all external factors that raise the hypothalamic threshold of sensitivity at the same time cause an acceleration of development and acceleration of aging, as well as age-specific pathologic disorders.

The peculiarity of the specific diseases of aging arises because these diseases are normal diseases that result from the implementation of the Law of Deviation of Homeostasis; at the same time they depend, more than any other disease, upon factors in the external environment.

However, the so-called factors of civilization, ie, stress of modern lifestyle, overeating, diminished physical activity, and chemical carcinogens, only determine within the ten normal diseases the choice of a disease and the rate at which one of these diseases is realized in a particular person. In other words, civilization does not cause the diseases of civilization, but it introduces the principle of uncertainty into the determined mechanism of the establishment of diseases of aging.

It may be suggested that the development of complex homeostatic systems in the course of evolution of higher animals (which by itself has

---

[1]Of course, random stochastic processes, such as somatic mutation or accumulation of errors on the posttranslational level, do contribute to the general picture of aging (see Chapter 23).

augmented the organism's freedom from the external enivornment and therefore has reduced mortality from external environmental causes) has given rise to another biologic phenomenon: regulatory death caused by internal factors, which in the course of implementation of the Law of Deviation of Homeostasis, inevitably disturbs the constancy of the organism's internal environment.

Taking into consideration the complex origin of the main diseases of man, they cannot be called, strictly speaking, either normal diseases (with the exception of climacteric, dysadaptosis, and age-connected adiposity when not induced by external factors) or specific diseases of aging. Therefore, when trying to classify the main diseases of man as a group, account should be taken of the key element in the pathogenesis of these diseases.

Since the elevation of the hypothalamic threshold is the driving gear of their mechanism, a compensatory stimulation of the peripheral elements of relevant homeostats occurs during aging and the diseases of aging. For example, the energy homeostat creates a compensatory rise in blood insulin level as a typical age-associated shift, which causes fat build-up and a predominant utilization of free fatty acids (FFA) for energy supply. This metabolic shift is typical of all diseases of aging. Considering the mechanism of their causation, the diseases caused by the elevation of the hypothalamic threshold were designated as diseases of compensation, and the mechanism of self-development as the elevational mechanism of development, aging, and specific age pathology formation (Dilman 1971).[1]

In contrast to diseases of adaptation, diseases of compensation develop gradually, independent of stress factors (see Chapter 19). A typical example of a compensation disease is the climacteric, in which a raised hypothalamic threshold of sensitivity to estrogen suppression with subsequent increased secretion of gonadotropins is countered, for a time, by increased ovarian function. The excess of ovarian hormones provides both the prolonged activity of menstrual function and, at the same time, exerts a pathologic influence on the reproductive organs (see Chapter 3).[2] But any diseases of compensation may develop at any age if the elevation of the hypothalamic threshold is caused by a pathologic rather than an aging process. The above argument favors the concept that aging is a

[1]From the viewpoint of the elevational model of development and aging, it is necessary to consider the following four stages of postnatal ontogenesis: growth or prediabetes, stabilization (in the female organism), prediabetes during which an active formation of diseases of compensation occurs, and involution when the development of the diseases of aging slows down (see Chapter 8).

[2]I should like to note that the interpretation of age-associated rise in gonadotropin secretion as one conditioned by the primary increase in hypothalamic activity (Dilman 1958, unpublished data) was a turning point in my studies aimed at the development of the elevation model of aging and age-associated pathology (see Chapter 23).

normal physiologic process and a disease, or rather a confluence of diseases of compensation (see Chapter 18).

This statement is essential for the evaluation of what, in the pattern of aging, is a norm and what is a disease. I believe that the so-called dynamic or age-associated norm, accepted now and formulated on the principle that the parameters of the norm change with every stage of aging, is actually nothing but a manifestation of the degree of deviation of the organism from the ideal norm, ie, it is a measure of the advancement of the diseases of homeostasis (see Chapter 10). Therefore, the level of physiologic indices in humans, right after the completion of body growth, should be called "an ideal norm." This means that the individual indices of the ideal norm parameters should be established in every healthy subject at 20–25 years of age. In other words the notion of an age-associated norm is a myth. The norm is a constant that is established at age 20, ie, on completion of growth. Any persistent deviation of physiologic characteristics from the levels set at age 20 is another milestone on the way to the formulation of specific diseases of aging. It is not enough to be fit, it is necessary to be normal.

Correspondingly, all the factors that accelerate the development of diseases of compensation, naturally accelerate their development and the natural process of aging. For example, intensification of the programmed disease of the pregnant organism caused by overweight or stress, results in the development of a large baby, which leads to accelerated development (see Chapter 21). Time goes by faster in overweight people, and the acceleration of development is also the acceleration of age pathology formation. Thus it becomes evident that it is necessary to consider the possible role of hypothalamic threshold elevation not only in the mechanism of body development, but also in the mechanism of aging and age pathology formation. In this context the similar metabolic pattern, intrinsic in pregnancy, normal aging, stress, and age-connected pathology, is easier to explain (Table 1-3).

The question arises: How can both laws, the Law of Constancy of Internal Environment and the Law of Deviation of Homeostasis, be realized simultaneously?

The Law of Constancy of Internal Environment limits the scope of the Law of Deviation of Homeostasis to three main homeostats that control the three main functions: reproduction, adaptation, and energy supply regulation. In other words the spectrum of specific age pathology is determined by the functional structure of the main homeostatic system or, more precisely, by the disturbance of regulatory processes in the energy, adaptive, and reproductive homeostats.

On the other hand, many fundamental physiologic parameters do not undergo regular aging-associated changes. For instance the concentrations of potassium (K) and sodium (Na) in the blood remain virtually

Table 1-3
Similarity of Hormonal-Metabolic Patterns in Pregnancy, Normal Aging, Stress, and Cancrophilia (Cancer)

Pregnancy	Normal Aging	Stress	Cancer (cancrophilia)
Hypersomatotropism caused by chorionic somatomammotropin secretion	Decreased level of biogenic amines in hypothalamus	Decreased level of dopamine in hypothalamus	Carcinogen-induced decreased level of biogenic amines in hypothalamus
	Resistance to feedback suppression in energy, adaptive, reproductive homeostats	Resistance to feedback suppression in energy, adaptive, homeostats	Resistance to feedback suppression in energy, adaptive, reproductive homeostats
Hypercorticism	Hypercorticism	Hypercorticism	Hypercorticism
Decreased glucose tolerance	Decreased glucose tolerance	Decreased glucose tolerance	Decreased glucose tolerance
Hyperinsulinemia	Hyperinsulinemia	Increased lipolysis	Hyperinsulinemia
Gain of body weight	Obesity		Obesity
Intensified oxidation of free fatty acids	Intensified oxidation of free fatty acids	Intensified oxidation of free fatty acids	Intensified oxidation of free fatty acids
Hypercholesterolemia	Hypercholesterolemia and hypertriglyceridemia	Hypercholesterolemia	Hypercholesterolemia and hypertriglyceridemia
Suppression of cellular immunity	Suppression of cellular immunity	Suppression of cellular immunity	Suppression of cellular immunity

unchanged during ontogenesis. This proves the maintenance of the Law of Constancy of Internal Environment. Correspondingly, the specific diseases of aging are not connected with the primary disturbance of K or Na balance. It is not the disturbance of the Law of Constancy of Internal Environment, but the exact implementation of the Law of Deviation of Homeostasis that determines the establishment of the diseases of aging. Moreover, if these diseases do not develop at a certain period in life, the natural course of development and aging has been disturbed.[1]

Several factors, interrelated in many respects, operating in the mechanism of elevation of the hypothalamic threshold of sensitivity to feedback control, can be discerned (see Chapter 18): a) age-associated decrease in the hypothalamic level of neurotransmitters, eg, biogenic amines, especially dopamine; b) reduction in the number of hormonal and neurotransmitter receptors and their binding capacity (this process may be partially determined by the decline in biogenic amine concentration)[2]; c) decline in the secretion of melatonin and pineal polypeptide hormones that can raise hypothalamic sensitivity to homeostatic stimuli; d) decline in glucose utilization in different areas of the brain, particularly the hypothalamus; and e) accumulation of body fat, which by itself, via the influence of glucose and FFA on the brain neurotransmitter system, is conducive to elevation of the hypothalamic threshold of sensitivity.

Although there are many uncertain aspects in the mechanism of diseases of aging, the elevational model of these diseases shows that curative treatment should be aimed at an "ideal norm," ie, the balance when the Law of Constancy of Internal Environment of the organism counteracts, in an optimal way, the influence exerted on the organism by realization of the Law of Deviation of Homeostasis.

As to the possibility of an artificial deceleration of aging, as well as of age-associated diseases, the caloric restriction in food intake and the administration of antioxidants are at present the most effective means for slowing down the development of age-related pathology and increasing the life span in experimental animals. These examples indicate that restriction in the accumulation or utilization of fat is essential. Hence, a

---

[1]For example, in hypophysectomized rats receiving the substitutional administration of glucocorticoids, no arteriosclerosis develops with age (Everitt et al 1976). The animals die in a healthy state, if we judge their state of health and age by the typical age standards for a rat.

[2]There is a consensus that aging involves a decline in the number of hormonal receptors in different tissues. Theoretically, such a phenomenon may be responsible for the age-associated elevation of the hypothalamic-pituitary threshold of sensitivity to the hormonal regulatory signals. At the same time it has been proposed that a decrease in hormonal receptor concentration may be a consequence of negative feedback regulation by circulating hormone (Roth et al 1975). Therefore, both the decrease and the increase in receptor concentration in the hypothalamus may be at some time the secondary event reflecting the hormonal modulation of hormone receptor concentration by the level of circulating hormones.

favorable influence can be expected, if we combine such influence with normalization of regulatory disturbances resulting in metabolic shifts.

Data will be presented throughout this book, showing that such drugs as phenformin, diphenylhydantoin, L-dopa, and pineal polypeptide extract (epithalamin), ie, preparations improving the hypothalamic sensitivity to homeostatic signals, can exert a favorable influence on various manifestations of aging and diseases of aging (see Chapter 23). The available data indicate that many factors promoting the development of age-associated pathology may be controlled, ie, in principle it is possible to slow down the development of diseases of aging and the very process of aging. And this is precisely why normal aging should conveniently lend itself to pharmacologic and other types of correction with a view to decelerating the development rates of aging and associated diseases.

At the same time, there is a tendency to draw a line between the mechanism of aging and that of diseases associated with aging. Such an approach has led numerous investigators to conclude that elimination of major diseases and even all the diseases of middle and old age might not have any effect on the mechanism of aging proper. It was claimed that an orientation toward therapy and elimination of basic diseases (atherosclerosis and cancer included) would have hardly any influence on the life span of *Homo sapiens* (Hayflick, 1976).

But this claim is somewhat misleading because it ignores the method by which the basic diseases of aging are to be eliminated. For instance, if cancer is to be cured by means of early diagnosis and timely surgery, then a substantial gain in life expectancy will hardly be assured because the factors promoting carcinogenesis play a key role in the formation of other pathologic processes. For example, the effect of hypercholesterolemia is not confined to promoting tumor cell division, but it also contributes to the development of immunodepression and atherosclerosis as well. If we succeed in preventing hypercholesterolemia or in rectifying incipient disturbances leading to it, we shall have a means for influencing a wider spectrum of diseases of aging and the mechanism of aging itself.

In particular, Figure 1-1 shows that phenformin prolongs the life span of C_3H strain mice, and decreases the frequency of mammary gland cancer. Figure 1-2 shows that pineal polypeptide extract prolongs the life span of rats and decreases the frequency of mammary cancer induced by a chemical carcinogen, dimethylbenzanthracene.

Consequently, an increase in life span does not necessarily result in a higher frequency of age-related disease; on the contrary, it is possible to secure both a longer life span and a less frequent occurrence of diseases linked with the mechanism of development and aging.

This book presents a description of a single mechanism for such

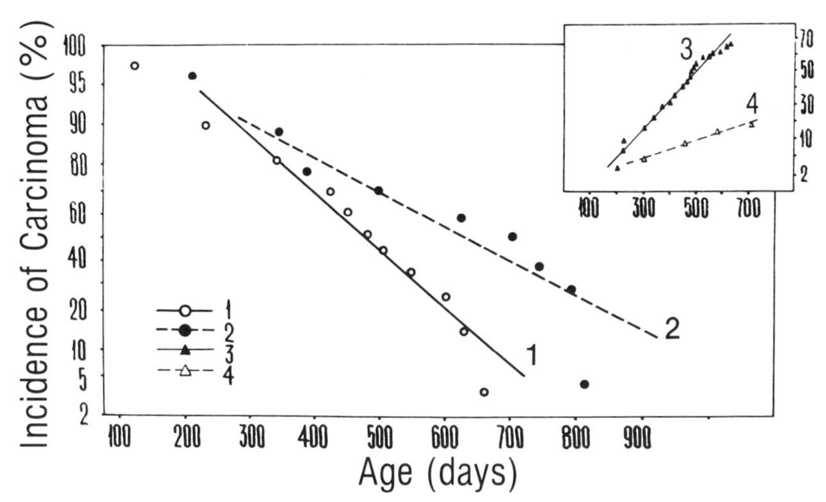

Figure 1-1 Influence of phenformin administration on life span of C_3H mice and incidence of mammary gland carcinoma. 1: Life span of control mice; 2: Life span of phenformin-treated mice; 3: Incidence of mammary gland tumors in control mice; 4: Incidence of mammary gland tumors in phenformin-treated mice.

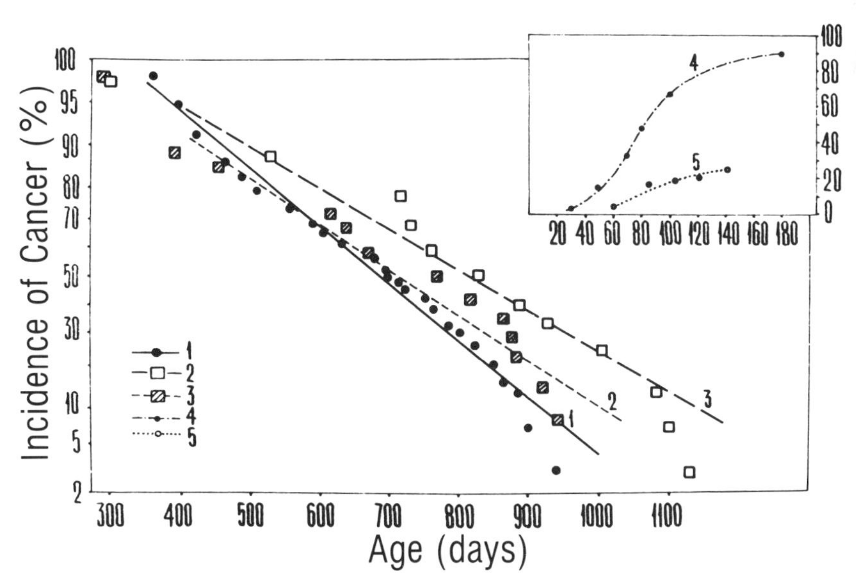

Figure 1-2 Influence of pineal polypeptide extract (epithalamin) on life span of rats and incidence of DMBA-induced cancer of mammary gland. 1: Life span of control rats; 2: Life span of epithalamin-treated rats (0.1 mg/day); 3: Life span of epithalamin-treated rats (0.5 mg/day); 4: Incidence of mammary gland tumors in DMBA-treated rats; 5: Incidence of mammary gland tumors in DMBA-treated and epithalamin-treated rats.

seemingly different physiologic and pathologic processes as the metabolic pattern of pregnancy, postnatal growth and development, age-associated switching-on and switching-off of reproductive function, the emergence of age-specific pathology, climacteric, obesity, dysadaptosis, maturity-onset prediabetes and diabetes mellitus, essential hypertension, atherosclerosis, metabolic immunodepression, autoimmune disorders, psychic depression, cancrophilia (metabolic conditions promoting carcinogenesis), and, finally, the natural death of the individual organism—all as a result of the implementation of the genetic program of normal ontogenesis in higher organisms, including humans.

The same mechanisms will be shown as the basis of the premature formation of age-specific pathology observed in recent decades. This mechanism will be shown to be responsible for the influence of external environmental factors (acute and chronic stress, excessive food intake and excessive illumination, some chemical carcinogens, etc) on the process of development, aging, and the appearance of aging-associated pathology.

In conclusion, it should be said that there is a common criterion that is often applied to evaluating any hypothesis. According to this criterion, the fewer the postulates set forth as the basis of a hypothesis and the more experimental findings that may be adequately interpreted in its terms, the greater its validity. In this connection it may be mentioned that the elevational model is based on one postulate only, and no other theory of aging joins such a great number of different data within one postulate: the Law of Deviation of Homeostasis (see Chapter 23).

It should be stressed that the regularities described by the Law of Deviation of Homeostasis do not exclude (but in many aspects explain) participation of other factors that exert influence upon the mechanism of aging and age-associated diseases (see Chapter 23).

The author will try to show that the Law of Deviation of Homeostasis allows the development of more generalized approaches to integrated medicine than has been possible until now. In particular, the concluding chapter of this book will enable the reader to decide to what degree the main diseases of humans, represented in Table 1-1, can be joined together in one integral mechanism.

Finally, if we suppose that the regulatory type of aging and natural death (Cannon 1942, Shock 1952, Verzar 1957, Comfort 1964, Timiras 1975, Finch 1976, Denckla 1977) is, so to speak, preceded by some more primordial mechanisms (the characteristics and manifestations of which we do not yet know, because regulatory factors cause death before we see the effect of the "primordial mechanism"), then it becomes apparent that the best we can do for the time being is to try to master the regulatory causes of aging and natural death. The elevational model of these phenomena provides a means for experimental testing of the problem.

2 Certain Peculiarities of Organization of the Neuroendocrine System

A hybrid of the nervous and endocrine systems, a junction of two worlds—internal and external environments—the hypothalamus is a wonder of Nature.

Maintenance of the constancy of the internal environment is of vital importance for the functioning of the living organism. According to Claude Bernard (1878) the constancy of the internal milieu is a necessary condition for free existence of the organism. Cannon (1925) coined the word homeostasis and identified its content.

In unicellular organisms homeostasis is attained mainly through a rapid change in intracellular metabolism produced by changes in the external environment. Therefore unicellular organisms are highly dependent on environmental conditions, and even relatively insignificant changes in these conditions may cause damage and death. Changes in external environmental conditions are thus generally the main cause of death in unicellular organisms.

The increased independence from environmental influences that has developed through a growing complexity and specialization of organisms in the course of their evolution has been, to a large extent, caused by the development of specialized regulatory systems, the nervous and endocrine systems, intended for the integration of the organism's functions. Their formation has ensured greater freedom of internal environmental factors. The development of the endocrine and nervous systems has also made possible the functioning of complex homeostatic systems, ie, component self-regulating systems capable of operating in such a manner as to ensure the maintenance of the equilibrium of the system as a whole. An illustration of such well-known homeostatic systems is the maintenance of a stable blood glucose level.

Feedback regulation is the basic principle which maintains the relative stability of the internal environment. Homeostasis deals with stability and freedom; feedback deals with the organization of processes (Yamamoto 1965). In other words, homeostasis is a biologic counterpart of a feedback control system, since it maintains some processes within or near desired values. The concept of feedback is derived from the operation of electrical networks, but the flavor of this idea has existed in physiology for a long time. The feedback principle operates at all levels, from the regulation of metabolism in a separate cell to the coordinated functioning of the neuroendocrine system. While there are two types of feedback mechanisms, positive and negative, the stability of any system is generally maintained through negative feedback.

The principle of negative feedback regulation consists in the maintenance of such a relationship between the initial and final products of the system that the accumulation of the final product suppresses the output of the initial one. The positive feedback mechanism, ie, the stimulation of the initial product output by the accumulation of the final product, and vice versa, is not typical of the maintenance of the constancy of the internal environment; however, it is vitally important for the impulse generation in a self-regulated system. Consider the simplest feedback regulation with two variables A and B. If $A = fB$ and $B = fA$, then a feedback relationship exists between the two. If the concentration or effect of A is increased when B increases, then positive feedback exists, whereas if A decreases when B increases, negative feedback exists (Rasmussen 1968).

The regulation of unicellular organisms is effected chiefly by means of the products of intracellular metabolism, which themselves undergo successive metabolic changes. However, there are specific intracellular regulators, such as cyclic nucleotides, most importantly cyclic 3′5′ adenosine monophosphate (cyclic 3′5′ AMP) (Sutherland 1970) and prostaglandins (Bergström et al 1968), synthesized from glucose and fatty acids, respectively. These specialized regulatory factors operate on the cellular level. For example, cyclic 3′5′ AMP regulates many metabolic processes in microorganisms, and thus this compound may be considered a primary hormone (protohormone) because the cyclic 3′5′ AMP performs a regulatory function but, unlike glucose, is not an intermediary product in energy metabolism. Therefore cyclic 3′5′ AMP, as well as the prostaglandins, may be considered to be the first level of a system of specialized regulation.[1]

One of the manifestations of tissue specialization is the formation of specific receptors on the cell membrane. As a result, the required type of specialized cell activity may be switched on or off when specific signals reach these receptors. Such a mechanism both coordinates the functions of separate cells and regulates their activity. To a large extent, hormones perform the regulatory function of such signals. The hormonal effect is often determined by the action on the receptor, which may switch on or off the synthesis of cyclic 3′5′ AMP. Specifically, this principle underlies the lipolytic and antilipolytic effects of hormones. The lipolytic hormones increase the rate of the lipase reaction by raising the level of cyclic 3′5′ AMP, whereas insulin, an antilipolytic hormone, slows this reaction by decreasing the cellular level of cyclic 3′5′ AMP.

Via different receptors, the plasma membranes regulate cell function. For instance, a cell will not enter the mitotic cycle unless the cholesterol level required for development of the membranes of daughter cells is attained (Chen et al 1975).

The peripheral hormones form the second level of hormonal regulation in the organism. It should be pointed out that negative feedback regulation also prevails at the second level. For instance, a decrease in blood calcium concentration results in an increase in parathyroid hormone secretion.

The functions of many endocrine glands are controlled by the pituitary, where a number of hormones regulating the activity of the peripheral endocrine glands are produced. Means for the integration and coordination of the functions of separate endocrine glands are provided at the pituitary level of the endocrine system. For instance, castration is followed by enhanced gonadotropin and ACTH secretion, which causes the synthesis of sex hormones in the adrenal cortex to increase, and consequently mitigates the postcastration hormonal insufficiency. Hence a third level of the endocrine control system is assured by the pituitary gland. At this level the relationship between the peripheral endocrine glands and the pituitary is also regulated by feedback mechanisms.

By regulating the function of numerous endocrine glands, the pituitary is "blind" to signals transmitted from the external environment. Therefore, it functions, to a considerable degree, as part of the hypothalamic-pituitary complex. Owing to its functional connection with the hypothalamus, pituitary activity is dependent both on signals generated by the variations in peripheral hormone level, and on the

[1]According to Sutherland (1970), cyclic 3′5′ AMP is designated as the second messenger, while hormones in an integrated organism may be defined as the first messengers.

abundant information supplied to the hypothalamus from the vegetative (autonomic) nervous system and from the organs of sense, and accordingly the central nervous system. Moreover, the hypothalamus has receptors that respond to variations in the blood level of some metabolites, eg, glucose concentration. In sum, the hypothalamus receives information both from the external and internal environments and adjusts the endocrine system activity to changing requirements. Hence the hypothalamus constitutes a fourth level of the organization of the endocrine system, since it is in the hypothalamus, which is part of the brain but possesses all the properties of an endocrine gland, where the activity of the entire endocrine system is integrated. As in other parts of the brain stem, the neurons of the hypothalamus form aggregates or nuclei. According to different classifications, 14–48 pairs of nuclei are distinguished.

As far as hypothalamic function is concerned, specific and nonspecific types of activity can be distinguished. The ability to secrete hypothalamic hormones may be referred to as specific activity, while the integration of sympathetic and parasympathetic effects may be considered largely nonspecific. The nonspecific activity of the hypothalamus may include the activity of specialized centers that regulate appetite, body temperature, water balance, blood pressure, heart rate, sleep, and emotional behavior. However, during sleep and emotional behavior the hypothalamus contributes only to the activity of other parts of the brain, namely the reticular formation, while other hypothalamic structures control gastrointestinal function, immune activities, etc.

It is difficult to describe separate effects of the hypothalamus in the nonspecific category, because the hypothalamus performs the integration of activities of all visceral systems, including sympathetic and parasympathetic control of the visceral organs and tissues. Therefore, irritation or injury to different regions of the hypothalamus may cause a variety of sympathetic and parasympathetic disturbances.

Numerous hormones are produced in the hypophysiotropic area of the hypothalamus by neurosecretory neurons. They are generally divided into two groups. The hormones of the first group act directly upon target tissues. For instance, vasopressin-antidiuretic hormone and oxytocin are produced in the supraoptic and paraventricular nuclei of the hypothalamus, to be then supplied to the posterior lobe of the pituitary by the neural hypothalamic-pituitary tract as a neurosecretory component. They are deposited here, to be drawn upon later, and reach terminal target cells by way of the general circulation.

The other group of hypothalamic hormones is composed of the so-called hypophysiotropic hormones that directly regulate the activity of the anterior lobe of the pituitary. They reach the median eminence of the hypothalamus, where a special portal system carries neurohormonal signals to endocrine way stations in the adenohypophysis. Accordingly, these hypophysiotropic factors were termed hypothalamic releasing and inhibiting hormones (Schally et al 1968). The existence of at least nine hypothalamic regulators of the pituitary gland is reasonably well established (Reichlin et al 1976). To date only three such hormones have been purified and characterized: gonadotropin (LH, FSH)-releasing hormone (LH-RH/FSH-RH); thyrotropin (TSH)-releasing hormone (TRH); and growth hormone (GH) release-inhibiting hormone (GH-RIH), or somatostatin (Besser and Mortimer 1974).

It is very likely that each pituitary hormone is controlled by two opposing hypothalamic hormones. The secretion of prolactin and probably melanocyte-stimulating hormone (MSH) is mainly regulated by the inhibiting hormones of the hypothalamus. The secretion of growth hormone, ACTH, thyrotropin and the gonadotropins is predominantly regulated by hypothalamic stimulating-releasing hormones.

However, some of the releasing hormones are not hormone-specific. For instance, thyrotropin-releasing factor (TRF) stimulates the secretion of thyrotropin, somatotropin, and prolactin (Besser and Mortimer 1974). This, in turn, makes the effect of some peripheral hormones on the hypothalamic-pituitary complex still more intricate.

At the same time, the influences of hypothalamic hypophysiotropic hormones are not limited to the anterior lobe of the pituitary. Recently, a number of laboratories have demonstrated behavioral changes following systemic administration of LH-RH/FSH-RH, TRH, or somatostatin. It has been shown that hypothalamic hormones may also play an integrated role in brain function, possibly as neurotransmitters (Luft et al 1978a). The hypophysiotropic hormones have also been found in peripheral blood. It is likely that some of hypothalamic hormones enter the general circulation. However, there is good evidence for somatostatin also being produced in gastrointestinal and pancreatic D cells. Moreover, it may be supposed that many hypothalamic hormones, if not all, are produced extrahypothalamically. In particular, tissue-corticotropin-releasing factor (CRF) was proposed to distinguish it from median eminence-CRF of hypothalamic origin (Brodish 1977).

Since the hypothalamus is the central element in the control hierarchy of the neuroendocrine system, the loops of the main homeostatic systems close there. Therefore, the rhythmic functioning of closed loop homeostatic systems and, to a considerable extent open loop systems, is governed by the hypothalamus automatically. This is illustrated by reproductive system regulation, in which its normal function is maintained by the hypothalamus without influencing the higher centers of the brain.

Considering the importance of the foregoing structural and functional features of the hypothalamus, it should be regarded as the main organ responsible for the maintenance of internal environment constancy as an indispensable factor of life. In addition, since information from the external environment is transmitted from different parts of the central nervous system, the hypothalamus plays a vital role in the organism's adaptation to the pressure of environmental factors.

A fifth level of neuroendocrine regulation is provided by the central nervous system, including the brain cortex. The activity of the hypothalamus as a brain area is controlled by numerous parts of the nervous system. It is well established that the hypothalamus responds to stimuli by liberating a corticotropin-releasing hormone. However, there is general agreement that the regulation of the circadian periodicity of ACTH content is under central nervous system control, and the hippocampus is thought to be inhibiting to ACTH release. It is also believed to be a site of corticosteroid feedback.

Moreover, it appears that the nerve endings of CNS neurons may also be target sites for glucocorticoid action and that the hormone may also rapidly regulate neurotransmitter metabolism. It must be stressed that some pituitary hormones, particularly ACTH, profoundly modify the electrical activity of the neuronal system of the brain, and that they may act as prohormones for the so-called opioid peptides (Guillemin 1976).

However, the extrahypothalamic CNS structures, including limbic structures, influence pituitary hormone secretion through the mediation of the hypothalamus.

Communication between neurons and endocrine cells in mammals is usually mediated by two types of chemical signals: neurotransmitters and neurohormones. The distinction between neurotransmitter and neurohormonal activities is not always clear. For example, somatostatin acts as a hormone and as a neurotransmitter (Luft et al 1978a). It is thought that the main neurotransmitters on the hypothalamic level are dopamine, noradrenaline, and serotonin (Smythe 1977). The role of acetylcholine, histamine, and γ-aminobutyric acid is obvious, too (Samorajski 1977). It is suggested that prostaglandins act as neurotransmitters in the central nervous system.

To summarize, all mediator systems take part in the regulation of hypothalamic function (Müller et al 1977). These authors undertook an analysis of the data suggesting that melatonin (a hormone produced by pineal parenchymal cells) may operate as a neurotransmitter. Also, interactions between melatonin and the serotonergic mechanism at the hypothalamic level have been observed. However, an ever-growing amount of data shows that the pineal gland produces polypeptides and even protein hormones (Benson et al 1972; Chazov and Isachenkov 1974).

It was suggested that at least some pineal polypeptides act as modulators, which change the threshold of hypothalamus sensitivity to regulatory endogenous stimuli (Dilman 1970a, 1971). It will be shown in different sections of this book that pineal polypeptide extract decreases the hypothalamic threshold to inhibition by estrogens and glucocorticoids (Ostroumova and Dilman 1972; Dilman et al 1973).

The role of some neurotransmitters in the regulation of numerous functions of the hypothalamus is not clear yet. An excellent review of this problem has been prepared by Müller, Nistricò, and Scapagnini (1977). One of the difficulties in this study is associated with functional interactions among the adrenergic, serotonergic, cholinergic, and other neurotransmitter systems in the CNS. Other aspects to this problem should be mentioned. There are conflicting results about the influence of L-dopa (precursor of dopamine) on the serum gonadotropin levels. Administration of L-dopa produces different shifts in blood-GH levels in normal subjects and in acromegalic patients. Perhaps, different physiologic states involve differences in the response of a relevant system to regulatory stimuli. For example, glucose loading produces a decrease in blood GH level in young subjects (Glick et al 1965) and, at the same time, a paradoxical increase in GH level in endometrial carcinoma patients (Benjamin et al 1969, Bobrov et al 1971). It should also be taken into account that the effects of this or that neurotransmitter on the secretion of some pituitary hormone, on the one hand, and on the threshold of sensitivity of the homeostatic system which controls the secretion of this hormone, on the other, are essentially different. Thus, neurotransmitters and hormonal receptors control the functional condition of the hypothalamus to a considerable degree.

But, finally, the hypothalamic neurons are typical of peripheral cell populations, generally, in that they are subject to the influence of an organism's internal environment. Primordial systems of regulation, relying on energy metabolites, cyclic 3′5′ AMP, and prostaglandins, also operate at this level.

The regulatory interaction of the hypothalamus and other parts of the endocrine system is also determined by a feedback mechanism that operates on several levels of the system. Of special physiologic importance is the relationship between the hormones of the peripheral endocrine glands and the hypothalamus. At present, this mechanism is identified as a long loop of feedback between the hypothalamus and the peripheral endocrine glands. To illustrate, when the level of a peripheral hormone, eg, cortisol in blood, is decreased, the activity of the hypothalamic nuclei producing corticotropin releasing factor (CRF) is enhanced. CRF, supplied to the anterior lobe of the pituitary through the hypothalamic-pituitary portal system, stimulates the secretion of ACTH, which in turn stimulates the output of cortisol in the adrenal cortex. When its concentration in blood reaches the critical level, the relevant center of the hypothalamus becomes inhibited through negative feedback, which eventually results in decreased stimulation of the adrenal cortex. It is in this way that the equilibrium of the hypothalamic-pituitary-adrenal system is maintained.

The long loop of the regulatory mechanism is complemented by a short loop of self-regulation. The latter term is used to designate the mechanism of action of pituitary hormones such as ACTH on the secretory activity of the relevant nuclei of the hypothalamus. For example, the treatment of adrenalectomized animals with exogenous ACTH has been reported to reduce pituitary weight, and to prevent the stress-induced fall in pituitary ACTH (Kitay et al 1959). Additional evidence for the function of a feedback system is provided by data from our laboratory showing the ability of acetylated ACTH, devoid of corticotropic and lipolytic activity, to inhibit the release of ACTH from the pituitary (see Chapter 24). The short loop feedback is probably important in the regulation of the output of the hormones that do not control the peripheral endocrine glands directly. For instance, the secretion of growth hormone may be inhibited by the injection of exogenous growth hormone (Sakuma and Knobil 1970). Finally, there is an "ultra-short loop" feedback by which the interaction between hypothalamic hormones and the relevant hypothalamic nuclei that produce these hormones occurs. It should be pointed out that the loops of the main homeostatic systems, which predetermine the functioning of the basic autonomic vegetative properties of higher organisms, close in the hypothalamus. In other words, the energy, reproductive, and adaptive homeostatic systems that control the abilities of a living organism to regulate the energy stream, to propagate, and to adapt have a common final pathway on the level of the hypothalamus. Therefore, the hypothalamus is the main structure for the maintenance of the Law of Constancy of Internal Environment.

Although each main homeostat is characterized by distinctive features, specific disturbances in self-regulation have been classified into three types of homeostatic failure:

1. Homeostatic failure may be caused by a decreased effect of the peripheral hormone at the hypothalamic-pituitary level. This results in diminished intensity of the negative feedback signal. Such a disturbance may be called the peripheral type of homeostatic failure. These disturbances occur, for instance, following a subtotal castration or a blocking of thyroid hormone synthesis.
2. Another type of homeostatic failure covers changes in the properties of secreted peripheral hormones. A disturbance of this kind is usually seen with a congenital enzyme defect, eg, the defect in hydroxylation of corticosteroids in congenital adrenal hyperplasia (Wilkins et al 1955). In another instance, the adrenal cortex may secrete, instead

of cortisol, androgen-like steroids primarily, which do not inhibit ACTH output adequately. Hence excessive ACTH is produced, thus stimulating the adrenals to release an excessive amount of androgen-like steroids that cause virilism. Such disturbances may be termed dysfunctional types of homeostatic failure.[1]

3. Homeostatic failure also develops when the primary setpoint of hypothalamic sensitivity to the regulatory effect of relevant peripheral hormones is elevated. In this case, the enhanced hypothalamic-pituitary activity is accompanied by increased activity of the peripheral link of the system which is subjected to an intensified stimulation. At the same time, the equilibrium of the homeostatic system cannot be regained due to a relative deficit of peripheral hormones, because their level is insufficiently high to overcome the increased hypothalamic threshold; this interferes with the operation of the self-regulation mechanism. For this reason, such a disturbance may be termed a central type of homeostatic failure. Such disturbances are observed in Cushing's syndrome where a much higher than normal dose of glucocorticoids (eg, dexamethasone) is required to inhibit the activity of the hypothalamic-pituitary system, and therefore the adrenal cortical activity (Liddle 1960).

It will be shown in different sections of this book that the central type of homeostatic failure is a key process in the implementation of the neuroendocrine program of development, aging, and age-linked pathology, leading eventually to the regulatory death of each individual organism in the course of normal ontogenesis.

Each homeostatic system maintains the stability of the internal environment by negative feedback, while at the same time its functioning is continually changing due to shifts in the setpoint of its central element. This is rather unusual from the viewpoint of classical cybernetics. The behavior of classic cybernetic systems is oriented toward maintenance of the homeostatic system parameter at a constant level. Therefore, the main tests for assessing the condition of the energy, adaptive, reproductive, and thyroid systems should characterize the threshold of sensitivity of the hypothalamic-pituitary complex to regulatory stimuli.

Considering certain peculiarities of the functional structure of the

---

[1]The study of qualitative alterations in the spectrum of secreted isohormones, when endocrine glands are subjected to intensive stimulation (Dilman 1968), is of interest. Changes occurring in the properties of some hormones may be a result of the influences of the internal environment on the posttranslational modification of protein hormones or the biotransformation of steroid hormones (Ryan et al 1972).

neuroendocrine system, it is necessary to specify some limitations of tests for identification of the type of homeostatic failure, predetermined by these peculiarities.

It might seem that the most reliable data could be obtained when only hypothalamic releasing or inhibiting hormones were tested. However, even if methodologic problems of testing these hormones were solved, an inevitable limitation would be that hypothalamic hormones are also produced by tissues other than the hypothalamus.

When assessing the condition of the main hypothalamic systems on the basis of changes of relevant pituitary hormones, consider that the buildup of the capacity of homeostasis is a function of both the secretory level of the pituitary hormone, and the magnitude of the compensating response of the peripheral element of the homeostatic system. For example, there is a discrepancy between ACTH and cortisol responses to insulin-induced hypoglycemia (Lindholm et al 1978), which signifies an overcapacity for ACTH action on the adrenal cortex.

Therefore, if the Law of Deviation of Homeostasis characterizes changes in the capacity of the homeostatic system, neither the central nor the peripheral element of homeostasis should be disregarded. Since hypothalamic sensitivity to homeostatic stimuli may depend on such factors as the concentration and metabolism of neurotransmitters, the concentration and properties of specific receptors of the membranes of neurons, as well as the plasma and extracellular fluids bathing the cells, the choice of a testing procedure may influence the results. The phenomenon of receptor "down regulation," namely, decreased hormone binding by specific receptors in response to elevation of hormone levels, has been well documented (Kahn 1976). Therefore, the decrease in receptor concentration in the hypothalamus and, hence, elevation of the threshold of sensitivity of the homeostatic system to regulatory stimuli, under certain conditions, may prove to be the result of a long-term administration of the test hormone.

Bearing this in mind, it may be suggested that obesity raises the basal level of insulin, thus leading to a decrease in insulin receptor concentration in the insulin-sensitive area of the CNS, particularly the hypothalamic area. This may cause a secondary elevation of the sensitivity threshold of centers that regulate body fat content via the basal level of insulin in cerebrospinal fluid (see Chapter 5).

It should be taken into consideration that the test hormone may influence the concentration of neurotransmitters both in the hypothalamus and in other areas of the neuroendocrine system, thus giving rise to changes in the original state of the homeostatic system as a whole. For example, the catechol estrogens (products of the conversion of estrogen to a catechol derivative) are potent competitive inhibitors of the

O-methylation of catecholamines by catechol-O-methyltransferase (Ball et al 1972).

Perhaps, even such a test as glucose loading may affect hypothalamic systems in a different manner, depending on the level of the metabolic processes. For example, the greater the carbohydrate tolerance decline, the higher the reactive insulinemia in response to glucose loading, and the greater the uptake of tryptophan by the hypothalamus (Fernstrom 1974). Therefore the serotonin concentration in this organ is higher. Hence, the testing procedure itself may cause additional changes in the system.

The following five chapters will explore the main results and hypotheses in support of the Law of Deviation of Homeostasis.

3 Age-Associated Disturbances in the Adaptive System A Normal Disease: Dysadaptosis[1]

In selecting between the internal and external environmental causes of natural death, the evolutional development of higher organisms has determined that to complete the specific life span and to die old and sick is to be preferred to death in young age and good health at any moment due to some external environmental factors.

Time is a natural stressor.

Outward appearance of many individuals undergoes characteristic changes, particularly after age 40. The face becomes moon-like and the trunk distribution of fat masses is further accentuated by relative reduction in fat accumulation on legs and arms. When pronounced, these signs suggest Cushing's syndrome. The symptoms indicate that aging is accompanied by the development of specific changes in the system of defense from damaging factors: the adaptive homeostat.

Adaptation to the action of damaging factors is inherent in the organism at all levels, including cellular and subcellular levels. But the majority of adaptational changes are effected by the neuroendocrine system and primarily by the hypothalamic-pituitary-adrenal cortex system. In this narrow context this system may be designated as an adaptive homeostat, although in stress reactions changes may also occur in

[1]It is better to define the disease described in this chapter not as "dysadaptosis," but as "hyperadaptosis," because the latter term more precisely characterizes its mechanism of development and its influence on the host.

other homeostatic systems, primarily the energy hoemostat. Moreover there are cortisol-sensitive neurons in regions of the brain other than the hypothalamus, such as the amygdala and hippocampus (Dafny et al 1973, Olpe and McEwen 1976). Thus, the limbic brain regions, long thought to be involved in mood, sleep, and emotional regulation, are also involved in hypothalamic-pituitary-adrenal regulation. Therefore neuronal pathways subserving the adaptive homeostat are widespread, but they finally converge on the hypothalamus. The hypothalamus, moreover, contains peptidergic secretory neurons, elaborating corticotropin-releasing factor (CRF), by which the information is transmitted to the anterior pituitary. The regulation of ACTH secretion occurs mainly by negative feedback, which ensures the rhythmic functioning of the system because of the reciprocal action of glucocorticoids (chiefly cortisol in humans) on the hypothalamus and accordingly on the production of CRF. As the blood cortisol level diminishes, the activity of the central (hypothalamic) element of the system is enhanced. This increases ACTH output, which in turn stimulates the adrenal cortex to increase the blood cortisol level. When its concentration in the blood is restored to normal, the latter inhibits the hypothalamic centers which govern the corticotropin-releasing hormone secretion. As a consequence equilibrium gradually is regained in the system. This mechanism of long loop negative feedback maintains the blood cortisol level within relatively narrow limits. Besides, the CRF effect may be blocked by corticoids. This demonstrates the existence of a feedback site at the pituitary level, apart from feedback receptors within the central nervous system.

However, there is presently no evidence for a pituitary feedback site for endogenous corticoids within the physiologic range. Our studies have previously shown that the administration of acetylated ACTH (which does not show adrenocortical activity) suppresses the release of ACTH from the adenohypophysis (Dilman et al 1974), which means that endogenous ACTH acts by a short loop feedback mechanism.

Cortisol concentration undergoes cyclic changes according to the so-called "diurnal circadian rhythm." Variations in CRF and ACTH output, and probably changes in the sensitivity of relevant hypothalamic centers and the CNS to the cortisol influence, underlie these rhythmic diurnal changes. With normal diurnal rhythm the blood ACTH level rises between 3 AM and 6 AM, with a subsequent increase in blood cortisol (Blichert-Toft 1975). This accounts for the maximum cortisol concentration in the morning, which later is gradually decreased, dropping to the minimal level by night. Under normal conditions, cortisol concentration in the morning is twice that at night. In practical terms the system is considered to be functioning normally if the blood cortisol level drops 40% to 50% from the basal value by 5 PM to 9 PM.

However, the results of the analysis of a 24-hour pattern of adrenocortical activity undertaken by Ceresa and colleagues (1970, 1972) provided arguments supporting the hypothesis that the hypothalamic mechanisms, which promote the circadian (impulsive) and basal ACTH activities, are different. Bearing this in mind, it is advisable to consider the literature and our own data on the age-associated changes in the adaptive homeostat in an attempt to identify the factor responsible for cushingoid sign development in the course of normal aging.

Table 3-1 shows that in the adaptive system the hypothalamic threshold of sensitivity to inhibition by glucocorticoids is elevated with advancing age. We observed this phenomenon in an experiment in which prednisolone was administered to female rats (Ostroumova and Dilman 1972). This experiment showed that, when rats are treated with prednisolone, young rats reveal a greater decrease in blood corticosterone level than adults.[1]

Table 3-1
Influence of Prednisolone Administration on Blood Corticosterone Levels in Rats of Different Ages

Body Weight (g)	Blood corticosterone (μg%)		Inhibition (%)
	Before Treatment	*After Treatment*	
100–200	7.9 ± 0.93	4.8 ± 1.05	39
150–170	15.4 ± 3.26	11.5 ± 3.26	25
200–220	20.9 ± 2.96	19.7 ± 3.37	6

These results may be interpreted as an indication of the age-associated elevation of hypothalamic sensitivity threshold to glucocorticoid suppression, which may also be suitably termed as a change in set point of hypothalamic sensitivity (Smelik and Papoikonamon 1973). In this connection, important results were reported by Riegle (1973), who showed that, in animals under stress, dexamethasone administration causes a much greater decrease in blood corticosterone level in younger animals than in older ones. Besides, ACTH administration diminished the response to stress in young rats, whereas this did not occur in older animals. This testifies to the age-associated increase in hypothalamic threshold of sensitivity to an increased corticosterone level (Hess and Riegle 1972).

Summing up, Riegle (1976) emphasized that "the most important age-related alteration in adrenocortical function is the decreased sensitivity

[1] It should be pointed out that, until sexual maturity, rats reveal a contrary tendency: they develop a certain resistance of the hypothalamic-pituitary complex to inhibition by dexamethasone (Ramaley 1975).

of the hypothalamic-pituitary adrenocorticotropin control mechanism in the aged rats."

It should be mentioned, however, that earlier, on the basis of his own findings, Riegle (1973) emphasized "the fundamental importance of changes occurring in this physiological control mechanism in aging processes in mammals."

A comparison of the conclusions of the latter author points to the following difference: in 1973 Riegle thought that the age-related elevation of the hypothalamic threshold of sensitivity is inherent in all mammals, while, in 1976, he limited this phenomenon to one mammalian species, the rat. Similar reasoning seems to appeal to Blichert-Toft (1978), who wrote: "...any clue suggestive of age-related elevation of hypothalamic threshold to feedback control as proposed by Dilman (1971) has not been provided in man."

It seems appropriate to ask whether the biologic differences between man and rat are so great. Age-associated elevation of the hypothalamic threshold in the adaptive system of rats has been definitely established. Similarly, reliable clinical evidence of age-associated formation of cushingoid signs has been obtained, which points to the central type of failure in the adaptive homeostat of man, a phenomenon experimentally established in rats. Let us look into the factors underlying these discrepancies.

In the studies of the threshold of adaptive homeostat sensitivity to feedback control at our laboratory, we employed two types of dexamethasone tests: a single dose or short-term test and a long-term test. In a short-term test, dexamethasone was administered in a dose of 0.5 mg at 11 PM, and samples of venous blood were taken at 9 AM the following morning. Table 3-2 shows that the dexamethasone treatment resulted in establishing equal levels of blood 11-hydroxycorticosteroid suppression in two different age groups of women.[1] However, when a long-term test was run, the administration of dexamethasone (0.125 mg, four times a day for two days) revealed an age-dependent difference in the efficiency of dexamethasone inhibition.

Long-term tests in women with breast cancer in stages I and II also showed that aging per se exerts some influence on the adaptive system (Table 3-3). These findings are consistent with the results of long-term dexamethasone tests in endometrial carcinoma patients (average age 51.2 ± 2.9 years). The levels of 17-hydroxycorticosteroid excretion before and after dexamethasone treatment were 4.8 ± 0.9 and 4.21 ± 0.9 mg/24 hrs (inhibition 12.8 ± 10%), respectively.

[1]These data differ from the data published in Dilman et al (1979), which show the difference in the percentage of inhibition in the short-term dexamethasone test between normal young and old subjects. The elderly subjects were observed under hospital conditions, while the young were observed as outpatients. However, the subjects under hospital conditions revealed a decrease of hypothalamic-pituitary complex sensitivity to dexamethasone inhibition like that caused by chronic stress.

Table 3-2
Comparison of Short- and Long-Term Dexamethasone Tests in Healthy Women of Two Age Groups

	Mean age (years ± SE)	
	35.4 ± 0.6	*50.6 ± 0.6*
Short-term dexamethasone test (blood 11-hydroxycorticosteroids in μg%) (N = 15)		
Before	13.9 ± 1.2 (n = 15)	15.0 ± 1.4 (n = 17)
After	4.6 ± 1.1	5.2 ± 1.3
Inhibition (%)	−67	−65
Long-term dexamethasone test (blood 17-hydroxycorticosteroids in mg/24 h)		
Before	4.7 ± 0.4 (n = 18)	4.86 ± 0.8 (n = 18)
After	2.5 ± 0.2	3.26 ± 0.2
Inhibition (%)	−42.7 ± 10	−24 ± 10
Significance *(p)*	0.001	NS

Table 3-3
Influence of Aging on Long-Term Dexamethasone Suppression Test in Breast Cancer Patients

		17-Hydroxysteroid Excretion Level (mg/24 h)				
Mean Age (± SE)	No. Cases	*Before Test a*	*After Test b*	*Difference between a and b*	*Inhibition (%)*	*Significance (p)*
36.5 ± 0.7	13	5.8 ± 0.7	2.14 ± 0.3	3.7 ± 0.6	58.7 ± 7.9	–
43.8 ± 0.3	39	5.3 ± 0.4	2.89 ± 0.2	2.4 ± 0.3	40.4 ± 6.0	NS
54.9 ± 0.5	22	5.3 ± 0.4	3.4 ± 0.5	1.9 ± 0.6	32.0 ± 11.0	< 0.05
68.4 ± 0.4	28	5.4 ± 0.4	3.4 ± 0.3	2.0 ± 0.4	34.0 ± 6.3	< 0.02

A more complicated pattern was observed after single dose dexamethasone tests in patients suffering from certain tumors and mental depression (Table 3-4). The patients with endometrial and prostatic cancer, as well as with mental depression, reveal both signs of the central type of homeostatic failure: a) elevation of the threshold of hypothalamic sensitivity to dexamethasone feedback suppression, and b) compensatory de-elevation of the basal levels of activity of the adrenal glands, which manifests itself in a rise in the basal level of 11-hydroxysteroids.

Table 3-4
Decrease in Sensitivity of Hypothalamic-Pituitary-Adrenal System to Dexamethasone Suppression*

Group	No. Cases	Mean Age (years)	Blood 11-hydroxycorticosteroids (μg% (mean ± SE) Basal Level	*After Dexamethasone*	Inhibition (%)
Control	17	56 ± 1.0	12.7 ± 1.1	7.5 ± 0.9	−39 ± 5
Endometrial cancer	29	59 ± 0.8	16.0 ± 1.7	10.7 ± 0.8†	−23 ± 8
Prostatic cancer	13	63 ± 2.0	20.8 ± 2.3†	14.8 ± 1.2†	−23 ± 9
Depressive illness	52	43 ± 1.8	20.6 ± 0.8†	16.5 ± 0.9†	−19 ± 5.0†

*Short-term dexamethasone test was used: administration of 0.5 mg dexamethasone at 11 PM was followed by an assay of 11-hydroxycorticosteroid level at 9 AM next morning to be compared with that measured at 9 AM on the day of dexamethasone administration.
†Difference is statistically significant ($p < 0.05$)

It is evident that a discrepancy exists in that, in certain states, a single dose test does not detect hypothalamic threshold elevation to feedback suppression, while the long test does (see Table 3-2). At the same time, these two types of tests may yield similar results, eg, in patients with endometrial carcinoma. In considering the possible causes of the said discrepancies, the two points should be taken into account. First, the impulsive activity may be elicited by a neural stimulus originating outside the hypothalamus (Ceresa et al 1970). This type of activity is easily inhibited by dexamethasone in the short-term test, whereas the basal activity may be controlled by a hypothalamic feedback that is relatively insensitive to corticoids. Second, the increase in the blood level of glucocorticoids can produce the decrease of sensitivity of the hypothalamic control mechanism because of negative feedback between blood hormone concentration and that of the receptors of this hormone (Kahn 1976, Finch 1976).

Bearing in mind these two points, it may be supposed that the impulsive neural mechanism is age-independent. This explains why dexamethasone, administered at 11 PM, ie, at the period of maximum sensitivity of the neural impulsive mechanism, suppresses the neural stimulus operating during sleep (impulsive activity) both in young and middle-aged subjects (see Table 3-2). However, the single dose dexamethasone test cannot provide an evaluation of the hypothalamic age-dependent basal feedback control mechanism. This supposition may account for the conclusion of Blichert-Toft (1978) that no age-related changes in the feedback control of the glucocorticoid-producing system have been proven.

However, his conclusion was based on the results of measurements of the diurnal rhythm of cortisol secretion. It is true that in most studies dealing with nyctohemeral (circadian, impulsive) regulation of cortisol secretion, no major disturbance of the rhythmic variation of cortisol level in plasma was seen in healthy, elderly people.[1]

On the contrary, the long dexamethasone test reveals the elevation of the hypothalamic threshold of sensitivity in the feedback mechanism that regulates the interaction between the hypothalamic-pituitary complex and the adrenal cortex, with increasing age.[2] It is worth mentioning in this connection that in obese subjects with signs of adrenocortical hyperfunction (similar to the hormone-metabolic pattern of aging) the dexamethasone test revealed an increase in the basal level with a normal impulsive activity (Ceresa et al 1970).

It is appropriate now to consider a situation in which resistance to dexamethasone is observed in both short- and long-term tests. If the hypothalamic threshold to inhibition is elevated, the central type of homeostatic failure will inevitably develop with an increased production of glucocorticoids and, particularly, an increased glucocorticoid basal level, as a consequence. In turn, the increase in glucocorticoid level in the internal environment may be supposed to lower the concentration of free cortisol receptors and, therefore, the sensitivity of hypothalamic-pituitary complex to inhibition by dexamethasone. This is because of the negative feedback between the concentration of the hormone bathing cells and that of the hormone receptors on the plasma membranes of hypothalamic neurons. This hypothesis is illustrated by the following data: It is known that serotonin stimulates the release of ACTH (Krieger and Krieger 1970). However, the administration of L-tryptophan during

---

[1] The stability of the level of this activity in aged subjects does not rule out changes which may be brought about by different factors, eg, stress. According to Blichert-Toft (1978), the disorders often present in old age such as insomnia, psychic distress, and cardiac insufficiency may be related to abnormal nyctohemeral rhythmic periodicity. Therefore, the results of such tests are subject to modification by many factors. For example, although Krieger et al (1971) demonstrated that age has no effect on the circadian pattern of plasma cortisol levels, their data show that the mean corticosteroid blood levels at 4 PM and 10 PM tended to be higher in the 30- to 40-year-old subjects than in the 15- to 20-year-olds. Also, Friedman et al (1969) showed that the nocturnal blood corticosteroid level was 6 μg% in the young subjects and 10.4 μg% in the older ones. There are, however, data testifying to the maintenance of the circadian rhythm in old age (average age 73.1 years) (Colucci et al 1975). But it should be remembered that this age is characterized by involution, when hypothalamic activity may decline (see Chapter 8).

[2] Friedman et al (1969) demonstrated in aged subjects normal adrenocortical suppressibility by giving 250 μg of dexamethasone orally, every six hours for two days. On the morning of the third day, 250 μg was given at 6 AM and blood taken for estimation of plasma control level at 9 AM. Hence, this study employed a dexamethasone dose over twice as high as the one used in our long-term test. Moreover, it should be taken into consideration that the average age of the subjects was 80 years.

five days was shown to potentiate the inhibitory action of dexamethasone (Ostroumova 1978). In other words, serotonin, an ACTH secretion-stimulating factor, promotes the re-establishment of equilibrium in the adaptive system. On the other hand, normal response to suppression by dexamethasone was elicited by the administration of an antiserotonergic agent, cyproheptadine, for a year, in a case of Cushing's syndrome (Krieger 1978). Considering the above data, it may be supposed that the decrease in blood cortisol level caused by cyproheptadine treatment improves the hypothalamic feedback mechanism by reducing cortisol concentration in a hypothalamus-bathing medium, which leads to the increase in the concentration of cortisol receptors in the hypothalamus and hypothalamic sensitivity to a dexamethasone suppression test.

This leads to still another supposition that the rise in the cortisol basal level, which causes the resistance of the hypothalamic feedback mechanism, may affect single dose test results. However, it is not clear if the increased basal level of cortisol induces resistance in the system of control of impulsive activity or if the considerable rise in the basal level of cortisol, in some situations, does mask changes in the impulsive control mechanism occurring as a result of dexamethasone treatment. For instance, in Cushing's syndrome, both the single dose test, for assessment of the impulsive activity of the adaptive homeostat, and the long-term test, for the basal hypothalamic mechanism of feedback, reveal resistance to inhibition in the adaptive homeostat.

Thus, if a differential approach to evaluation of the available data is used, similar age-associated changes in the adaptive homeostat in the rat (Riegle 1973; Ostroumova and Dilman 1972) and man may be identified.[1] The above suggests a hypothesis on three types of disturbances in the rhythm of adaptive homeostat functioning:

1. Hypothalamic type, which is characterized by the elevation of the threshold of sensitivity to inhibition by dexamethasone in the basal system of the feedback mechanism (normal aging, android obesity, Cushing's syndrome). These disturbances may be detected by the long-term dexamethasone test; age-associated changes will not be identified unless a minimal dose of dexamethasone that proves to be an effective inhibitor in a given population of young subjects is found. In our study this dose was found to be 0.125 mg, every six hours for two days.
2. Extrahypothalamic type involves the rise in the threshold of sensitivity to inhibition by dexamethasone in the im-

[1]We used single dose dexamethasone tests for rats in the morning (see Table 3-1), ie, at a period other than the critical one for circadian rhythm regulation. In these circumstances, this test actually evaluated the basal hypothalamic feedback mechanism.

pulsive (circadian) system of the adaptive homeostat. Such disturbances are mostly related to shifts in the circadian rhythm of cortisol secretion and in single dose dexamethasone tests made in depressive patients.[1]

3. Combination type is related to the primarily hypothalamic or extrahypothalamic rise in the sensitivity threshold in the adaptive homeostat that results in the increase in the basal level of cortisol, thus causing the secondary elevation of the threshold of hypothalamic-pituitary complex sensitivity to inhibition by cortisol. Resistance to dexamethasone is revealed in such cases both in short- and long-term dexamethasone tests. Although this type of homeostatic failure has not been sufficiently proven, in my opinion, it is characteristic of Cushing's syndrome as well as all those pathologic processes accompanied by a persistent rise in basal blood cortisol levels. It may be suggested that a similar situation occurs in endometrial and prostatic cancer patients, too.

Thus, the dexamethasone suppression test demonstrates the operation of the Law of Constancy of Internal Environment and its counterpart, the Law of Deviation of Homeostasis, at the same time. Whenever we follow events taking place in a young animal (or human) as a result of the long-term dexamethasone test, we see the Law of Constancy of Internal Environment in operation, and this process is ensured in the young organism by a reliable mechanism of negative feedback. Yet, the same test performed in an older organism indicates the lack of stability with time (ie, with aging) and the inhibitory effect, which is well pronounced in the young, diminishes with time, and thus we see the Law of Deviation of Homeostasis.

Naturally, a question arises whether age-related regulatory changes can cause disorders observed in normal aging. Theoretically, the age-associated elevation of the hypothalamic threshold of sensitivity results in the formation of a "normal disease" of regulation in the adaptive homeostat system. This disease may be designated as dysadaptosis. Dysadaptosis is actually a disease because, strictly speaking, a disease is any persistent disturbance of homeostasis (see Chapter 1). Simultaneously, dysadaptosis is a normal disease because it forms inevitably in the course of aging, regardless of external, random causes. Now, it is appropriate to ask if the signs of dysadaptosis, ie, a normal disease of the

[1]Carroll et al (1976) administered a large dose of dexamethasone (2 mg) in their study of the sensitivity of the adaptive homeostat to inhibition by this drug, but did it at a critical period, ie, they studied impulsive activity. It was found that depressed patients had an abnormally early escape from dexamethasone suppression.

adaptive homeostat "blue-printed" by normal aging, really exist and, if they do, what they are.

The similarity of Cushing's disease to many manifestations of aging in the rat and Pacific salmon (Wexler 1971, 1976) and in man (Dilman 1961, 1971; Wexler 1971) attracted the attention of researchers years ago. It was mentioned above that many middle-aged subjects develop mild (subclinical) cushingoid features.[1] Although Cushing's syndrome involves a raised level of blood cortisol, the hypothalamic-pituitary complex does not become inhibited by negative feedback, and such a hyperfunctioning homeostatic system does not regain equilibrium spontaneously. This explains why a similar, although less pronounced, picture is observed in the course of normal aging, which is also characterized by the central type of homeostatic failure.

However, the actual situation seems to be more complicated. In man the 17-oxysteroid blood level does not significantly increase with advancing age. According to Grad et al (1967), the blood oxysteroid levels were 12.7 ± 1.1 μg% in 24-year-old women and 12.4 μg% in women at age 70. In men at those ages they were 12.9 ± 1.3 μg% and 14.6 ± 1.1 μg%, respectively. At the same time it is known that the production of other corticosteroids, particularly 17-ketosteroids, declines both in males and females with advancing age (Borth et al 1957, Abbo 1966). The cause of the dissociation in the age-related dynamics of corticosteroid production is not clear. Since the secretion of both groups of hormones is controlled by the hypothalamus-ACTH complex, the differences are likely to be caused by factors relating to the adrenal cortex itself. Therefore, it may be suggested that the lack of a compensating increase in blood oxysteroid level, which should be expected at an elevated hypothalamic set point, is conditioned by the general decline of adrenal activity in the course of aging. Ultimately, however, the level of 17-oxysteroids becomes relatively higher than that of 17-ketosteroids. Table 3-5 shows that the 17-ketosteroid/17-hydroxysteroid secretion level ratio progressively declines with increasing age in both healthy males and females. Therefore, relative hypercorticism develops in human organisms in the course of normal aging.

This shift may be illustrated by Table 3-6 which shows that the age-associated decrease of tolerance to carbohydrates and some other metabolic disturbances is, to a considerable degree, caused by excessive glucocorticoid action.

The same dose of prednisolone was administered to all age groups. Therefore, the age-associated decrease in glucose tolerance in this test

---

[1] It should be noted that as early as 1964, Blumenthal reported that pituitary-corticotropin content does not decrease with age. A number of investigators reported an age-associated elevation of the basal corticosteroid level in blood in rats (Barnett and Phillips 1976).

Table 3-5
The Ratio of Secretion of 17-Ketosteroids to 17-Hydroxycorticosteroids in Control Subjects and Breast Cancer Patients of Different Age Groups

	Ratio of 17-ketosteroids/17-hydroxycorticosteroids		
	Control Subjects		*Breast cancer patients*
Age Group	*Men*	*Women*	
20–29	2.26	2.10	–
30–39	1.34	1.43	1.38
40–49	1.25	1.38	1.20
50–59	1.27	–	0.98
60+	0.83	0.78	0.80

Table 3-6
Relationship between Mean Blood Glucose Level during Prednisolone-Glucose Test and Age in Male Patients with Ischemic Heart Disease*

	No.	Blood Glucose Level (mg%)	
Age Group	Cases	*1 hr*	*2 hr*
Under 50 years	25	197.9 ± 7.2	144.2 ± 7.1
50–59 years	31	220.4 ± 8.2	169.6 ± 6.3
More than 60 years	17	244.8 ± 7.7	203.6 ± 5.8

*15 mg of prednisolone was administered 8.5 and 2 hr before intake of 100 g of glucose.

may be accounted for by the growing diabetogenic influence of endogenous glucocorticoids with advancing age. Similar results are reported by other authors (Pozefsky et al 1965). This has motivated some investigators to establish different limits of the norm for each successive decade after age 40 to avoid admitting that nearly all middle-aged and old people have latent chemical diabetes (Pozefsky et al 1965).

Thus the relatively greater output of 17-oxysteroids compared with 17-ketosteroids in aging seems to be pathogenic. Bulbrook et al (1971) expressed this relation as an index of discrimination: 17-oxycorticosteroids (mg/24 hours) + etiocholanolone (μg/24 hours). They showed that a discrimination index less than unity indicates a predisposition to breast cancer (Bulbrook 1972).

Later, similar results were reported in studies of endometrial cancer (De Waard et al 1969) and lung cancer (Rao 1972). (In the latter case androsterone level was determined instead of etiocholanolone.) It should be noted that the negative index of discrimination also has been found in patients with ischemic heart disease. A high blood cortisol level is also observed in coronary-prone individuals (Friedman et al 1970).

Thus the enhanced glucocorticoid influence predisposes an organism to the development of age-specific pathology. Moreover, clinical evidence shows that a relatively small but long-term rise in the blood cortisol level caused by hypothalamic resistance to inhibition appears to have a substantial effect on a tumor process. For instance, the cases with a rapid progress of the disease revealed elevated cortisol production matched by an insufficient decrease caused by dexamethasone (Saez 1974). Besides, plasma cortisol levels were lower in patients who had a positive immunoresponse to tuberculin than in patients with a negative response (MacKay et al 1971). Similarly, we showed in our laboratory a negative correlation between levels of excretion of 17-oxysteroids and 17-ketosteroids in breast cancer patients with a dinitrochlorobenzene (DNCB) skin test (Table 3-7). At the same time, those patients who showed a positive reaction tended to have a better prognosis.

Table 3-7
Levels of Excretion of 17-Hydroxycorticosteroids and 17-Ketosteroids in Breast Cancer Patients with Positive and Negative DNCB Skin Test

Group	17-hydroxy-corticosteroids (mg/24 hr)	17-keto-steroids (mg/24 hr)	Coefficient 17KS/17-OHS
DNCB-positive	4.3 ± 0.7	6.4 ± 0.5	2.3 ± 0.5
DNCB-negative	7.5 ± 1.3	3.5 ± 1.1	0.5 ± 0.1
	($p < 0.05$)	($p < 0.05$)	($p < 0.02$)

Thus, the blurred distinction between the mechanism of normal aging and the pathogenesis of specific age pathology is a peculiar feature of the pathophysiologic processes that are promoted by the age-associated drift of the hypothalamic threshold of sensitivity. In this context, specific age-associated pathology may be regarded as an intensified aging, while the process of normal aging, in this case, dysadaptosis, is regarded as a disease. Since the aging of a population inevitably results in increased numbers of overweight individuals and those suffering from prediabetes, latent adult-onset diabetes mellitus, atherosclerosis, mental depression, etc, ie, states characterized by an elevated output of glucocorticoids, it may be said a priori that a sufficiently strict distinction between normal age-associated shifts and those related to age-connected pathology is not feasible. As a consequence, the results of the studies of age-associated changes in the adaptive homeostat may vary from population to population.

It is easy to see a striking similarity between dysadaptosis and the changes that develop in chronic stress, eg, in chronic stress caused by an increased density of animal population (Christian 1976). But the chief distinction of dysadaptosis from diseases of adaptation is that the former is induced by internal factors that cause changes in adaptive homeostat regulation rather than by external stressors. In other words, dysadaptosis is bound to develop even under ideal conditions, as a result of time. As far as dysadaptosis is concerned, time is a natural stressor. Moreover, dysadaptosis is not merely a "normal disease of aging" that introduces features of chronic stress into an organism that functions normally when there is no stress. Whenever a stress situation develops, it takes the dysregulated adaptive system longer than usual to regain equilibrium; therefore, its overall response to stress becomes excessive. Of particular interest are the data that show that middle-aged patients respond to surgical stress by a longer rise in blood 11-hydroxycorticosteroid level than younger ones (Blichert-Toft 1975). The organism pays a higher price for protection from stress in old age than in youth and it is forced to do it by the Law of Deviation of Homeostasis.[1]

An evaluation of the commencement of the changes inherent in normal aging, as well as specific age pathology, suggests several hypotheses for the possible mechanism of elevation of hypothalamic threshold in the adaptive homeostat.

At present, there is equal evidence to support both the role of catecholamine and of serotonin deficit in the brain in the pathogenesis of endogenous depression (Schildkraut 1965, Mass 1965). On the other hand, age advancement involves a decline in the hypothalamic level of biogenic amines both in man and in the rat (Robinson et al 1972, Robinson 1975, Anisimov et al 1977). This phenomenon is accompanied by a rise in monoamine oxidase activity (Robinson et al 1977). Therefore, it is possible to suggest that the age-associated elevation of hypothalamic threshold of sensitivity in the adaptive homeostat is caused by the age-related decrease in the hypothalamic levels of biogenic amines. This suggestion can be supported by some direct and indirect evidence. Table 3-8 shows that L-tryptophan, phenformin, and L-dopa treatment potentiated the inhibitory action of dexamethasone (Ostroumova et al 1978).

Of particular interest are the data demonstrating that phenformin, an antidiabetic biguanide, raises the sensitivity of the hypothalamic-pituitary complex to feedback inhibition by dexamethasone. It is probable that phenformin is capable of raising the receptor affinity for

[1]Blichert-Toft (1978) reported that on the day of surgery the increment in plasma cortisol concentration was significantly higher in elderly patients than in the young. Throughout four postoperative days, the evening level of plasma cortisol was significantly higher in elderly than in young patients. Taking into consideration the duration of these observations (five days) and that the rise in urinary 17-KGS excretion was also generally higher in elderly than in young. The higher level of blood cortisol cannot be accounted for by the slowed metabolic disposal of cortisol with age, as Blichert-Toft believes. His results point to the elevation of the hypothalamic threshold to inhibition by endogenous cortisol in the aged patients both before and after operative stress.

Table 3-8
Effects of L-Tryptophan, L-Dopa, and Phenformin on Dexamethasone Test Results in Humans

	Treatment*			
	L-Tryptophan (n = 20)	*L-Dopa (n = 14)*	*Phenformin (n = 16)*	*Phenformin (n = 12)*
Test hormone	11-hydroxy-steroids (μg%)	11-hydroxy-steroids (μg%)	17-hydroxy-steroids (mg/day)	17-keto-steroids (mg/day)
Steroid level before treatment				
Basal level	20.2 ± 1.5	20.6 ± 1.8	7.5 ± 1.1	6.3 ± 0.6
After dexa-methasone	12.0 ± 1.5	11.5 ± 1.4	4.3 ± 0.6	4.5 ± 0.6
Inhibition (%)	−40 ± 7	−39 ± 7	−46 ± 9	−21 ± 15
Steroid level after treatment				
Basal level	20.0 ± 1.9	19.3 ± 1.9	6.6 ± 0.8	8.5 ± 1.0
After dexa-methasone	8.2 ± 1.4†	6.1 ± 1.9†	3.8 ± 0.7	3.8 ± 0.7
Inhibition (%)	−59 ± 4†	−51 ± 10	−60 ± 6	−41 ± 12†

*L-Tryptophan (3 to 6 g daily) and L-dopa (1 to 3 g daily) during one week were administered to depressive illness patients and healthy controls. Phenformin (100 mg daily) was given to patients with coronary atherosclerosis for 2.5 to 3 months.
†Difference is statistically significant.

its specific hormone, as suggested by Muntoni (1974). It should be mentioned, in this respect, that some tissues have been found to have lower concentrations of receptors of glucocorticoids (Roth and Livingston 1976), as well as a decline in the corticosterone-stimulated induction of certain enzymes with increasing age (Adelman 1976).[1] It is quite possible that similar development may also occur in the hypothalamus. It is also possible, however, that phenformin produces inhibition of monoamine oxidase activity in the brain, as it does in the pancreas (Feldman and Durchen 1975). Moreover, there are some weighty arguments suggesting a correlation between the condition of "hypothalamic threshold" and metabolic processes occurring in the body. These interrelationships may provide explanations for the phenformin-induced decrease in the threshold of hypothalamic sensitivity to inhibition by dexamethasone.

In acute stress, dexamethasone fails to cause an adequate suppression of corticosterone level in rats (Zimmerman and Critchlow 1969, Ostroumova 1978). But it is known that stress entails a decrease in the biogenic amine level in the hypothalamus (Scapagnini et al 1973, Vermes

[1]The age-associated decline in receptor concentration and, particularly, changes in the inductive synthesis of enzymes may be caused by age-dependent shifts in the internal environment.

et al 1973). It is also supposed that the decrease in the hypothalamic level of catecholamines annuls the tonic inhibition of ACTH secretion, thus causing the blood level of this hormone to rise (Gruen 1978). Simultaneously, the decline in the biogenic amine level is likely to result in the elevation of the hypothalamic threshold to inhibition. The latter hypothesis explains why the elevation in glucocorticoid level in response to stress takes longer in older age both in humans (Blichert-Toft 1975) and in rats (Riegle 1973). It seems that stress, which causes the decline in biogenic amine level, adds to the effect of the age-associated decrease in the hypothalamic concentration of the biogenic amines. It is well known that stress may accelerate normal aging (Selye and Tuchweber 1976) or bring about mental depression. This phenomenon may also be explained by a correlation between the decrease in biogenic amine level and elevation of the hypothalamic threshold.

Thus, the age-associated elevation of hypothalamic threshold in the adaptive system may come about as a result of the decrease in biogenic amine concentration in the brain, and, probably more precisely, in the hypothalamus.

The influence of the pineal gland is yet another factor affecting hypothalamic sensitivity to homeostatic inhibition in the adaptive homeostat. Pineal polypeptide extract apparently raises the sensitivity of the hypothalamic-pituitary complex to inhibition by dexamethasone

Table 3-9
Effect of Pineal Polypeptide Extract (Epithalamin) and Phenformin on Dexamethasone Suppression Test and Epithalamin on Stress-Induced Corticosterone Surge

Preparation	No. Animals	Corticosterone Blood Level (μg%) *Basal*	*After Dexamethasone*	Changes (%)	*p*
Control	17	7.2 ± 1.2	5.0 ± 0.8	−31	> 0.05
Epithalamin (1 mg/day)	17	6.8 ± 0.9	3.9 ± 0.5	−42	< 0.02
Control	12	7.1 ± 0.7	5.1 ± 0.6	−28	< 0.05
Phenformin (5 mg/day)	12	7.4 ± 0.7	3.7 ± 0.4	−50	< 0.001
Stress + saline	30	57.7 ±2.8	...	...	...
Stress + epithalamin (1 mg/day)	30	46.4 ± 3.0	...	...	< 0.05

Note: Pineal polypeptide extract (epithalamin) was injected subcutaneously for 5 days. Animals were subjected to ether stress 2 hours after the last injection of preparation (1 ml ether/liter of vessel volume for 2 minutes). Blood was sampled before stress application and 20 minutes after. Phenformin was injected intraperitoneally for 5 days.

(Table 3-9). Similar results were obtained when pineal polypeptides were used in conjunction with prednisolone (Ostroumova and Dilman 1972).

In conclusion, it should be mentioned that all pathologic shifts induced by age-associated disturbances in the adaptive system are determined by the physiologic role of the adaptive homeostat. Moreover, adaptation would not take place at all unless the hypothalamic threshold to inhibition were elevated, because hormonal-metabolic shifts indispensable for protection, including a rise in levels of blood cortisol, glucose, and free fatty acids, would inhibit the hypothalamic-pituitary complex by negative feedback and arrest the mechanism of protection. In the final analysis, this promotes the formation of age-associated pathology (see Chapter 18).

Thus, I think that the development of complex homeostatic systems in the course of the evolution of higher animals (which, by itself, has reduced the organism's dependence on the external environment and, therefore, the incidence of death from external environmental causes) has given rise to another biologic phenomenon: regulatory death caused by intrinsic factors, which, in the course of homeostatic system self-development, inevitably disturb the constancy of the internal environment of the organism.

4 Age-Associated Changes in the Reproductive Homeostat A Normal Disease: Climacteric

Climacteric is both a natural process and a disease; it is a norm because the climacteric develops in the course of natural aging, and it is a disease because the climacteric is the result of a persistent disturbance of constancy of internal environment of the organism, which eventually results in a certain decline in the longevity of the organism. Climacteric is, therefore, a normal disease of the reproductive homeostat.

The reproductive system may be influenced by many factors of the external and internal environment, but in a regulatory respect the reproductive homeostat functions as a closed loop system, ie, as a homeostatic system which does not need specific signals generated by other systems in order to maintain its function.[1]

An essential feature of the reproductive homeostat is its age-associated switching-on, but equally essential is the age-associated switching-off of the reproductive function. Hence, it would be of particular interest to learn the mechanism of these phenomena, since it would allow penetration into the processes by which the genetically programmed development and aging of an organism are implemented. In this chapter our aim is to show the presence of a single mechanism of

[1]Strictly speaking, the reproductive system is, of course, not a closed loop system, since the processes taking place in the open system of the energy homeostat are needed for the functioning of the reproductive homeostat. For example, the age-related fat accumulation determines, within certain limits, the age when the reproductive function is switched on (Frisch 1973).

age-related switching-on and switching-off of the reproductive function. This consideration is important to our argument that age-associated disturbances in the regulation of the main homeostatic systems are the result of implementation of the Law of Deviation of Homeostasis.

Functional Organization of the Reproductive Homeostat

In primates the reproductive homeostat is a closed loop system that functions independently of external stimuli. In the female organism this system functions cyclically, whereas in the male organism it operates constantly. However, it has been observed experimentally that animals possess a tendency toward the formation of the cyclic (female) type of functioning soon after birth, irrespective of sex. Boys then develop the noncyclic, continuous type of functioning from the influence of androgens (see Chapter 9). These androgens operate on the hypothalamic level, where the "sex center" is located. The existence of such a center in the brain was suggested as early as the 1930s (Hohlweg and Döhrn 1931). At present there are known to be two such centers in the hypothalamus: the tonic center that regulates the constant secretion of gonadotropins, and the cyclic center which is responsible for the mechanism of ovulation. The hypothalamic FSH/LH-releasing hormone that controls the secretion of both the follicle-stimulating and luteinizing hormones of the pituitary has been synthesized (Schally et al 1972). However many data indicate that the two gonadotropic hormones are secreted independently of one another. This probably is caused by a self-regulatory mechanism that operates both on the hypothalamic and pituitary levels.

Cyclic gonadotropin secretion is also associated with numerous brain structures outside the hypophysiotropic zone of the hypothalamus. It appears that the ovulatory mechanism is influenced by impulses from the limbic system associated with olfactory and tactile signals, whereas the epithalamus-pineal gland complex exerts its effect in response to light signals. Although the reproductive homeostat normally is a closed loop system, it also is exposed to the influence of signals from the external environment. These signals either contribute to the optimization of reproductive system functioning or promote a quick switching-off of reproductive functioning if the organism is exposed to unfavorable external conditions. In the final anaylsis, however, all these influences register at the level of the hypothalamic-pituitary complex.

The neurons that secrete gonadotropin-releasing hormone have receptors capable of binding sex hormones. The receptors for estrogens have received the most study, and like uterine receptors they are a specific protein. The basic systems of neurotransmitters in the hypothalamic part of the reproductive homeostat are dopamine and noradrenaline. They belong to the adrenergic system, whereas the antagonistic system operates chiefly by means of serotonin, melatonin, and perhaps some polypeptide hormones of the pineal gland. Mediation of catecholamines is of vital importance for the transmission of impulses from the cyclic center to the tonic one, which regulates the secretion of FSH/LH-releasing hormone (Kamberi 1973). Taking into account these and some other data, it may be supposed that the cyclic secretion of gonadotropins is stimulated by noradrenaline, while the tonic secretion of gonadotropins seems to be stimulated by noradrenaline and inhibited by dopamine (Fuxe et al 1972; Anisimov 1975). The fact that low doses of L-dopa stimulate gonadotropin secretion, while high doses inhibit it, may be accounted for by the limiting activity of dopamine-β-hydroxylase, dopamine being accumulated as a consequence of large doses of L-dopa.

The inhibitory action of tuberoinfundibular dopamine neurons on peptidergic neurons in the median eminence secreting LH/FSH-RH was inferred. The negative feedback action of estrogens seems to be effected through the dopamine system (McCann et al 1973). For example, estradiol, at doses inhibiting LH secretion, markedly increases dopamine turnover in the hypothalamus (Fuxe et al 1974).

The rise in serotonin levels in the hypothalamus seems to provide one of the factors inhibiting reproductive function. A similar influence is exerted by melatonin, and the effect of melatonin is mediated by serotonergic neurons.

Some data indicate that cholinergic mechanisms are involved in the transmission of inhibitory stimuli from the amygdala and septum to different areas of the hypothalamus. Finally, some data prove that histamine, prostaglandins and γ-aminobutyric acid are involved in the mechanism of hypothalamic regulation of the reproductive homeostat (Müller et al 1977).

In addition to the receptors sensitive to sex hormones, the hypothalamus contains receptors responsive to pituitary gonadotropins. These findings are consistent with the results of our investigations which showed that acetylated FSH, deprived of gonadotropic effect, can inhibit the compensatory hypertrophy of the ovary caused by unilateral castration (Table 4-1).

Table 4-1
Inhibitory Effect of Ovine Acetylated Hypophyseal FSH on the Biological Action of Endogenous FSH in Rats Following Unilateral Ovariectomy

Group	Dose (mg/day)	No. Animals	Compensatory Hypertrophy of Ovaries (%)	
Control	–	39	80.5 ± 1.24	
Acetylated FSH*	1.5	35	41.8 ± 1.19	$p < 0.001$

*Acetylated FSH was administered for ten days.

The inhibitory effect of acetylated FSH is based on the short loop mechanism of negative feedback. In addition, the reproductive system of the hypothalamus features an ultra-short loop feedback that is based on self-inhibition of FSH/LH-releasing hormone production. Therefore three types of negative feedback loops may be distinguished within the reproductive homeostat.

Estrogens exert both stimulating and inhibitory effects on gonadotropin secretion, ie, by positive and negative feedback. This biphasic pattern is dependent largely on the dosage level of the estrogens (Yen and Tsai 1971), and it is possible that both negative and positive feedback mechanisms are switched on simultaneously following estrogen administration. It also is probable that castration, which involves a sharp fall in estrogen level, is followed initially by elimination of the positive feedback effect. Therefore ovariectomy results in an initial decline in serum gonadotropin level that persists for one to five days (Monroe et al 1972). Small doses of estrogens stimulate FSH and LH secretion (Monroe et al 1972), while large doses inhibit them (Franchimont et al 1972). Data showing that an ovulatory surge of LH may be induced by moderate doses of estrogens support a positive feedback influence on the cyclic center. On the other hand the inhibition of gonadotropin secretion by large doses of estrogens is effected at the tonic center level by negative feedback.

The Ovulatory Cycle

FSH promotes the maturation of ovarian follicles. Accordingly the blood FSH level rises in the premenstrual period after a sharp decrease in estrogen output. Estrogens are then synthesized in the ovaries under the joint control of FSH and LH, and as the follicle grows in size the blood concentration of estrogens, mainly estradiol, increases. At a later stage of follicle formation the blood FSH level is decreased, falling to the minimal value 12 to 18 hours before the ovulatory surge of gonadotropin secretion. The preovulatory decrease in FSH level (Ross et al 1970) has not been interpreted from the physiologic point of view. It seems to be caused by the inhibitory influence of estrogens, which act on the tonic center through negative feedback. This effect is a manifestation of the normal level of sensitivity in the tonic center of the hypothalamus, ie, an indicator of the level of sensitivity at which ovulation may be induced.

The ovulatory peak of estrogen secretion occurs immediately before the ovulatory release of gonadotropins. The estrogen peak is responsible for the ovulatory surge of gonadotropins, because ovulation does not occur unless the blood estrogen level is increased. At this stage estrogens operate through positive feedback, stimulating the cyclic center, probably by a catecholamine mechanism, to produce a sharp increase in blood FSH and LH levels. This condition is referred to as the ovulatory surge. Thus, in the mechanism of ovulation the key role lies in the sensitivity of the hypothalamus to the positive feedback effect of estrogens. As it has been shown, progesterone and 17-hydroxyprogesterone secretion, which starts rising in the preovulatory period, is essential in modulating the threshold of hypothalamic sensitivity.

The rupture of a mature follicle and ovulation take place under the influence of LH. Some authors claim that the surge of FSH secretion is required then for the preparation of follicles for the next cycle (Mougdal et al 1974). The surge of gonadotropins subsides quickly as the estrogen concentration falls below the level that immediately preceded its surge. Later, as the corpus luteum starts functioning, the estrogen level rises again, and at the same time the concentration of progesterone in the blood begins to rise. As a result of the action of sex hormones the endometrium develops first proliferative changes and then the secretory changes required for the nidation of the fertilized ovum. Estrogens and progesterone contribute to the gradual inhibition of gonadotropin secretion, particularly LH, which controls the function of the corpus luteum. The inhibition of LH secretion switches on mechanisms, among them prostaglandins, which are responsible for the regression of the corpus luteum. This results in a sharp decrease in estrogens and progesterone and, finally, in menstruation. A decrease in estrogens releases the hypothalamus from inhibition, thus leading to an increase in FSH secretion and a repeat of the reproductive cycle.

Mechanism of Age-Associated Switching-On of Reproductive Function

The mechanism of age-associated switching-on of the reproductive function seems to be determined by a decrease in the sensitivity of the hypothalamic-gonadotropic system to inhibition by estrogens (Donovan and Van der Werff ten Bosch 1959). This conclusion is based on data (Hohlweg and Döhrn 1931, Byrnes and Meyer 1951, Ramirez and McCann 1963, Eldridge et al 1974) pointing to the age-associated elevation of resistance in the hypothalamic "sex center" to inhibition by estrogens; this leads to an increase in gonadotropin production, stimulation of the sex glands, and eventually to puberty and the switching-on of the ovulatory cycle in the female organism (Donovan and Van der Werff ten Bosch 1959).

According to the current model, which distinguishes between two separate sex centers, tonic and cyclic, the mechanism of switching-on of the reproductive cycle in the female organism should be modified as follows (Dilman 1974a).

The decrease in hypothalamic sensitivity to inhibition by estrogens (the elevation of the set point) seems to originate in the tonic center. Thus the output of FSH/LH-releasing hormone, and accordingly the secretion of FSH and LH, increases gradually, which results in an increased production of estrogens by the ovaries.

It has been shown that blood levels of FSH and LH increase with those of estradiol (Jenner et al 1972). Considering that estradiol inhibits the tonic production of gonadotropins by negative feedback, the situation points first to the phenomenon of age-associated elevation of the hypothalamic threshold of sensitivity to inhibition by estrogens and, second, to the phenomenon of a compensatory increase in estrogen secretion. These features are inherent in the central type of homeostatic failure, which is responsible for the development of the potential of the overall system (see Chapter 1).

However, the switching-on of reproductive function in the female organism is dependent on the activity of both the tonic and cyclic centers of the reproductive area of the hypothalamus. This calls for a refinement of the model (Dilman 1974a).

It may be suggested that reproductive function is switched on in a female organism when estrogen concentration has reached a critical level as a result of the above mechanism, and triggers the stimulation of the cyclic area of the sex center by positive feedback (the so-called Hohlweg effect). Such an effect was observed in an experiment in which premature puberty and estrus were induced in rats by administering estrogens one week before the physiologic switching-on of the reproductive function (Döcke and Dörner 1965). This mechanism of positive feedback gradually develops during ontogenesis, which is matched by the age-associated dynamics of estrogen uptake by the hypothalamus (Presl et al 1973). This process is likely to be partially controlled by the steroids of the adrenal cortex (Forest et al 1973, Sizonenko and Pannicz 1975).

In the rat, estrogen action to induce ovulation seems to be effected by means of the intensification of catecholamine secretion, which stimulates the cyclic center directly. This stimulation causes an ovulatory surge of gonadotropins, thus switching on the reproductive cycle. According to this model of the switching-on of the reproductive function, the elevation of the hypothalamic threshold originates in the tonic center. This increases the production of sex hormones, which eventually results in the stimulation of the cyclic region of the hypothalamic sex center. In this sequence the tonic center is released gradually from inhibition by estrogens and subsequently stimulates their production. But this activity must continue for several years before estrogen levels become sufficiently high to stimulate the cyclic center and induce ovulation.

Mechanism of Age-Associated Switching-Off of the Reproductive Cycle

It is generally believed that the age-associated switching-off of reproductive function is caused by a decrease in the hormonal activity of the ovaries and a gradual reduction in the quantity of primordial ova. However, this point of view does not account for the regression of follicles, the quantity of which is by far in excess of that required for reproductive function. Nor is it clear why the estrogen output of the ovaries is decreased, particularly considering that the climacteric onset is characterized generally by a so-called "polyfolliculine" stage when estrogens are excessive (Zondek 1935). Moreover during aging and menopause it is possible to observe hyperplasia of the thecal tissues of the ovaries, ie, the tissues in which ovarian steroids are synthesized. Years ago I developed a concept in which the switching-off of reproductive function is caused by a primary increase of hypothalamic activity, rather than by a decline in the functional activity of the ovaries (Dilman 1958, unpublished data).[1] At that time it was known that both menopausal women and ovariectomized women have a high level of excretion of total gonadotropins, particularly FSH. It was believed that the menopause develops because of the primary ovarian failure.[2] In essence, this point of view is still maintained. Mills and Mahesh (1978) note that "the most obvious explanation for the elevated levels of gonadotropins in the menopause is that the senescent ovary secretes insufficient steroid to suppress gonadotropin production. In this respect, the menopause is similar to the dynamics in gonadotropin secretion which follow ovariectomy," ie, it is a consequence of the peripheral type of homeostatic failure (see Chapter 2).

Rakoff and Nowroozi (1978) also support a concept according to which "the climacteric is caused by physiological ovarian failure attributable to a progressive loss of functioning ovarian tissue."

However, in 1955 (Dilman, unpublished data) I suggested that the high level of FSH, characteristic of the menopause, is caused by hypothalamic shifts, and that the rise in FSH excretion should start prior to the onset of the climacteric because of the primary elevation of hypothalamic activity. From that hypothesis it followed that the origin of the menopause should be sought in the hypothalamus, rather than in the ovaries.

Albert (1956) showed that the excretion of total gonadotropins in females with normal menstrual cycle nearly doubles during ages 30–39 years, as compared with 20–29 years, ie, in a period when there is no substantial age-associated decrease in estrogen secretion.

Subsequently, similar results also have been reported by others

---

[1]Later, Sheehan (1968) noted that the subventricular nucleus of the hypothalamus undergoes marked hypertrophy in approximately one-third of postmenopausal women, and moderate hypertrophy in another third.

[2]The findings of Costoff and Mahesh (1975) showing the presence of normal primordial follicles in menopausal patients seem to negate this popular theory.

(Christiansen 1972, Tajic and Longhino 1968) who pointed to an approximately threefold increase in gonadotropin excretion in females aged 41–45 compared with a group aged 17–40 years. Sherman et al (1976) showed that in women aged 45–56 years with regular cycles there was a striking increase in FSH content throughout the cycle, while LH remained in normal range. Long before that, Henderson and Rowlands (1938) noted an increase of gonadotropin level in the pituitary during aging. Even earlier, Fluhman (1931, 1956) reported an increase of gonadotropin excretion prior to the onset of the climacteric. However, the authors of these notable studies did not abandon their concept of the primarily ovarian origin of the climacteric (Dilman 1958, 1968, 1974a). In particular, analysis was undertaken of the reasons why Loraine and associates (Brown et al 1958) had first negated the increase of gonadotropin excretion prior to the onset of the climacteric, while later they reported that urinary gonadotropins were elevated in the perimenopausal years before the cessation of ovulatory function (Adamopoulos et al 1971). Another serious obstacle toward accepting the idea of the hypothalamic origin of the climacteric was the numerous data indicating that, with aging, the excretion of classic estrogens declines in women. Moreover, it was known that, two years after onset of menopause, the ovaries secrete practically no classic estrogens. Nevertheless, that obstacle seemed vulnerable in many respects.

First, the incidence of cancer of the reproductive system rises in the postmenopausal period. This is particularly true of endometrial carcinoma, which occurs in conjunction with endometrial hyperplasia in about 75% of cases. Moreover this hyperplasia cannot be the result of the low level of classic estrogen secretion characteristic of the postmenopausal period. What can be offered as an explanation for this discrepancy? A further development of my hypothesis was based on an evaluation of the age-associated changes of the excretion of not only total gonadotropins and FSH, but also of the excretion of total phenolsteroids.

Generally the hormonal activity of the ovaries is assessed on the basis of the production of the so-called "classic estrogens," estradiol, estrone, and estriol. Based on determinations of these estrogens most authors have concluded that the ovarian production of classic estrogens is decreased in the course of aging, and practically ceases approximately two years after menopause (Judd et al 1974). As a rule the total excretion of classic estrogens does not exceed 10 μg/24 hours in the postmenopausal period.

However, it has been established during the last decade that in addition to the three classical estrogens a large number of other phenolsteroids are produced in the human organism. Of these, 2-methoxyestrone, 2-methoxyestradiol, 16-epiestriol, 17-epiestrone, 16,17-epiestriol, 18-hydroxyestrone, and 16-hydroxyestrone have received the most study. If these hormones are designated as nonclassic estrogens, total phenolsteroids may be regarded as the sum of classic and nonclassic phenolsteroids. Then the magnitude of nonclassic phenolsteroid excretion may be obtained from the difference in the levels of total phenolsteroids and classic estrogens. However, it is not yet clear whether the group of nonclassic phenolsteroids is limited to the hormones known at present. At the same time, all total phenolsteroids were believed to be metabolites of classic estrogens (Diczfalusy and Lauritzen 1961). If the climacteric were connected with a decline in the production of classic estrogens, then it was believed that by studying total phenolsteroids it was impossible to get additional information on the mechanism of the climacteric. However, I suggested that the nonclassic phenolsteroids are produced independently of classic estrogens, at least partially (Dilman 1961, 1968). Table 4-2 shows that excretion of total gonadotropins, FSH, and total phenolsteroids increases with advancing age (Dilman and Pavlova 1963). These data indicate that in the process of aging the same disturbance of homeostasis is observed in the reproductive homeostat, which is typical of the mechanism of the age-associated switching-on of reproductive function. In fact, since the rise in gonadotropin excretion occurs concomitantly with elevation of total phenolsteroid excretion, it may be inferred that the cause of homeostatic failure is the elevation of the hypothalamic threshold to the suppressive effect of phenolsteroids, ie, the central type of homeostatic failure.

Table 4-2
Age-Associated Dynamics of Excretion of Total Gonadotropins, FSH, and Total Phenolsteroids

	Normal Menstrual Cycle			
Hormones	*20–29 years*	*30–39 years*	*40–49 years*	Menopause
Total gonadotropins (mouse units/24 hrs)	7.0 ± 4.2	41.0 ± 7.5	81.0 ± 10.2	220.0 ± 14.8
FSH*	1.05 ± 0.1	–	5.4 ± 0.4	12.7 ± 0.5
Total phenolsteroids (μg/24 hrs)	38.6 ± 4.12	46.0 ± 4.84	55.6 ± 3.7	38.4 ± 2.7

*FSH testing was performed by the method of Steelman and Pohley (1953). FSH was determined by the difference in ovarian weight (mg) in experimental and control groups of rats with reference to one hour equivalent of diurnal diuresis.

In this context I suggested a common model of both the age-related switching-on and the age-related switching-off of reproductive function (Dilman 1974a).

According to the revised model, the elevation of the hypothalamic threshold of sensitivity to inhibition by sex hormones takes place first in the tonic center, which is chiefly controlled by negative feedback. This results in the age-associated elevation of gonadotropin production and stimulation of sex gland functioning. The blood sex hormone levels rise accordingly.

The estrogens act on the cyclic center by positive feedback. Therefore, it may be supposed that the rise in blood estrogen concentration, because of the increase in the tonic center resistance to inhibition, finally reaches a level at which the cyclic center is stimulated by estrogens. The cyclic center acts on the tonic center via the neurotransmitter mechanism, resulting in the ovulatory release of gonadotropins that induce ovulation. Therefore, the genetic program of the development of the organism, ie, the reproductive system in our case, is implemented because of the elevation of the hypothalamic threshold to inhibition in the tonic region of the sex center.

Meanwhile, the elevation of the sensitivity threshold to the action of sex hormones continues in the tonic center after the switching-on of reproductive function. This results in the age-associated rise in gonadotropin output; ovarian hyperstimulation is an inevitable consequence. From this point of view, the increase in nonclassic phenolsteroid output is a compensatory reaction, which takes place in response to the elevation of the hypothalamic threshold to inhibition. Thus, two alternative hypotheses of the mechanism of age-associated switching-off of reproductive function may be proposed.

According to the first one, the shift in the spectrum of secreted estrogen-like isohormones causes the predominant excretion of nonclassic phenolsteroids and, therefore, a decrease in blood estradiol level. This leads to a situation in which the concentration of this hormone proves to be insufficient to stimulate ovulation by acting on the cyclic center by positive feedback. Such a mechanism would be a manifestation of peripheral homeostatic failure.

According to the second hypothesis, the elevation of the hypothalamic threshold of sensitivity commences in the cyclic center, too, after the switching-on of the reproductive cycle. This means, however, that as the hypothalamic threshold rises steadily, ovulation will not be induced unless blood estrogen concentration is increased at the same time. In other words, if the estrogen level does not reach the threshold of sensitivity of the cyclic center, reproductive function will be switched off and the regulation of gonadotropin secretion during this menopausal period will be effected predominantly in the tonic center.

It seems likely that the elevation of the sensitivity threshold of the cyclic center is compensated for a long time by a simultaneous increase in ovarian function. This follows inevitably from the age-connected enhancement of gonadotropin secretion, leading to hyperstimulation of the ovaries. Such a compensatory process preserves the mechanism of positive feedback despite the gradual age-associated elevation of the sensitivity threshold.

In the context of this proposed model reproductive function is switched off when, despite the compensatory increase in ovarian hormone production, the level of estrogen proves insufficient to induce ovulation because the set point of the cyclic center has become extremely high.

Therefore, according to the elevational model, both the age-associated switching-on and the switching-off of reproductive function are effected by the same mechanism, ie, the elevation of the threshold of sensitivity to homeostatic stimuli both in the tonic and cyclic centers of the reproductive homeostat. The switching-on of the cycle is caused by increased resistance of the negative feedback of the tonic center, whereas the switching-off is caused by increased resistance of the positive feedback of the cyclic center.

This model has to be tested experimentally. Numerous data indicate that the changes of hypothalamic sensitivity to sex hormones occur during a period directly associated with sexual maturity. However, the problem remains of whether hypothalamic sensitivity continues to change in the mature animal, ie, after reproductive function is switched on. To provide an answer to this problem, we used estrogen-induced suppression of compensatory ovarian hypertrophy caused by hemicastration in rats. Application of this method provides an assessment of the condition of the hypothalamic-pituitary complex that predominantly controls the secretion of FSH (Benson et al 1969, Müller et al 1972; Butcher 1977). Figure 4-1 demonstrates that, as age advances, an ever-increasing dose of estrogens is required to suppress the compensatory hypertrophy of the ovaries. It should be emphasized that this relationship persists after sexual maturity (Anisimov et al 1974). Recently, McPherson and colleagues (1977) showed that with increasing age there is a decreased pituitary and/or hypothalamic sensitivity to the feedback action of estradiol. However, since the age-connected gain of body weight may influence the distribution of exogenous estrogens in the animal's body, producing a misleading impression of hypothalamic threshold elevation, we conducted experiments involving the injection of estradiol-17 β into the third ventricle of the brain of hemicastrated rats. Figure 4-2 shows that in 14-to 16-month-old rats the dose of estradiol required for suppression of the compensatory ovarian hypertrophy by 50% and 100% was four to five times greater than in younger, three-month-old rats. This increase may be interpreted as an indication of the constantly rising hypothalamic threshold to inhibition in the tonic center of the reproductive homeostat.[1]

[1]There is some evidence that in old rats the sensitivity of the neurons to electric impulses is reduced in the hypothalamic preoptic and arcuate areas (Babichev 1973).

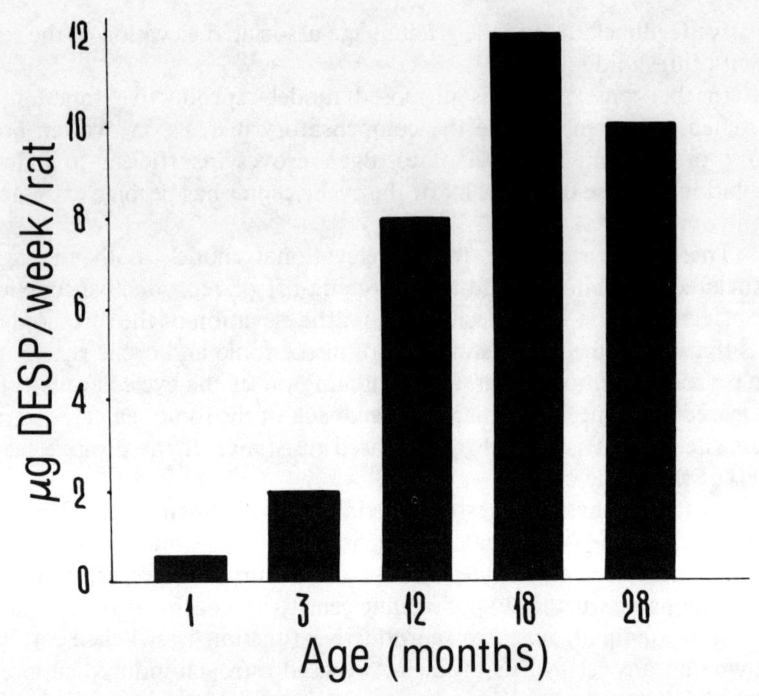

Figure 4-1 Correlation between dosage of diethylstilbestrol propionate (DESP), required for suppression of compensatory ovarian hypertrophy, and age of rat. Subcutaneous injections of DESP were started on the day of hemicastration. Rats were sacrified on the eighth day of the experiment.

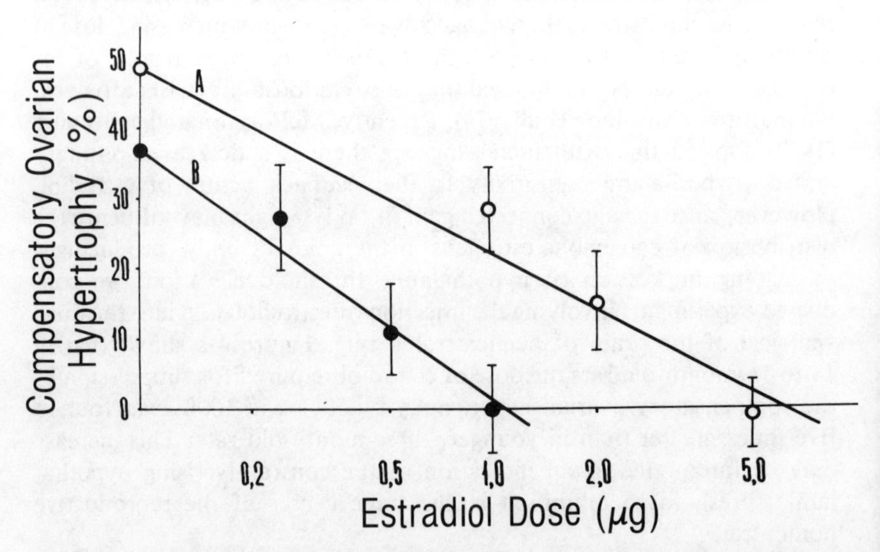

Figure 4-2 Correlation between dosage of estradiol-17β (intracisternally) required for suppression of compensatory ovarian hypertrophy, and the age of rat. A: 14- to 16-month-old rats; B: 3- to 4-month-old rats.

At the same time, it should be emphasized that my idea dating back to 1955 (Dilman, unpublished data) (according to which elevation of hypothalamic activity, or, to be more exact, elevation of hypothalamic threshold of sensitivity to homeostatic stimuli, is the mechanism implementing the age-related switching-off of reproductive function in the female organism) for a long time had no support among other researchers.

Consider the experimental and clinical data that support the elevational model of climacteric mechanism, ie, the concept of a reduced sensitivity of the hypothalamic-pituitary axis to hormonal feedback in aged females and males. First, the elevation of the hypothalamic-pituitary axis to the inhibiting effect of estrogens has been well documented only with respect to the rat; however, analogous data have been obtained on the changes in human beings. The blood gonadotropin level in prepubertal girls is suppressed by 2 μg of ethinylestradiol and by 10 μg in pubertal girls (Kelch et al 1973).

On the whole there are weighty arguments in favor of the idea that in humans from birth to puberty there occurs "the elevation of the threshold of sensitivity of the gonadostat to the negative feedback of steroids" (Forest et al 1976).

It should be noted that data are contradictory on the changes taking place after the reproductive function has been switched on. These changes are estimated on the basis of the influence of estrogens upon the blood level of gonadotropins in women in the reproductive and the menopausal periods. In particular, some researchers have been unable to find an elevation of the threshold of sensitivity of the hypothalamic-pituitary system to the inhibitory effect of estrogens in menopausal women (Franchimont et al 1972b, Wise et al 1973).

At the same time, Franchimont et al (1972) observed that although doses of 20 to 25 μg of ethinyl estradiol lowered gonadotropins in perimenopausal and postmenopausal women, doses as large as 50 μg were ineffective in restoring levels of the premenopausal period. Bolton et al (1975) also showed that 50 μg of ethinyl estradiol inhibits LH levels, although not to the level in premenopausal women. Another group reported that "the implantation of 50 mg estrogen pellets in postmenopausal women resulted in a steady level of serum estradiol of 167 ± 26 pg/ml and estrone of 110 ± 15 pg/ml. Whereas these levels of blood estrogens are very effective in suppressing RSH and LH in premenopausal women, the estrogen pellets lowered, but did not suppress, elevated gonadotropins in postmenopausal women even 11 weeks after implantation" (Mills and Mahesh 1978). Isaacs and Havard (1978) give similar information (Table 4-3).

The failure of suppression of gonadotropins to premenopausal level, despite restoration of premenopausal estrogen levels, supports the concept that in postmenopausal women there exists a central type of

Table 4-3
Effect of Long-Term Administration of Estrogens on Blood Levels of LH, FSH, Estrone, and Estradiol in Menopausal Women

	LH (units/liter)	FSH (units/liter)	Estrone (pg/ml)	Estradiol (pg/ml)
Before estrogen treatment	57.0 ± 5.4	25.8 ± 2.0	59 ± 6	14 ± 3
After estrogen treatment	50.3 ± 3.3	16.5 ± 1.5	528 ± 70	83 ± 10

Source: Isaacs and Havard 1978.

homeostatic failure in the reproductive homeostat. By comparing the available data it may be deduced that the postmenopausal decline of estradiol blood level will probably increase the sensitivity of the hypothalamic-pituitary axis to the inhibitory effect of estradiol, in accordance with the mechanism of negative feedback between the concentration of the hormone and the number of its hormone receptors (see Chapter 2). This is why only prolonged administration of estrogens to restore the premenopausal level can create conditions of the sensitivity threshold in the hypothalamic-pituitary axis to the inhibiting effect of estradiol, in postmenopausal women, that can be detected. When attempting to analyze the causes of the present contradictions, note that data should be obtained from women of different ages who still exhibit normal menstrual cycles because menopause, which involves a long-term shortage of estrogens, may affect their hypothalamic threshold of sensitivity. On the other hand, it should be taken into account that estrogen administration at the proliferative stage of the menstrual cycle may induce an ovulatory release of gonadotropins that will interfere with the evaluation of the inhibitory effect of estrogens. A rise in gonadotropin secretion is observed even in menopausal females following estrogen treatment (Yen and Tsai 1971).

However, there are insufficient data on the age-related changes taking place on the level of the cyclic center. Recently it was shown that aging involves elevation of the hypothalamic threshold to the action of estrogens by positive feedback in the female rats (Meites et al 1978). Studying the influence of photoperiods on reproductive functions in female mammals, Hoffmann (1973) also concluded that the ovulatory surge threshold rises with age in the rat.

This information is an essential contribution toward the elevational model of the age-related switching-off of the reproductive function (Dilman 1974a), since that element of the model has not been previously supported experimentally.

Gosden and Bancroft (1976) believe that the reduced magnitude or surge levels of LH found in old compared to young ovariectomized rats after treatment with gonadal steroids is consistent with the hypothesis that hypothalamic dysfunction in reproductive homeostat would result from a progressive age-related elevation of the threshold of feedback control by gonadal steroids. Some indirect evidence points to a similar conclusion. It is known that the cyclic center in rats can be disturbed with a neonatal administration of testosterone; this causes constant estrus (Barraclough and Haller 1970, Hendricks 1969). In many respects this action resembles age-associated changes in the reproductive system. In particular, it has been shown that androgenized animals exhibit a fresh corpus luteum after noradrenaline treatment (Flerko 1974).

However, some peculiarities of the functioning of the reproductive homeostat in the rodent allow interpretation of these data as not due to aging changes in women. Most authors agree that the menopausal female apparently remains sensitive to the positive feedback of estrogens. However, as with analyzing the data on the negative estrogen-hypothalamic-pituitary feedback, we need to select carefully the dose of estrogen loading, since the cyclic center retains its capacity to be stimulated by estrogens. For example, Wise et al (1973) showed that the progestin-stimulated gonadotropin surge occurred in postmenopausal women after pretreatment with a daily dosage of 400 μg of ethinyl estradiol but not after 20 μg ethinyl estradiol per day. Meanwhile, such doses as 20 to 25 μg of ethinyl estradiol lowered gonadotropins in perimenopausal and postmenopausal women (Franchimont et al 1972).

Thus, an age-related elevation of hypothalamic threshold to the inhibiting effect of estrogens has been strictly proven for women as well as for rats. In addition, it has been proven that the same phenomenon, with respect to the stimulating effect of estrogens upon the cyclic center, is discovered in old female rats, the estrogens acting in accordance with the positive feedback mechanism. Elevation of the sensitivity threshold to the homeostatic effect of estrogens, both in the tonic and in the cyclic regions of the sex center, provides experimental proof of the elevational model of the age-related switching-on and -off in the rat.

At the same time, Meites and associates (1978) offer a somewhat unexpected conclusion on the differences in the mechanisms of the age-related switching-off of reproductive function in the female rat and the human female. They write: "Thus, the primary cause for termination of menstrual cycles in women appears to lie in the ovaries, whereas in female rats termination of estrous cycles lies in the hypothalamo-pituitary system."

This categorical conclusion seems unexpected primarily because the mechanisms of the age-related switching-on of reproductive function in the female rat and in the human female are analogous. What are, then, the differences in the mechanisms of the age-related switching-off of reproductive function in rats and in women? Meites et al (1978) believe that the greatest difference is that the ovaries of women show exhaustion of ova and follicles and nonresponsiveness to gonadotropic hormone stimulation, whereas the ovaries of aging female rats retain some ova and follicles and some capacity to respond to gonadotropins until the end of their life.

I believe it a matter of principle to state some suggestions referring to the present problem, since the search for ways and means aimed at restoring or prolonging the reproductive period will certainly depend upon this point.

In the rat, the problem is soluble, in principle, by using drugs affecting the hypothalamic threshold of sensitivity. In women, it should be emphasized that although there was a dramatic decline in the number of primary oocytes with age, a significant number of these structures were present at the onset of menopause (Block 1953). However, why these remaining follicles do not respond to elevated gonadotropins in the menopause is not clear. It is possible that the lack of response of the postmenopausal ovary to gonadotropins is due to decreased gonadotropin receptors in the aged ovaries (Mills and Mahesh 1978).

For my part, I believe that the decline in the number of receptors (and probably even the rate of decline in the number of oocytes) is determined by the increased blood level of gonadotropins.[1] In particular, it has been shown (Jones and Krohn, 1961) that hypophysectomy in the mouse significantly retards the normal progressive loss of oocytes from the ovary.

Besides, the essential difference between the rat and the woman, with respect to the age-related changes in the reproductive system, lies in the fact that aged female rats showed a reduced capacity to secrete FSH and LH (Meites et al 1978), while in women during aging the hypothalamic-pituitary system responds with a marked elevation in secretion of both FSH and LH. These differences appear to be caused by the fact that in rats dopamine acts as a stimulator of LH release (Kamberi et al 1970), whereas in humans dopamine acts as a suppressor of gonadotropin secretion (Rakoff et al 1978). In humans as well as in rats, dopamine concentration in the hypothalamus declines with advancing age (Finch 1973, Robinson 1975); this can result in the opposite-directed changes in the level of gonadotropins, though in rats the decline of dopamine concentration in the hypothalamus is responsible for the elevation of the hypothalamic threshold of sensitivity to estrogens, and it cannot be excluded that in humans the result is the same.[2]

Therefore, in order to find out whether human ovaries really stop responding to gonadotropins, it is necessary, with the help of pituitary

---

[1] The exposure of ovaries to LH for 16 hours in vitro abolished the hormone's responsiveness without any alteration in sensitivity to prostaglandin E_1 (Zor et al 1976).

[2] It is of interest to find out whether the differences in the neurotransmitters controlling the reproductive functions in rats and in humans can be connected with the differences in the diurnal pattern of activity of these two species.

inhibitors (eg, a combination of estrogens and progestins), to suppress firmly, the natural secretion of gonadotropins, and only after that administer the exogenous gonadotropins. It is probable that this very principle determines the resumption of cyclicity of the menstrual cycle in women during the perimenopausal period, which is frequently observed after a few months of cyclic administration of estrogens and progestins (Dilman 1961, 1968). Moreover, it should be taken into account that during aging there is an essential change of the LH to FSH ratio in the blood, in favor of the latter (Adamopoulos et al 1971). It is probable that an excess of FSH harmfully affects the follicular tissue of the ovaries, whereas an excess of LH, by causing hyperplasia in the thecal tissues of the ovaries, changes the spectrum of the hormones produced by the ovaries. As has been shown by Weiss et al (1977), in subjects with catecholamine blockade, an LH surge can be induced by estrogen treatment. This contrasts to results obtained in rats and suggests that the control mechanism of LH surge production differs in rodents and humans. This circumstance may be responsible for the differences in the age-related dynamics of the LH level in rats and in women. It is also probable that the practical means of modulating hypothalamic activity should be different for rats and for humans, if this modulation is based on the change of concentration or turnover of biogenic amines. However, bearing in mind the role played by neurotransmitters in the functioning of the CNS, the species-specific differences can by no means exclude the participation of hypothalamic neurotransmitters in the mechanism of the age-related switching-off of reproductive function in the female organism. Consequently, I believe that both the menopausal gonadotropins and chorionic gonadotropin are of little help in stimulating the hormonal activity of the ovaries.

Now, proceeding from the concept that the differences in functional alterations of the hypothalamic regulation of the reproductive homeostat in rats and in women cannot be called essential, we shall consider the most vulnerable position of the elevational model. This is that, in the course of aging there develops, during the reproductive period, a compensatory elevation of hormonal activity of the ovaries, caused by the elevation of the threshold of sensitivity to the inhibitory effect of estrogens on the tonic region of the sex center.

From the physiologic point of view the formation of the central type of homeostatic failure should result in stimulation on the peripheral part of the system. Data in Table 4-2 show that the age-associated increase in gonadotropin excretion is accompanied by a simultaneous rise in excretion of total phenolsteroids. This may be a manifestation of the process of compensation that appears to maintain the reproductive cycle under conditions of constantly growing hypothalamic activity (see Chapter 1).

Such an approach offers an explanation for the so-called polyfolliculine phase of the climacteric described by Zondek (1935). However, the hypothesis of an age-associated compensatory elevation of ovarian function may meet with certain objections, because it is based on the determination of total phenolsteroids instead of classic estrogens. Therefore it is necessary to cite some data proving that by testing total phenolsteroids it is possible to get additional information that cannot be obtained by studying classic estrogens.

Earlier studies in our laboratory revealed that gonadotropin excretion is increased following ablation of menopausal ovaries, although the excretion of classic estrogens remains at the same level (Dilman and Pavlova 1963, Dilman 1968). This may be evidence that menopausal ovaries produce hormones other than classic estrogens, and their elimination by means of ovariectomy causes gonadotropin production to increase through negative feedback. A similar conclusion can be derived from analysis of data reported in other studies. For instance, there is a study of ovarian function in menopausal women (Procopè 1969) that used the Brown method of determining classic estrogens and found that in some cases this method does not account for a full range of ovarian hormonal activity. To illustrate, the level of classic estrogen excretion before and after ovariectomy was 2.6 μg and 4.5 μg/day, respectively (see summary, Table 1, case no. 7 in Procopè 1969), which means that ovariectomy did not result in a decrease in the excretion of these hormones. This is interpreted by the author as an indication of the cessation of hormonal activity in the ovaries. However, the excretion of total gonadotropins showed a sharp increase following ovariectomy. (Similar changes may be observed in case nos. 11 and 56 in Procopè's report.)

Some findings reported by Charles et al (1965), also may be interpreted from this point of view. After ovariectomy, six out of nine patients with endometrial carcinoma revealed a compensatory increase in the function of the adrenal cortex, although the excretion of classic estrogens did not decrease. This means that the menopausal ovaries produced some other hormones that cannot be determined by the Brown method. Such data are consistent with the conclusion that the compensatory elevation in activity of the reproductive homeostat is implemented by an elevation in the organism of the level of nonclassic phenolsteroids. Of course, there have long existed data on the presence of a number of other estrogen-like phenolsteroids. However, even now, nonclassic phenolsteroids are thought to be derivatives of the classic estrogens, estradiol and estrone (Diczfalusy and Lauritzen 1961). It is believed also that if estradiol production is decreased considerably, as in menopause, the determination of nonclassic phenolsteroids, metabolites of estradiol, may be neglected. However data in Table 4-4 show that the excretion of total phenolsteroids may change, whereas that of the classic estrogens does not. On the basis of these data, I suggested earlier that in the human organism the production of a part of the nonclassic phenolsteroids is possible, independent of the production of the classic estrogens (Dilman 1961, 1968). This hypothesis is supported further by the results of a study on the excretion of classic estrogens and total phenolsteroids before and after x-ray inhibition of ovarian function in women of reproductive age (Table 4-5).

Table 4-4
Prednisolone Effect in Excretion of Total Phenolsteroids, Classic Estrogens, and 17-Ketosteroids

Group*	Total Phenol-steroids (μg/24 hr)	Classic Estrogens (μg/24 hr)	17-Keto-steroids (μg/24 hr)
Before prednisolone	56.0 ± 4.85	5.3 ± 1.57	7.8 ± 1.129
After prednisolone	26.4 ± 2.70	4.6 ± 1.60	3.2 ± 0.65

*Prednisolone was administered in dosage of 20 mg/day for ten days.

Table 4-5
The Effect of Radiation Treatment on Excretion of Classic Estrogens and Total Phenolsteroids in Patients with Cervical Carcinoma

	Classic Estrogens (μg/24 hr)		Total Phenolsteroids (μg/24 hr)	
Menstrual stage	*Before treatment*	*After treatment*	*Before treatment*	*After treatment*
Proliferative phase	24.3 ± 1.0	5.1 ± 0.8	39.0 ± 3.6	70.0 ± 3.6
Secretory (luteal) phase	20.6 ± 1.8	4.0 ± 0.3	58.2 ± 7.8	105.0 ± 18.5

When ovaries are removed that have been pretreated with x-rays it is possible to observe a decrease in total phenolsteroid excretion without any changes in the excretion of classic estrogens, and the excretion of total gonadotropins rises concomitantly (Table 4-6).

On the basis of these data an hypothesis may be put forward on the nature of factors that determine the predominant production of non-classic phenolsteroids. Radiation treatment is known to destroy ovarian follicles. At the same time exposure to certain doses of radiation results in hyperplasia of the interstitial tissue of the ovaries. It is known that the synthesis of ovarian steroids starts in the interstitial tissue, where androgens form initially. It may be supposed that their aromatization and conversion to estrogens are accomplished by the enzymatic systems of

Table 4-6
The Effect of Ovariectomy on Excretion of Total Phenolsteroids, Classic Estrogens, and Total Gonadotropins in X-Ray Castrated Patients

Treatment	No. Cases	Average Age (years)	Total Phenol-steroids (μg/24 hr)	Classic Estrogens (μg/24 hr)	Total Gonado-tropins (muu/24 hr)*
X-ray castration	10	40	72.5 ± 7.4	5.2 ± 2.2	138 ± 44.9
X-ray ovari-ectomy	10	40	35.8 ± 3.5	6.0 ± 1.6	325 ± 50.1

*muu—mouse uterine units.

the follicular tissue (or theca interna of the ovarian follicles). When this tissue is destroyed by x-ray castration this stage of biosynthesis is disturbed, and the ovaries begin to secrete mostly androgens and probably certain nonclassic phenolsteroids.

The process of normal aging reveals similar changes that culminate in this case with menopause. It is probable that the age-associated elevation of gonadotropin output, and particularly LH, results in hyperplasia of the ovarian interstitial tissue (Sommers and Teloh 1952, Dilman 1968). However, disturbances in the cyclic secretion of gonadotropins are conducive to a developmental disorder of the follicular tissue of the ovaries. All these factors lead to a situation similar to that after radiation castration.

Now the problem can be considered in a different light, but the general conclusion on the role of nonclassic phenolsteroids will probably retain its importance. It is known that the main estrogen in the postmenopausal period is estrone. Estrone production results from aromatization of C_{19} steroidal precursors and accounts for the greater portion of total estrogens. Androstenedione is the predominant precursor in extragonadal conversion to estrone (MacDonald et al 1967, Grodin et al 1973, Poortman et al 1973). Consequently, even if the nonclassic phenolsteroids are not produced directly by the ovaries during the postmenopausal period, they can be formed as a result of biotransformation of the ovarian androgens in different tissues and, in particular, in the fat tissue where the aromatization of androgens is intensive. With advancing age, an increase in the efficiency of conversion of androstenedione to estrone was demonstrated by Hemsell et al (1974). This rate of conversion is markedly altered by obesity (Vermeulen and Verdonck 1978). Correspondingly, many factors within the system of the energy homeostat can probably affect the spectrum of nonclassic phenolsteroids produced in the organism extra-ovarially. This probably causes the elevation of level and the change of spectrum of the nonclassic phenolsteroids in patients with cancer of the uterus (for whom considerable adiposity is a characteristic feature) (Dilman et al 1968). It is possible, however, that apart from androstenedione there is an additional precursor of plasma estrone (Vermeulen and Verdonck 1978).

Thus the advancement of age is accompanied by an increase in the excretion of total phenolsteroids that may be responsible for the compensation taking place in the reproductive homeostat. It should be pointed out that overstimulation of an endocrine gland is a factor responsible for changes in the spectrum of secreted isohormones (Dilman 1968). Many findings demonstrate that long-term overstimulation of an endocrine gland may involve a redistribution in the spectrum of relevant isohormones. This effect has been disclosed in the secretion of different isohormones of FSH following ovariectomy (Peckham et al 1973). Such an effect seems to be a general phenomenon, and in menopause or following radiation castration it assumes the form of a predominant output of nonclassic phenolsteroids that may be regarded as isohormones of estrogens (Dilman 1968).

Hence classic estrogen production is a precise means for the evaluation of ovarian function during the reproductive period. On the other hand the importance of nonclassic phenolsteroids grows steadily in the course of aging, particularly after menopause. Therefore, in the postmenopausal period it is inadequate to evaluate the hormonal activity of the ovaries on the basis of classic estrogen determination.

It should be mentioned that, apart from the ovaries, precursors of nonclassic phenolsteroids also are produced in the adrenal cortex. The data in Table 4-4 show that prednisolone administration to ovariectomized patients with breast cancer brings about a decrease in total phenolsteroid excretion without appreciably affecting the level of classical estrogen excretion.

Particularly, cortisol can be converted to estrogens by peripheral tissues (Ganis et al 1974).[1] Finally, the possibilities of androstenedione conversion to nonclassic phenolsteroids have not actually been studied.

The group of total phenolsteroids is not likely to be homogeneous as far as the intensity and spectrum of biologic action are concerned. However, in some cases this action is similar to the effect of classic estrogens. The antigonadotropic effect of nonclassic phenolsteroids observed in ovariectomized menopausal patients already has been noted. The nonclassic estrogens also exert some influence on the peripheral level.

Table 4-7 shows a correlation between the estrogen-stimulated type of response of the vaginal epithelium and the level of total phenolsteroid excretion in menopausal patients with endometrial carcinoma.

---

[1] Fishman and Norton (1975) established a biochemical link in the CNS between estradiol and catecholamines through the intermediacy of the catecholestrogens, which in principle must be classed with the nonclassic phenolsteroids.

Table 4-7
Correlation between Excretion Levels of Total Phenolsteroids and Classic Estrogens and Type of Response of Vaginal Epithelium in Menopausal Patients with Endometrial Carcinoma

Hormone	Excretion Level	Vaginal Smear *I and II*	Vaginal Smear *III and IV*
Classic estrogens	high	0	2
	normal	11	10
Total phenolsteroids	high	3	10
	normal	8	1

Source: Berstein et al 1969.

Changes that occur in the reproductive homeostat cause a number of shifts in sex hormone pattern. The shift to predominant synthesis of nonclassic phenolsteroids involved in the central type of homeostatic failure also occurs at the expense of classic estrogens (Dilman 1968, 1974b). At the same time the inhibitory effect of nonclassic phenolsteroids on the hypothalamic-gonadotropic system becomes less than that of classic estrogens. For example, following x-ray castration, despite an excess in nonclassic phenolsteroids, the excretion of gonadotropins is enhanced, although generally it stays below the postovariectomy level. The overstimulation of the ovaries is perpetuated by excessive gonadotropins, which in turn further shift the balance in favor of nonclassic phenolsteroids, thus promoting the formation of the dysfunctional type of homeostatic failure (see Chapter 2). Finally the decrease in classic estrogen output, a consequence of the above changes, results in a situation typical of the peripheral type of homeostatic failure. Thus all three main types of homeostatic insufficiency develop in the reproductive system in the normal course of aging. Mills and Mahesh (1978) noted that Dilman's finding of an increase in both gonadotropins and estrogens in the perimenopausal period have been confirmed in a few women by Netter and Lambert (1975). These investigators found very high serum estradiol and urinary estrogens in several perimenopausal women in association with high serum and urinary FSH and LH. Later, van Look et al (1977) showed that the FSH and LH levels in some perimenopausal women were elevated despite the presence of circulating 17 β-estradiol levels in the early-mid follicular phase range.

Therefore, when the function of the ovaries during the menopausal period is estimated only by the output of classic estrogens, an impression is formed that the mechanism of the menopause is equivalent to the changes developing after ovariectomy, ie, that the primary cause for termination of reproductive function is different in the human and the rat. Moreover, it should be stressed that there is a sufficiently complete coincidence of the age-related changes in the reproductive homeostat during prepuberty in the rat and in the human female. From my point of view, this is an argument in favor of the concept that the switching-off of reproductive function is implemented in these higher organisms by principally the same mechanism; that is why experimental data on the problem are of considerable interest. The experiments involving heterochronic transplantation of the ovaries from old animals to young (resulting in the resumption of cyclic activity of the ovaries), and from young animals to old (resulting in the functional failure of the ovaries) show that the switching-off of the estrous cycle is not caused by a depletion of the gonads (Aschheim 1964–1965, Kushima et al 1961).

Proceeding from the viewpoint that elevation of the hypothalamic threshold may be responsible for age-associated switching-off of cyclic function, let us consider some data relating to the mechanism of hypothalamic threshold elevation proper.

Stoll (1972) suggested that elevation of the hypothalamic threshold to homeostatic inhibition by estrogen, by negative feedback, is associated with the age-dependent decrease in dopamine level in the hypothalamus. This hypothesis is supported by our findings (Dilman and Anisimov 1975). Figure 4-3 shows that L-dopa raises the sensitivity of the hypothalamic-pituitary complex to inhibition by estrogens, ie, it lowers the hypothalamic threshold of sensitivity. At the same time, it is known that age advancement is accompanied by a decrease in the hypothalamic level of catecholamines, particularly the concentration and metabolism of dopamine, whereas the latter, characteristics of the serotonergic system, are susceptible to changes to a lesser degree (Finch 1973, 1976;

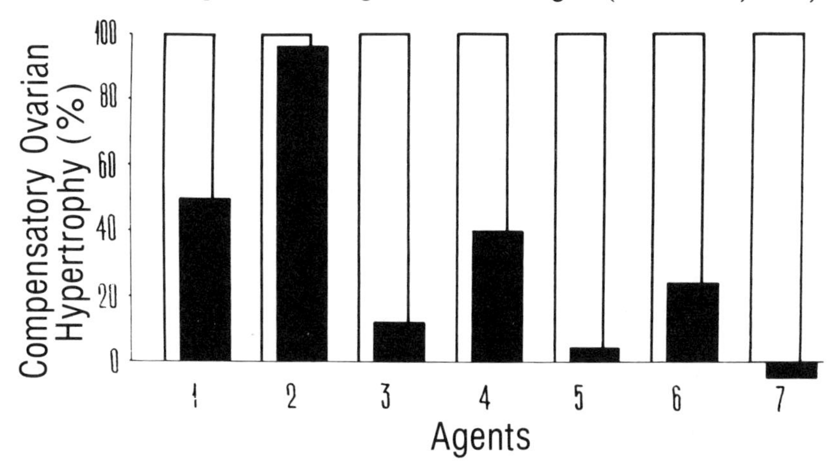

Figure 4-3 Effect of some drugs on hypothalamic-pituitary complex threshold to diethylstilbestrol as determined by suppression of compensatory ovarian hypertrophy. Agents: 1: Control (3 mos); 2: Control (18 mos); 3: L-dopa; 4: Dilantin; 5: Epithalamin; 6: Phenformin; 7: Succinate.

Robinson 1975; Segall and Timiras 1976; Anisimov et al 1977). We obtained similar results when catecholamine, serotonin, and histamine levels were assayed at the same time (Table 4-8). Therefore, the above results point to a positive correlation between the decrease in biogenic amine levels and elevation of hypothalamic threshold to inhibition by estrogens.

Table 4-8
Levels of Biogenic Amines in Hypothalamus of Male Rats of Different Ages*

Biogenic Amines (ng/g wet tissue)	Age (months)				
	1 (n = 32)	*2 to 3 (n = 72)*	*6 (n = 32)*	*13 to 15 (n = 28)*	*36 (n = 12)*
Noradrenaline	1142 ± 70†	1466 ± 63	1393 ± 152	1256 ± 73 ‡	1216 ± 60 †
Dopamine	319 ± 58‡	486 ± 34	390 ± 65	261 ± 54‡	543 ± 134
Serotonin	721 ± 79	810 ± 97	625 ± 94	778 ± 71	671 ± 143
5-HIAA	737 ± 64	814 ± 121	751 ± 72	894 ± 198	662 ± 79
Histamine	608 ± 56†	1067 ± 111	802 ± 94	853 ± 289	758 ± 167

*Rise in biogenic amine levels between one and two to three months is probably associated with the process of the hypothalamus development.
†Difference from value for two- to three-month old rats is statistically significant, $p < 0.01$.
‡$p < 0.05$.

Some indirect evidence also suggests that the age-associated changes taking place in the cyclic center are caused by similar shifts in biogenic amine levels. The administration of L-dopa, or iproniazid, an inhibitor of monoamine oxidase, and progesterone results in the resumption of ovarian cyclicity in old female rats with constant estrus (Quadri et al 1973, Huang and Meites 1975, Lehman et al 1978). According to Aschheim (1976) cycling rats reveal an elevated ability to respond by pseudopregnancy to estrogen treatment with advancing age. This is a manifestation of the age-associated decline in the hypothalamic threshold of sensitivity. It is possible that this effect is associated both with the age-related decrease in the hypothalamic level of dopamine and estrogen ability to lower catecholamine levels in the hypothalamus and, thus, to stimulate prolactin secretion. The same phenomenon, age-connected decrease in the hypothalamic level of catecholamines, may produce two opposite directed effects in the reproductive system proper and the system that controls prolactin secretion.

In addition to the adrenergic system, the serotonergic and cholinergic systems take part in the implementation of elevation of the hypothalamic threshold of sensitivity to estrogens (Figure 4-4). The effect of the serotonergic system, is particularly pronounced during stress or continuous lighting (Kledzik and Meites 1974, Takahashi et al 1973).

The decreased binding of a hormone by the receptors of the target tissue may be one of the factors that determine hypothalamic sensitivity to homeostatic stimuli. Peng and Peng (1973) reported a decreased uptake of ^{3}H-labeled estradiol by the anterior hypothalamus, pituitary, and uterus in old female rats with spontaneous constant estrus. Table 4-9 shows that the uptake of ^{3}H-estradiol-17β by the anterior and mediobasal hypothalamus decreases with advancing age even before the onset of age-associated disturbances in ovarian cyclicity, and this decline becomes apparent at earlier stages than similar changes in the pituitary gland or uterus. The administration of L-dopa, on the other hand, raises the hypothalamic uptake of ^{3}H-estradiol, producing no marked effect on its binding in the pituitary or uterus (Table 4-10), which points to a certain causality between the hypothalamic levels of biogenic amines, and binding ability of the hypothalamic receptors of estrogens, and the elevation of the hypothalamic threshold of sensitivity. Apart from the levels of biogenic amines and the functional state of hormone receptors in the hypothalamus, some metabolic factors seem to affect the age dynamic of the hypothalamic threshold, too. For example, Kennedy and Mitra (1963) demonstrated that the age-associated switching-on of reproductive function in rats is correlated with the body weight of the

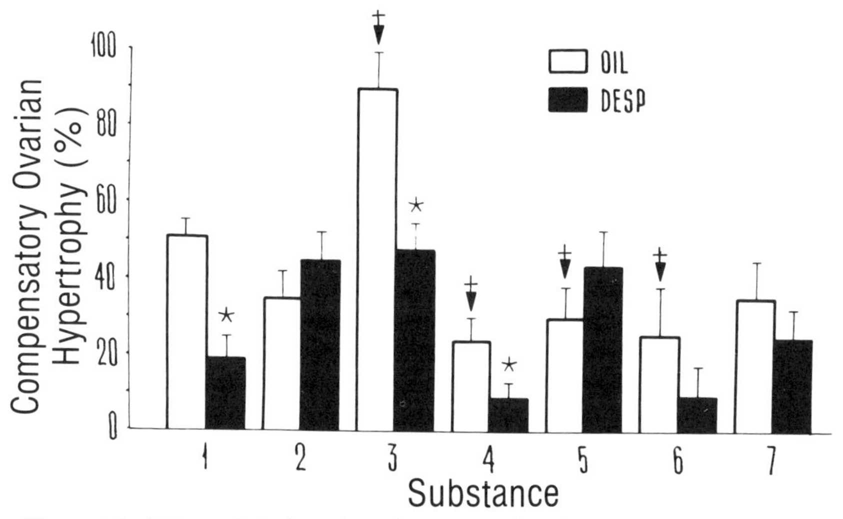

Figure 4-4 Effect of cholinergic and serotonergic substances on compensatory ovarian hypertrophy and its inhibition by diethylstilbestrol propionate (DESP) in young rats. Blank columns: treatment with substance and oil. Solid columns: treatment with substance and DESP. Substances: 1: Control; 2: Arecoline (3 mg/kg, ip); 3: Nicotine (2 mg/kg, ip); 4: Metamizyl (20 mg/kg, sc); 5: IEM-506 (5 mg/kg, sc); 6: L-tryptophan (100 mg/kg, ip); 7: Typindole (10 mg/kg, ip). *Significant difference from the rats of the same group, treated with oil, $p < 0.05$. †Significant difference from control, $p < 0.05$.

animal and that this function may switch on at an earlier stage if the animal is fed a fat-rich diet. This finding is corroborated by the statistical data of Frisch (1973) on the relationship between body weight and age of menarche. Since the switching-on of reproductive function is associated with elevation of the hypothalamic threshold, it may be inferred that this phenomenon in the reproductive system is regulated by processes that occur in the energy system ("the metabolic control of puberty," according to Donovan, 1974).

Table 4-9
Uptake of ^{3}H-Estradiol-17β (Specific Radioactivity in dpm/mg) by Tissues of Hypothalamus, Cerebral Cortex, Adenohypophysis, and Uterus in Rats of Varying Ages*

	Age of Animals (months)				
	2 *(n = 4)*	*6* *(n = 4)*	*10* *(n = 2)*	*16* *(n = 10)*	*24* *(n = 3)*
Anterior hypothalamus	103 ± 15	109 ± 27	80 ± 4	61 ± 7†	60 ± 14†
Mediobasal hypothalamus	119 ± 22	110 ± 32	92 ± 10	43 ± 6†	54 ± 8†
Posterior hypothalamus	77 ± 10	69 ± 10	66 ± 7	73 ± 11	59 ± 5
Cerebral cortex	70 ± 3	57 ± 4	70 ± 20	50 ± 8	66 ± 4
Adenohypophysis	261 ± 46	251 ± 26	254 ± 30	263 ± 29	161 ± 16†
Uterus	503 ± 85	537 ± 141	347 ± 18	332 ± 33	261 ± 122†

*Rats with regular estral cyclicity (2 to 16 months) and a spontaneous constant estrus (24 months) were ovariectomized one week before the experiment. On the first day of the experiment, rats were killed one hour after intraperitoneal administration of 0.2 μg/100 g body weight of ^{3}H-6.7 extradiol-17β (specific radioactivity 10.2 mCi/mM). Radioactivity of tissues was measured in a liquid scintillation counter, Mark II (Nuclear Chicago, USA).
†Difference with the indices for six-month-old rats is statistically significant, $p < 0.05$.

Table 4-10
The Effect of Treatment with L-dopa on Uptake of ^{3}H-Estradiol-17β (Specific Radioactivity in dpm/mg) by Tissues of Old Rats

	Control (n = 15)	L-dopa* (n = 9)
Anterior hypothalamus	72 ± 10	133 ± 18†
Mediobasal hypothalamus	74 ± 8	251 ± 57†
Dorsal hypothalamus	43 ± 5	101 ± 20†
Cerebral cortex	35 ± 2	72 ± 12†
Adenohypophysis	170 ± 16	168 ± 26
Uterus	237 ± 21	292 ± 28

*L-dopa was injected intraperitoneally 100 mg/kg, 30 minutes before ^{3}H-estradiol.
†Differences statistically significant, $p < 0.05$, for L-dopa vs control.

In view of this it is noteworthy that the sensitivity of the hypothalamic-pituitary complex to inhibition by estrogens was restored in our experiments by the administration of phenformin (phenethylbiguanide), succinic acid, and Dilantin (diphenylhydantoin), which influence different levels of metabolism (Dilman and Anisimov 1975). However, unlike L-dopa, phenformin and Dilantin failed to increase the uptake of estradiol by the hypothalamus, which means that metabolic factors exert their effects on hypothalamic threshold by a pathway other than biogenic amines. It was shown in our laboratory that phenformin and Dilantin decrease the output of gonadotropins both in the rat and in the human (Dilman 1974a, Dilman et al 1975). It cannot be excluded that the decrease can result in a normalization of FSH/LH ratio (because of elimination of the factor of hyperstimulation of the system), which, along with the decrease in the level of gonadotropins, can increase the sensitivity of the ovaries to the effect of gonadotropins and restore their ovulatory effect. Thus, according to our data, in rats aged 16–18 months, constant estrus was observed in 23% of the animals, and pseudopregnancy in 15% of cases (ie, disturbance of estrous cycle was observed in 38% of female rats); on the other hand, when buformin, Dilantin, or pineal polypeptide extract were administered, the figures for the same disturbance in the rats (developed by the same time of life) were 9%, 4%, and 7%. Correspondingly, buformin administered to rats with constant estrus was responsible for resumption of cyclic estrus in 11 out of 16 animals. It is noteworthy that most animals retained the cyclic activity of ovaries for two weeks after buformin administration had been discontinued. Four out of 15 animals developed pregnancy terminating in parturition. Administration of Dilantin was responsible for resumption of estrous cycle in 5 out of 15 animals.

The pineal gland contributes to the formation of the phenomenon of age-associated elevation of hypothalamic threshold of sensitivity to homeostatic stimuli, too. It was suggested earlier that, apart from their direct inhibition of the hypothalamic-pituitary system, some pineal factors are capable of raising hypothalamic sensitivity to homeostatic stimuli (Dilman 1970a). This hypothesis is supported by our data on the improvement of sensitivity of the hypothalamic-pituitary complex to estrogens and glucocorticoids, as a result of pineal polypeptide extract administration (Ostroumova and Dilman 1972, Ostroumova 1978, Dilman and Anisimov 1975). Table 4-11 shows that the administration of pineal polypeptide extract in old animals returned hypothalamic sensitivity to inhibition by stilbestrol to normal. It should be noted that the administration of pineal polypeptides caused the resumption of cyclicity of ovarian activity in old rats with constant estrus (Anisimov et al 1973a, Figure 4-5). This means that pineal polypeptides raise hypothalamic sensitivity to homeostatic stimuli both in the tonic and cyclic centers of the reproductive homeostat. However, in contrast to the effect produced by buformin and Dilantin, which normalize the hypothalamic threshold of sensitivity to estrogens and reduce the gonadotropin secretion, cessation of pineal polypeptides resulted in a quicker loss of cycle.

Table 4-11
Effect of Polypeptide Extract of Pineal Gland on Sensitivity of Hypothalamic-Pituitary System to Inhibition by Stilbestrol

Animals	Treatment	Compensatory hypertrophy of the ovary (%)
Three-month-old rats	Control	59.8 ± 6.9
	Estrogens	33.9 ± 6.0
	Estrogens and pineal extract	30.9 ± 16.4
16-month-old rats	Control	26.0 ± 9.6
	Estrogens	18.3 ± 6.5
	Estrogens and pineal extract	0.4 ± 7.0

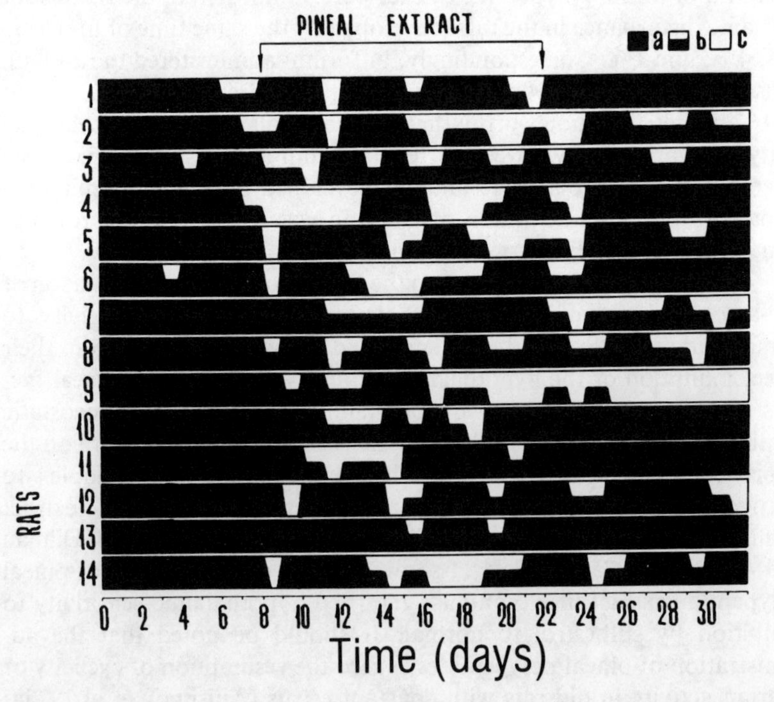

Figure 4-5 Effect of treatment with pineal polypeptide extract (epithalamin) on estrus cyclicity in old rats. a: Estrus; b: Pro- or metaestrus; c: Diestrus. Epithalamin administered in dose of 1 mg/day.

Elevation of hypothalamic sensitivity to homeostatic stimuli induced by pineal polypeptides throws some light on the role played by the elevation of hypothalamic threshold in the adaptation of reproductive function to the action of external environmental factors. It was reported that constant lighting accelerates the switching-on of reproductive function in sexually immature rats (Wurtman 1970). Considering that maturity of the reproductive homeostat is associated with elevation of the hypothalamic threshold of sensitivity to the action of estrogens, it may be expected that such a phenomenon can be easily established in an experiment involving the use of continuous lighting. It is clear from Figure 4-6 that continuous lighting results in elevation of the hypothalamic threshold of sensitivity to inhibition by estrogens in young animals, which must result in an elevation of level of endogenous estrogens. Accordingly, the continuous light accelerates an estrogen-induced precocious sexual maturation in female rats (Piacsek and Streur 1975).

On the basis of the data on the influence of continuous lighting on the reproductive system, Hoffman (1973) concluded that the hypothalamic threshold of sensitivity to positive feedback rises during exposure to continuous light. Continuous lighting, like aging, decreases

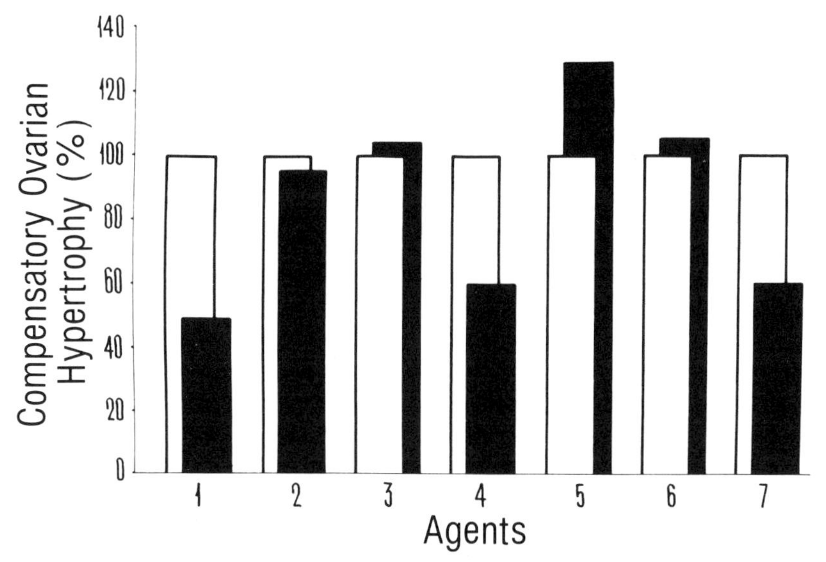

Figure 4-6 Effect of carcinogens, exposure to light, and transplanted tumor on hypothalamic-pituitary complex threshold to diethylstilbestrol, as determined by suppression of compensatory ovarian hypertrophy. Blank columns: agent plus oil. Solid columns: agent plus diethylstilbestrol. Agents: 1: Control (3 mos); 2: Control (18 mos); 3: Treatment with carcinogens (20-methylcholanthrene, nitrosodiethylamine, nitrosoethylurea, DDT, 1,2-dimethylhydrazine; 4: Treatment with anthracene; 5: Continuous exposure to light; 6: Transplantation of Walker carcinoma 256, Pliss lymphosarcoma, sarcoma 45; 7: Transplantation of muscle.

estrogen uptake by the rat's hypothalamus (Illei-Donhoffer et al 1974). This gives a clue as to why continuous lighting induces constant estrus in mature rats, ie, it leads to the switching-off of reproductive function.

Apart from continuous lighting, some other factors raise the hypothalamic threshold of sensitivity to inhibition by estrogens. They include, for example, some chemical carcinogens and the transplantation of tumors (see Figure 4-6). It is necessary to point out that normal development and aging, continuous lighting, neonatal administration of androgens, and some chemical carcinogens all cause similar changes in the reproductive system (Dilman 1974a).

Therefore, I believe that elevation of the hypothalamic threshold of sensitivity to inhibition plays a key role not only in the mechanism of age-associated switching-on and switching-off of reproductive function, but also in the adaptation of reproductive function to the influences of a number of unfavorable factors of the external and internal environment. Also, the factors that can raise the hypothalamic threshold (neonatal administration of androgens, continuous lighting, and some chemical carcinogens) accelerate the processes of maturing and aging in the reproductive system. Thus, the elevation of the hypothalamic threshold of sensitivity to homeostatic stimuli depends upon such factors as the age-associated decline in the hypothalamic level of catecholamines, decreased binding of sex hormones by the hypothalamic receptors, decreased activity of the pineal gland, and a shift in energy metabolism toward predominant utilization of free fatty acids for energy supply. Resumption of cyclicity of the reproductive system as a result of medication provides an additional argument in support of the hypothesis on the regulatory mechanism of aging and, particularly, the aging of the reproductive system.

Age-Associated Changes in the Reproductive System of the Male Organism

After maturity, the functioning of the reproductive system of the male organism is noncyclic. The masculine type of functioning of the hypothalamic sex center develops as a result of androgen influence in the first days of postnatal ontogenesis (Barraclough and Haller 1970, Hendricks 1969). Data show that the age-associated switching-on of the male reproductive system occurs in the same manner as that of the female organism. As in female rats, much higher doses of testosterone (three to four times as great) are required for the suppression of LH secretion in adult male rats than in younger animals (Ramirez and McCann 1963, Bloch et al 1974, Sharpe and Shahamanes 1974). However testosterone has been found to raise LH-releasing hormone secretion in immature rats, which illustrates testosterone action by positive feedback (Shin et al

1974). Such findings should be considered when the hypothalamic threshold is determined in young animals.

There is clinical evidence that the dose of clomiphene citrate required for the inhibition of gonadotropic function in the male organism rises from 1 mg in prepuberty to 5 mg in puberty and up to 500 mg in adult men (Kulin et al 1972). Some data indicate that sexually immature children need fewer estrogens than adults in order to suppress gonadotropins (Kulin and Reiter 1972). The age-associated rise in the hypothalamic set point also is shown indirectly by data on gradually increasing blood FSH and LH levels. This process begins long before puberty (Lee et al 1974) and continues until 61–70 years of age. Since the testosterone level does not decrease significantly within this period, these data may be interpreted as a symptom of the development of the central type of homeostatic failure. It should be noted, however, that as far as the central type of homeostatic failure is concerned, a compensatory increase in the output of testosterone should be expected, since testosterone is a hormone of a peripheral endocrine gland. Yet blood testosterone level starts to decrease after age 50, although a high level of testosterone, typical of young men, is often observed in men 80 or even 90 years old (Vermuelen et al 1972). To explain this discrepancy it might be suggested that a relatively stable level of testosterone in old age probably is determined by two opposite processes: the elevation of hypothalamic-pituitary activity, which stimulates testosterone production; and the regression of the functional tissue of the sex glands, inherent in aging. It should be emphasized that the age-associated decline in free testosterone concentration is caused (among other factors) by the increased binding capacity of a specific testosterone-binding globulin (Vermeulen et al 1972). Mice reveal a stable blood testosterone level from puberty to old age (J.F. Nelson, K.R. Latham, and C.E. Finch, personal communication, 1975). However, analysis of this relationship is more difficult because it is postulated that an inhibiting factor (inhibin or factor X) is secreted by the Sertoli cells and inhibits gonadotropin production.

Hence age-associated changes in the male reproductive system are characterized by certain distinctive features. First, the cyclic center does not function in the male organism. Second, although the reproductive function is switched on by a mechanism in the hypothalamus, no mechanism is provided for switching it off. Therefore phenomena similar to the climacteric (interpreted as a mechanism of switching-off of reproductive function) do not occur in the male organism. The noncyclic functioning of the male reproductive homeostat suggests a greater likelihood of fertilization than the female reproductive system, considering the limitations imposed by the cyclic functioning of the female system. The age-associated decrease in the reproductive ability of the male organism is caused by the lowered level of sex hormones, leading to diminished potency.

Spermatogenesis continues until old age and never ceases completely. This peculiarity is expressed by less pronounced age-associated changes in gonadotropin and sex hormone secretion in males than in females. Because of different changes in the reproductive homeostats of female and male organisms, age-associated metabolic shifts develop at different periods for the female than for the male (see Chapter 9).

The Female Climacteric

By definition, the climacteric is the mechanism of age-associated switching-off of the reproductive function (Dilman 1968); menopause is a persistent discontinuance of cyclic activity of the ovaries, caused by the climacteric; and climacteric neurosis is a hypothalamic syndrome that is not directly connected with the mechanism of the climacteric but merely coincides with it in time. For example, one of the key elements of the mechanism of climacteric is the elevation of blood levels of FSH, but this shift is not related to one of the key elements of climacteric neurosis, hot flashes (Baranov and Dilman 1949, Isaacs and Havard 1978).

During ontogenesis the reproductive homeostat functions at a constantly rising rate; reproductive function is switched on and off as age advances. There are two factors of primary importance in this program: elevation of the hypothalamic threshold, and a compensatory increase in sex hormone production (Dilman 1958, 1968, 1971). Target tissues of the reproductive system are overstimulated as a result of this increase of gonadotropic and sex hormones. Increased hyperplasia of the thecal tissue of the ovaries results from increased gonadotropin secretion; proliferative changes occur in the reproductive organs because of the excess production of sex hormones. Thus, intensified ovarian function, which develops regularly in the course of aging as a compensation for the rise of the hypothalamic threshold, also becomes the cause of certain pathologic disturbances in the organs of the reproductive system.

This is a typical manifestation of diseases of compensation. The process of converting age-related physiologic processes to pathologic ones is aided here particularly by follicular persistence, one of the elevating mechanism's primary means of switching off the reproductive cycle. This develops when the estrogen level becomes too low to induce ovulation, but it often causes pronounced hyperplasia of the endometrium and "climacteric bleeding." The age-dependent increase in the activity of the ovaries is actually a compensatory process that counteracts the premature switching-off of reproductive function with steady elevation of the hypothalamic threshold. A prolonged reproductive period, consistent with the Law of Constancy of Internal Environment, is implemented in accordance with the Law of Deviation of Homeostasis. In this context, dysfunctional climacteric bleeding is an attempt by the organism to delay the onset of menopause. Hyperestrogenization in the postmenopausal period is not likely to be caused by the action of classic estrogens because their excretion does not exceed 10 μg/24 hours in persistent menopause (Dilman 1968). Nonclassic phenolsteroids form the greater portion of estrogens during age-connected compensation, and their elevated level also causes hyperplasia of the endometrium in menopausal patients, with endometrial carcinoma in some cases. Accordingly, hyperestrogenization in menopausal women has been reported repeatedly on the basis of both clinical signs and the magnitude of total phenolsteroid excretion (Klotz and Jayle 1951, Smith and Emerson 1954). Therefore, the more pronounced the process of compensation, the higher the age of onset of menopause.

Note that the age-connected switching-off of reproductive function takes place 1½–2 years later in patients with breast cancer or endometrial carcinoma than in healthy women (McMahon et al 1973). We may interpret this as further evidence of the role of the elevating mechanism in the climacteric. When such cancer develops, more ovarian hormones are produced than usual; this allows the reproductive homeostat to keep pace a while longer with the steady elevation of the hypothalamic threshold. Indeed, these diseases involve increased production of both gonadotropins and nonclassic phenolsteroids, factors that seem to determine the rate of tumor incidence in the reproductive system in pre- and postmenopausal periods. Therefore late-onset menopause, which traditionally is regarded as a manifestation of unusually prolonged normal functioning of the reproductive system, signals possible cancer risk. Thus the climacteric is both an age-associated physiologic normal process, and a typical disease of compensation, as well as a factor of the inevitable development of some pathologic states. This can also be illustrated by the fact that a stable elevation of the gonadotropin level in rodents results in the development of tumors of the ovaries (Lipschutz 1957). At the same time, the human female shows a manifold increase of gonadotropin secretion between 25 and 50 years of age. If it is true that hyperproduction of gonadotropins, by increasing the proliferating pool of cells in the target tissues, increases the probability of carcinogenesis, then in the female organism this condition is always fulfilled in the course of normal aging. The relationship of the developmental process with the climacteric, and the relationship of the climacteric with climacteric bleeding, the higher frequency of tumors in the reproductive system, as well as a deficiency of classic estrogens in the organism—all show the double-faced pattern of the climacteric as both a norm and a disease, ie, as a pattern of a normal disease.

The elevating mechanism of the climacteric is also responsible for a certain nonspecificity of this process. Any factor causing elevation of the hypothalamic threshold simultaneously accelerates the climacteric. This effect may be produced by psychic stress for instance, often resulting in amenorrhea with all the signs of the climacteric. Similarly, some other factors may cause a follicular persistence and polyfolliculine uterine bleeding. All these are manifestations of a relationship between the climacteric as a typical disease of compensation, and external environmental stimuli that intensify the normal, genetically-programmed process of development and aging.

Finally, the climacteric syndrome may develop as part of more complex diencephalic disturbances with a concomitant increase in hypothalamic activity (Zondek et al 1948). Hence the climacteric regarded as a specific age-related phenomenon, and the climacteric regarded as a symptom of other more complex syndromes, have a common feature determined by the elevating mechanism. Similarly climacteric neurosis, which often is identified incorrectly with the climacteric or menopause, is actually a manifestation of elevated hypothalamic activity, though it is pathogenically independent of the development of these states. Hot flashes, a typical symptom of climacteric neurosis, may occur even when the menstrual cycle is still undisturbed (Baranov and Dilman 1949, Dilman 1968). However, the often observed chronologic coincidence of the climacteric and climacteric neurosis is caused by the increase of hypothalamic activity in both, with its resulting deficiency of classic estrogens. It is interesting to note that the arguments proving that hot flashes are independent of an increase in the production of gonadotropins (Baranov and Dilman 1949) were recently supported by Isaacs and Havard (1978).

The mechanism of the age-related switching-off of reproductive function is practically an irreversible process, although it is based on functional hypothalamic changes. Meanwhile, reproductive function may be restored in the female organism as a result of a spontaneous decrease in hypothalamic activity or by an increased effect of compensation, as evidenced by the cases of pregnancy in menopausal women described in the literature. In experiments in which the condition of the hypothalamus is returned to normal, cyclic activity of the reproductive system may resume, as in the administration of pineal gland extract and L-dopa. As noted in this chapter, I suggest a hypothesis that if, by administration of some drugs, we retard the elevation of the hypothalamic threshold of sensitivity and the production of gonadotropins, maintaining it at the level characteristic of women aged 20–25 years old, this must lead to a considerable suppression of the rate of development of the climacteric and of all pathologic processes associated with it.

All the foregoing evidence favors the hypothesis that age-associated switching-off of the reproductive cycle is caused by the primary elevation of the hypothalamic threshold to the homeostatic influence of estrogens.

This suggests the existence of the same mechanism for age-connected switching-on and switching-off of the reproductive function. Hence the elevation of the hypothalamic threshold in the course of aging should be regarded as a key mechanism in the implementation of the genetic program of development and aging of the human organism. At the same time, the unity of the age-related switching-on and -off of reproductive function is a stumbling block that remains unnoticed by most researchers and is ignored in most theories of aging (see Chapter 23).

5 Age-Associated Changes in Appetite Regulation and Obesity as a Normal Disease of Aging

Obesity is not a problem of this century, it is the problem of all times.

With advancing age, the satiety center in man is "led astray."

According to current concepts excessive food intake results in the development of age-connected overweight and all the ensuing metabolic consequences. Such a view attributes the pathogenesis of age-associated weight gain to the sole influence of exogenous factors. But the problem is oversimplified when the causes of obesity are sought only in the interplay of those factors which promote the formation of so-called diseases of civilization. There exists a rigid homeostatic system of appetite regulation that ensures a stable maintenance of body weight in normal subjects aged 20–25 years of age, which shows that body weight is regulated by rather precise mechanisms. After all, age-connected obesity is not a specific feature of humans. The age of rats generally is estimated on the basis of weight, since there is a positive correlation between these two parameters. In many cases there is conclusive evidence for the increase of appetite as a consequence of regulatory disturbances. According to the most popular concept, the hypothalamus incorporates two interdependent centers which regulate appetite: a satiety center, located in the ventromedial area, and a feeding center, in the lateral hypothalamus (Mayer and Arees 1970). The satiety center has glucoreceptors, which affect its functional condition, depending on the metabolism of glucose. Hyperglycemia is thought to activate the satiety center, which inhibits the feeding center (Mayer 1965). Besides, there is evidence that brain cells, in particular cells within the ventral hypothalamus, are sensitive to insulin. The insulin causes glucoreceptors to take in glucose more rapidly and to respond as if glucose levels were suddenly elevated (Debons et al 1969). Therefore, when the blood sugar level (or, according to some authors, insulin level) is increased, food intake is decreased. Experimentally induced disorders of these mechanisms, for example, administering gold thioglucose, which destroys the satiety center, lead to hyperphagia and obesity. The hypothalamic system controlling food intake can be denoted as "the tactical center of appetite," since the system "measures out" the necessary amount of energy-producing substrates, but it cannot control the factors providing for such prolonged processes as maintenance of a stable body weight.

As stated by Woods and Portė (1978) the hypothalamic weight regulatory system is controlled by insulin levels in the blood (more preceisely, in the cerebrospinal fluid). Basal blood insulin level is very highly correlated with the degree of adiposity. An increase of insulin in CSF is hypothesized to be a signal indicating an increase of adiposity that causes the ventromedial hypothalamus to reduce meal size and to mobilize stored fuels, and vice versa. This hypothalamic system can be denoted as "the strategic center of appetite," owing to which animals rigorously defend and maintain a particular level of adiposity, ie, body weight set point, according to the terminology of Woods and Porte (1978). These authors, however, present their model of regulation of body weight as one nearly excluding the hypothalamic model of "tactical regulation" of appetite. However, neither of these two concepts of appetite regulation answers the question about the cause of age-associated increase in body weight, ie, the cause of disturbance of homeostasis in these systems. Woods and Porte (1978) write: "Although it is not clear whether insulin levels determine adiposity or whether adiposity determines insulin levels, it is clear that there is no a priori method for determining which is causative." I believe it possible to suggest a hypothesis that both eliminates the necessity to answer this question and takes into account the existence of the two interrelated systems of hypothalamic regulation of calorie homeostasis—the system regulating the appetite and the one regulating body fat content.

Considering that postprandial hyperglycemia level rises with advancing age (see Chapter 6), it may be concluded that hypothalamic sensitivity to regulation by glucose declines with age (Dilman 1958), or that in terms of the above concept on appetite regulation, the threshold of sensitivity of the satiety center is elevated.[1]

Indeed, since the satiety center is controlled by blood glucose and insulin levels, and since postprandial hyperglycemia and hyperinsulinemia are increased with aging, the feeding center should be progressively inhibited with the advancement of age. This would bring about a decrease in body weight. However, clinical experience attests to the fact that body weight does not decrease with aging. On the contrary, it increases, with the exception of the period of involution (see Chapter 8). Therefore it would appear that age-associated changes in appetite are conditioned either by elevation of the set point of the satiety center, which results in its insufficient stimulation in postprandial hyperglycemia, or by a resistance to the inhibition of the feeding center itself.

Thus disorders of this system of appetite regulation represent a central type of homeostatic failure with advancing age. According to the hypothesis under consideration, because of elevation of the set point of the satiety center, stimulation of this center is checked. This creates a situation where a human subject (or a rat fed ad libitum) has time to eat more food than is actually needed. Bearing in mind that with advancing age utilization of glucose in the muscle tissue declines (see Chapter 6), excess glucose, resulting from overeating, causes an accumulation of fat. If a person does not realize that, with aging, the satiety center is "led astray" and if he keeps on controlling his food intake only by appetite, then his body weight will inevitably increase with age.

Unfortunately, even if food intake is controlled precisely, ie, if the energy supply exactly equals the energy expenditure, this will not prevent the development of age-associated obesity; according to the hypothesis, the disturbance in the control of appetite results in a disturbance in the system of body weight regulation. In fact, if an increased appetite is responsible for obesity, then obesity in turn is responsible for an elevation of the basal level of insulin in the blood (and in CSF). This is a rule without exceptions, and in every model of experimental obesity insulin levels are increased. At the same time, overfeeding, even if determined by exogenous factors, leads to endocrine-metabolic changes that are observed in spontaneous obesity (Sims and Horton 1968). In particular, the number of receptor sites in target tissues is inversely correlated with the

[1] In my earlier hypothesis (Dilman 1958, unpublished data) the elevation of hypothalamic activity was considered to be the key factor of the age-associated disturbances of appetite regulation. From that point of view it was possible, at that time, to give an explanation as to why the age-related hyperglycemia does not result in a lower food intake (lack of appetite) in middle-aged subjects.

level of fasting plasma insulin (Kahn 1976). Therefore, the decreased insulin binding is a characteristic feature of insulin resistance in obesity. There are no reasons to believe that the hypothalamus could be an exception to this regularity, because the self-regulation of membrane receptor concentration appears to be one of the major mechanisms responsible for the desensitization of many target cells. Thus, the following chain of events can be imagined:

Age-associated food intake → increased storage of fat in the body (adiposity) → increased level of insulin in the blood (and CSF) → decline of the set point of the body weight control center → stabilization of obesity → progressive shift of the set point for body fat regulation.

Apparently, this chain of related events leads to a concept that the age-associated obesity cannot be prevented by the system of "strategic control of body weight." Table 5-1 shows the age-associated dynamics in increasing the storage of body fat in healthy men and women.

Table 5-1
Age-Associated Increase in Content of Body Fat in Healthy Men and Women

	Percentage of Fat in the Body	
Age	*Women (n = 215)*	*Men (n = 192)*
20–29	27.3 ± 0.5	13.9 ± 0.4
30–39	32.2 ± 0.5	17.6 ± 0.4
40–49	36.4 ± 0.4	19.7 ± 0.5
50–59	38.7 ± 0.5	20.4 ± 0.8
60–69	36.1 ± 0.3	22.3 ± 0.8

It should be pointed out that it is possible on the basis of current knowledge to attribute the elevation of the sensitivity threshold of the satiety center to the decline in the levels of noradrenaline (Saller and Stricker 1976) and serotonin (Breisch et al 1976) in the hypothalamus, since a decline in the concentration of these neurotransmitters controlling food intake takes place in the hypothalamus with advancing age.

Data available on the effect of emotions on appetite throw some light on age-related changes in appetite regulation. In the young, negative emotions generally inhibit appetite. By contrast it has often been reported that the same negative emotions increase appetite and body weight in middle-aged persons (Johnson 1947). A decrease in appetite in response to emotions may be interpreted as showing the normal sensitivity of the hypothalamic centers to the action of glucose, the level of which is known to rise in stress. In middle age, however, the satiety center becomes more resistant; therefore, stress-induced hyperglycemia fails to exert a regulatory effect. Instead it results in a paradoxical reaction similar to glucose load, which brings about a paradoxical increase in growth hormone secretion when the hypothalamic centers show a resistance to suppression (see Chapter 6). Stress as such causes a decreased concentration of biogenic amines in the hypothalamus (see Chapter 19). It is probable that when the influence of aging and of chronic stress combine, this can result in an escape of the feeding center from the inhibitory influence of the satiety center. In other words, the increase of appetite in response to negative emotions is an indication of intensification of aging. Let us imagine that the set point of the satiety center is not elevated with aging. In that case, a very young baby and an adult ought to be taking in the same amount of food, since an attempt to increase the amount of food with age would have resulted in an inhibition of appetite, or the adult would never be hungry, since the levels of glucose and insulin in an adult are always higher than those in a baby. The programmed "error" of the satiety center serves, in essence, to implement the program of development and growth of the organism. In particular, fat storage is needed to realize the growth spurt at the corresponding stages of ontogenesis (Tanner 1973). In light of the above concept, the age-associated storage of fat is a normal disease, in the same way as the climacteric and dysadaptosis.

However, a strong objection can be foreseen against treating adiposity in such a way. If restriction of food intake can prevent the development of adiposity, then may we really class the age-associated adiposity with the normal diseases of the regulatory system? In this respect it should be noted that the fat content in the body increases with age even in those cases where body weight remains stable (Dudl and Ensinck 1977).

In the next chapter a model will be considered in which fat storage is caused by alterations in the energy homeostat, which leads to the appearance of the lipid shunt. The lipid shunt can provide for a higher metabolism of glucose into fat and for the development of adiposity even if the food intake is properly balanced. Fat storage, in its turn, will cause a higher blood level of insulin, thus "forcing" the hypothalamic center of body weight regulation to function incorrectly, ie, in accordance with the elevation of the body weight set point.[1]

According to the classic point of view, general distinction can be made between regulatory obesity, in which the impairment is in the central mechanism regulating food intake, and metabolic obesity, in which the primary lesion is an inborn or acquired error in the metabolism of

[1]It cannot be excluded that elevation of the hypothalamic threshold of sensitivity takes place both in the satiety center and in the center regulating the body fat. Both parts of this hypothesis are to be checked experimentally.

tissue per se. In the first case habitual hyperphagia may lead to secondary metabolic abnormalities. And in the second case, peripheral metabolic dysfunction may in turn interfere with the function of the central nervous system (Mayer 1965). Thus, normality of thc age-associated adiposity is determined by both the elevation of the set point of the satiety center and the age-related changes in the energy homeostat, which result in a shift toward an intense storage and utilization of fatty acids. It is probable that, with aging, man first gains weight and, consequently, starts taking in more food than he actually needs, and naturally keeps on gaining more and more weight. With aging, man starts putting on weight not because he eats more, but he eats more because he stores fat. In the next chapter the development of age-related disturbances in the system of energy homeostasis will be considered, as well as the course by which these disturbances promote a self-reproducing mechanism of obesity.

6 Age-Associated Changes in the Energy Homeostat

"Fats burn down in the flames of carbohydrates," but carbohydrates do not burn down in the flames of fats.

It is generally believed that ancient man fed on carbohydrates only, and that omnivorousness, which led the man to eating meat and animal fat, was a decisive factor in the development of all modern diseases of men. However, this statement is not quite true. Contrary to existing opinion, both ancient man and man-like primates had always used glucose and fatty acids as energy substrates. The myth of herbivorousness of our ancestors is associated with the fact that ancient man actually obtained the energy substrates from vegetable food, using glucose and fructose as the chief fuel supply. However, irrespective of the kind of food, if an excess of glucose appears in the blood, it is metabolized in the liver and adipose tissue into fat.

Thus, whatever kind of food man might have eaten, he actually used both carbohydrates and animal fat as fuel, ie, as energy-producing substrates. Between these two sources of energy supply there exists an antagonism that provides for two types of energy processes.

Glucose and free fatty acids (FFA) are the basic energy substrates. During lipid β-oxidation, acetyl-CoA is formed, which in turn may oxidize in the citric acid cycle, generating energy, or may enter into various reactions and take part in the synthesis of acetoacetate, fatty acids, cholesterol, steroids, or in acetylation processes. Pyruvic acid formed in the oxidation of carbohydrates (and to a lesser degree amino acids) also may serve as a source of acetyl-CoA. Hence while the metabolism of energy-producing substrates differs in its initial states, the oxidation of common substrates formed in the metabolism of carbohydrates, fatty acids, and proteins (gluconeogenesis) terminates mainly in the citric acid cycle.

However some relations between the processes of energy untilization of carbohydrates and fat are highly antagonistic. The utilization of carbohydrates decreases that of FFA, and vice versa (Randle 1965, Wahlqvist et al 1973, Balasse and Neef 1974). The mechanisms of such antagonistic relationships are not the same, however.

The elevated glucose metabolism suppresses fat mobilization by providing increased amounts of γ-glycerol phosphate for triglyceride synthesis by the fat cell, as well as by decreasing the activity of the triglyceride lipase resulting from the rise in insulin levels. Accompanying the decrease in fat mobilization, the liver, muscle, and other extrahepatic tissues that use FFA as a major energy-producing substrate switch to glucose and its oxidation products as the chief substrates for producing Krebs cycle intermediates (Felber et al 1977).

By contrast, the organism's energy requirements during starvation are satisfied mainly by the utilization of fatty acids (Schlierf and Dorow 1973). The inhibition of glucose metabolism in increased lipolysis is achieved mainly in the "fatty acid-glucose cycle" (Randle 1965, Weber et al 1966, Coleman 1969). Glucose and free fatty acid utilization compete at another level as well: the level of hormonal interplay. Glucose and fatty acid concentrations are not only regulated by hormones; both these metabolic substrates exert a regulatory effect on secretion of insulin and growth hormone that plays a key role in energy homeostasis.

In the metabolic regulating mechanism, growth hormone secretion is influenced by changes in the concentration of glucose, fatty acids, and amino acids in the blood. As the glucose level rises, the growth hormone secretion is inhibited (Glick et al 1965), while even a 10–15 mg% decrease in the blood sugar level is followed by an increase in growth hormone secretion (Luft and Cerasi 1968). Such a high sensitivity of the hypothalamic glucoreceptors that govern growth hormone secretion is a manifestation of the key importance of the hypothalamic-growth hormone-glucose system in the regulation of the two rhythms of utilization of the energy substrates in energy homeostasis.

An increase in blood FFA level causes a fall in growth hormone level in man and in monkeys (Cryer et al 1972, Hertenlendy and Kipnis 1973), while a decrease in fatty acid level following administration of nicotinic acid results in an increase in the level of growth hormone (Quabbe et al

1977). Accordingly total lipoatrophy involves an extremely high concentration of growth hormone (Tzagournis et al 1973). It should be pointed out that increased FFA concentration inhibits the elevation of growth hormone level in insulin hypoglycemia (Blackard et al 1969). These observations and the influence of FFA on growth hormone secretion during sleep suggest the hypothesis that the utilization of fatty acids affects the hypothalamic receptors that control growth hormone secretion.

An increase in the level of amino acids in the blood (or in high protein diet) causes a rise in insulin and growth hormone secretion (Sukkar et al 1967). The stimulating effect of amino acids on growth hormone secretion can be inhibited by glucose administration. In a high carbohydrate diet the arginine-induced growth hormone secretion is suppressed completely (Merimee et al 1973). These observations testify to the substantial physiologic importance of the glucose-regulated hypothalamic mechanism of growth hormone secretion.

The precise role of growth hormone in the elevation of fatty acid level in fasting is not known. This factor seems to act as the primary starting mechanism, later inhibited as the fatty acid concentration grows, though some data show an unmistakable rise in growth hormone level during prolonged fasting (Merimee and Fineberg 1974). According to Cahill et al (1966) on the sixth day of fasting, growth hormone level rises from 0.3 ± 0.3 ng/ml to 6.0 ± 2.9 ng/ml. On the other hand an excessive intake of carbohydrates is followed by a persistent decline in growth hormone secretion, and the reactive release of growth hormone in response to the administration of amino acids is also inhibited (Merimee et al 1973). This inhibitory effect is observed even in cases of isocaloric diet with excessive carbohydrates.

Considering that growth hormone is a powerful antagonist of insulin the better utilization of glucose that occurs in a high carbohydrate diet is accounted for by the suppression of growth hormone secretion that also takes place.

The stressor mechanism of growth hormone regulation is not controlled by blood glucose level.

Growth hormone regulation of another type occurs at different stages of sleep. This neurogenic stimulation is thought to be caused by the limbic structures of the brain. Surges in growth hormone secretion are observed at the slow wave stage of sleep (Sassin et al 1969). They result in an increase in hormone concentration up to 50 ng/ml. The nocturnal secretion of growth hormone is not inhibited by glucose (Parker and Rossman 1971) and is independent of insulin and cortisol levels (Lucke and Glick 1972), but partially inhibited by a high FFA level (Lucke et al 1972) and by melatonin. The cycle of growth hormone secretion is repeated every night in a manner peculiar to each individual. It has been suggested that the nocturnal rise in growth hormone level promotes amino acid entry into protein synthesis (Llanos 1973). It should be noted also that nocturnal peaks are more pronounced in childhood, when anabolic processes prevail.

Apart from these three types of regulation by the long loop of negative feedback, the energy system has a mechanism responsible for the inhibition of growth hormone secretion as its blood concentration rises. This effect probably is exerted by short loop negative feedback. For example, the administration of an analog of growth hormone, devoid of its metabolic effects, inhibits the growth of bone and cartilage (Dilman and Kovaleva 1964).

As a result of growth hormone administration a considerable quantity of insulin is released in response to glucose and amino acid loading (Rabinowitz et al 1967, Mitchell et al 1970). Administration of growth hormone also affects the pattern of hyperinsulinemia. As a result the maximum level is reached at later stages, and the total increase of insulin concentration is augmented. Such a response is often referred to as a delayed reaction. These changes in insulin secretion are generally observed in cases of prediabetes and early stages of maturity-onset diabetes, obesity, and atherosclerosis.

Some investigators believe that the numerous metabolic effects of growth hormone, including the influence on the metabolism of glucose, fatty acids, and amino acids, are interdependent. In an attempt to explain this interaction, Weil (1965) claims that the lipolytic effect of growth hormone is of primary importance, since it determines all other growth hormone-dependent energy processes. Though the normal fatty acid level is generally below 500 μEq/liter and as a rule does not exceed 700–800 μEq/liter after moderate fasting, such an increase points to a great influx of fatty acids into muscle tissue because the half-life of FFA is as short as two to four minutes (Laurell 1972). Fatty acid concentration in the tissues is increased considerably as a result of speedy metabolism during fasting.

The effect of insulin in the energy homeostat is antagonistic in many ways to that of growth hormone. One of the basic physiologic effects of insulin is the stimulation of the glucose and amino acid flux across the cell membrane (Fritz 1972).

Another basic property of insulin consists in its antilipolytic action. Such small concentrations are required to produce this effect that they practically fail to affect glucose utilization and are of great physiologic importance, since most hormones are lipolytic. Insulin secretion is stimulated by many metabolic and hormonal substances, including glucose, fructose, ribose, amino acids, ketone bodies, glucagon, growth hormone, ACTH, glucocorticoids, thyroxin, estrogens, secretin, pancreozymin, gastrin, prolactin, placental lactogen, 3′5′-cyclic AMP, potassium ions, and by vagus excitation.

Normally a rapid rise in blood insulin level is observed after glucose loading, which is considered to be a result of the release of insulin from the stores in β-cells of the islets. But insulin secretion is decreased generally as a result of catecholamine action and fasting.

Variations in growth hormone and glucose levels play a very important role in the regulation of insulin secretion. At the same time changes in fatty acid and ketone body concentrations also affect insulin secretion. As the fatty acid concentration is increased, reactive hyperinsulinemia after glucose loading also occurs (Balasse and Ooms 1973). Finally it should be pointed out that somatostatin both inhibits the growth hormone secretion of the pituitary, which reduces reactive hyperinsulinemia, and exerts a direct inhibitory effect on insulin secretion (Daughaday et al 1976). Notwithstanding, the fundamental importance of the energy homeostat and, correspondingly, of the vast and complex system of its realization, data now available suggest a four-component model of the energy homeostat; in terms of that model we can consider the relationships forming a basis for energy homeostasis both in the fed state and in the fasting state.

The energy homeostat was determined to be a four-component system that regulates the relationships between the two main energy-producing substrates, glucose and free fatty acids, and two main hormones controlling the utilization of these substrates, insulin and growth hormone (GH) (Dilman 1974a). Their interaction is shown schematically in Figure 6-1. During the day when food is eaten, it is mainly glucose

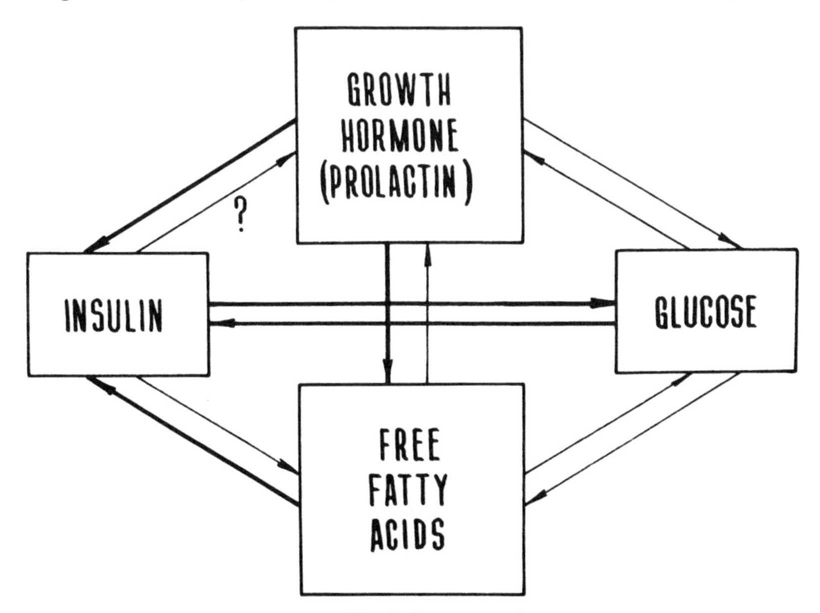

Figure 6-1 Four-component model of the energy homeostat.

and, to a lesser degree, FFA, that are used for the energy supply of the body. It is natural that when these food substrates are consumed, it is not necessary to draw upon the reserves of energy materials that are mainly stored in fat depots as triglycerides. Therefore, the postprandial rise in the blood levels of glucose and FFA, via suitable hypothalamic receptors, inhibits by negative feedback the secretion of GH, a lipolytic hormone, which is controlled by the blood level of energy substrates. At the same time, glucose stimulates the secretion of insulin, which exerts an antilipolytic effect on the one hand, and ensures the utilization of glucose on the other. As a consequence, optimal conditions for the uptake of glucose by insulin-dependent tissues are created.

Conversely at night, when no food is eaten, the energy supply is switched over to the predominant utilization of FFA, instead of glucose (Schlierf and Dorow 1973).

This switching-over mechanism operates as follows: since no food is taken in, the blood glucose level is decreased, thus leading to a rise in blood GH level and a decline in blood insulin concentration. As a result, the lipolytic action of GH on adipose tissue is enhanced and the antilipolytic effect of insulin is diminished simultaneously. This boosts the blood level of FFA, which is chiefly taken up by muscle tissues for energy supply. At the same time, FFA suppress glucose uptake by muscle tissue (Randle 1965) thus contributing to a better supply of nervous tissues with glucose.

Thus, there are two methods of providing the organism with the energy substrates. They may be conventionally designated as nocturnal and diurnal types. Numerous other regulatory effects on energy processes are exerted eventually, either through this four-component system or through an influence identifical to that of one of these components. For instance the effect of glucocorticoids is similar to that of growth hormone, both effects being exerted simultaneously. The same applies to the action of prolactin, which like growth hormone and cortisol reduces glucose uptake by muscle tissue. All these factors stimulate insulin secretion and contribute to fat accumulation, simultaneously intensifying lipolysis.

Figure 6-1 shows each component of the energy homeostat to be directly or indirectly correlated with the other components of the system. For example, when food is ingested, hyperglycemia produces several effects simultaneously, including the stimulation of insulin secretion, inhibition of growth hormone secretion, and suppression of lipolysis (Felber et al 1977). The latter effect is dependent both on glucose action and insulin level increase, and a decline in growth hormone level. These shifts develop the optimal conditions for glucose utilization. The energy homeostat with its perfect system of regulation would seem to be able to ensure the stability of energy homeostasis. Meanwhile, it is known that disturbances in lipia-carbohydrate metabolism are inherent in aging.

These changes are manifested by fat accumulation (age-connected body weight gain); glucose intolerance; increased blood cholesterol, triglyceride, β-lipoprotein, and insulin levels; and particularly, an increase of reactive hyperinsulinemia, which develops after glucose loading. Table 6-1 illustrates the age-dependent dynamics of these parameters in healthy men.

Table 6-1
Age-Associated Changes in Metabolic Parameters in Healthy Men

Test	Age Groups				
	4–19	*20–29*	*30–39*	*40–49*	*50–59*
Blood sugar (mg%)					
Basal	76.0±2.5	80.0±1.5	84.0±2.6	84.0±4.2	85.0±3.4
1 hour	83.0±3.3	100.0±4.3	117.0±9.9	131.9±9.2	141.0±8.0
2 hours		84.0±4.9	96.0±6.8	104.0±9.5	117.0±10.9
Blood insulin (μu/ml)					
Basal	19.0±2.4	23.0±3.7	19.0±2.9	25.0±6.0	37.0±13.0
1 hour	37.0±2.9	58.0±15.4	63.0±11.0	98.0±20.0	88.0±16.0
2 hours		43.0±12.9	64.0±17.0	118.0±8.0	84.0±10.5
Body weight (% deviation from norm)	−3.4±6.3	−8.3±2.5	+1.2±3.0	+3.3±3.1	+2.3±2.4
Cholesterol (mg%)	189.0±11.9	172.0±7.6	204.0±8.6	216.0±7.9	229.0±12.5
Triglycerides (mg%)	93.0±9.0	100.0±6.5	119.0±8.5	132.0±8.6	150.0±9.1

It is generally explained that such age-related metabolic changes are caused by external factors such as excessive food intake, low physical activity, and stress. And it is true that all play a decisive role in these metabolic disturbances. However, it is difficult to agree that external environmental factors alone determine such changes in energy regulation. Therefore, the question arises as to why the energy homeostat fails to maintain the stability of the internal environment. One probable answer to this question is that the process of normal aging causes a disturbance in the rhythm of functioning of the energy homeostat, which results in the central type of homeostatic failure.

It is clear from Table 6-2 that a glucose load of 40 gm/m^2 body surface results in a considerable fall in GH level in young subjects, which manifests normal functioning of the energy homeostat. At the same time, subjects in the middle-age group respond to glucose loading by an insignificant decrease in blood GH concentration. We obtained similar results when a less efficient method of GH testing was used (Dilman 1971). These data illustrate the central type of homeostatic failure, ie, an elevation of the threshold of sensitivity in hypothalamic structures toward the inhibiting effect of glucose. In normal conditions, the inhibiting effect of glucose must result in the switching of the energy homeostat from the "nocturnal" type of energy supply, with its characteristic predominant utilization of FFA, to the "diurnal" type, in which glucose is used as the chief fuel. Any disturbance in the switching-over mechanism must result in a situation characteristic of the normal course of aging, when a metabolic plethora, because of the antagonistic relationship between FFA and glucose, causes a metabolic pattern that gives certain properties of a disease to the normal aging process. Before we proceed to the age-associated model of metabolic shifts, mention should be made of one unexpected circumstance that does not fall into line with the general notion on the development during aging of the central type of homeostatic failure in the energy homeostat.

Table 6-2
Age-Associated Decrease in Inhibition (%)
of Blood Growth Hormone Level (ng/ml) by Glucose Load

	Average Age (years)	
	15 ± 1 (n = 22)	*48 ± 1 (n = 27)*
After fasting	2.4 ± 0.5	1.0 ± 0.1
One hour after glucose load	1.2 ± 0.2 (−50%)	0.9 ± 0.1 (−10%)
Two hours after glucose load	0.9 ± 0.2 (−62%)	0.9 ± 0.1 (−10%)

The development of age-associated resistance to inhibition by glucose by negative feedback should inevitably result in a rise in blood GH concentration. However, it is clear from Table 6-2 that the basal level of GH in middle age is much lower than that in younger subjects. Numerous other reports present convincing evidence that age advancement is accompanied by a decline in the basal level of GH and its diurnal output (Finkelstein et al 1972). At present these shifts are attributed to the effect of the age-associated gain in body weight (Dudl and Ensinck 1977) or, more precisely, the increase in the body fat mass, which leads to an intensified spontaneous lipolysis and, hence, a rise in the blood level of FFA. Such a conclusion is in keeping with those experimental and clinical data that show that a rise in blood FFA level inhibits GH secretion (Quabbe et al 1977). This is corroborated by data on the rise in growth hormone level following a loss of body weight (Londono et al 1969, Crockford and Salmon 1970). However, a low level of growth hormone is observed in diabetes with combined hyperglycemia and obesity. Hyperglycemia alone does not significantly inhibit growth hormone secretion (Stephen et al 1973). It should be pointed out that the level of growth hormone rises very high (nearly ten times the normal concentration of growth hormone) in total lipoatrophy, ie, on depletion of fat deposits (Tzagournis et al 1973). It is generally accepted now that obesity is associated with a diminished growth hormone response to a variety of stimuli. The return of growth hormone sensitivity after weight reduction has led to the conclusion that the blunted growth hormone responses are secondary to the accumulation of fat. In particular a strong negative correlation has been observed between the peak growth hormone levels, after arginine is administered, and the degree of obesity (Dudl et al 1973). This seems to explain the fact that some investigators have failed to observe an age-associated decrease in basal growth hormone level, since this phenomenon may depend on the specific features of the examined population.

The age-associated decrease in basal growth hormone level does not, however, depend on the decline of functional activity of the hypothalamic-pituitary complex. Some evidence indicates that hypoglycemia may cause similarly pronounced, if not higher, rise in growth hormone in elderly subjects (Pitis et al 1973, Kalk et al 1973, Root and Oski 1969, Sachar et al 1971). However a reduced response to insulin administration also has been reported (Dudl et al 1973, Bazzarre et al 1976). These data on FFA levels are indispensable for the assessment of the controversy. Besides, Muggeo et al (1975) believe that, since the insulin hypoglycemic effect becomes less rapid with aging, this could, in part, explain the progressive decline in the growth hormone response to insulin.

Considerable hypersecretion of growth hormone caused by insulin-induced hypoglycemia has been observed in cases of breast cancer (Carter et al 1967) and in endometrial carcinoma (Benjamin 1974), ie, in those pathologic processes which, similar to aging, are characterized by a resistance in the hypothalamic-growth hormone system to inhibition by glucose (see Chapter 17). In breast cancer patients, growth hormone concentration has been found to rise eighteenfold despite resistance to insulin (Carter et al 1967, 1975).

Although some authors report that the release of growth hormone stimulated by arginine is diminished in elderly subjects (Dudl and Ensinck 1972), arginine infusion does not reduce blood fatty acid level, ie, it fails to eliminate the "fatty" inhibition of growth hormone secretion.

Thus, the condition of the hypothalamic-growth hormone-glucose system should be tested preferably when lipolysis is inhibited. For this purpose infusions of nicotinic acid may be recommended. Such data seem to necessitate the identification of not only two types of body energy supply (nocturnal and diurnal), but also two systems of metabolic homeostatic regulation of GH secretion, one of these systems being controlled by the hypothalamic sensitivity threshold to inhibition by glucose, and the other by the hypothalamic sensitivity threshold to FFA.

In this connection, another factor is of interest. In children, particularly in prepuberty, the blood FFA level is higher than after onset of sexual maturity (Corvilain et al 1961). However, the GH level is higher in children than in adults, which means that children are characterized by an elevated hypothalamic threshold of sensitivity to inhibition by FFA. These data suggest that the age-associated changes in the hypothalamic threshold of sensitivity to inhibition by glucose and FFA are oriented in opposite directions. Children reveal a high level of sensitivity to inhibition by glucose (see Table 6-2), and resistance of the hypothalamic centers to inhibition by FFA. On the contrary, age advancement involves a high sensitivity to inhibition by FFA and resistance to inhibition by glucose. Thus, the domination of the glucose or diurnal type of regulation is gradually superseded by the domination of the fat or nocturnal type of regulation (Figure 6-2).

It is shown that insulin-induced hypoglycemia causes a considerable rise in blood GH level in a 29-year-old woman, which persists even after fat loading. This is a manifestation of the predominance of the glucose type of regulation in young age. On the other hand, a 46-year-old woman with signs of moderate obesity reveals a low basal level of GH secretion, which points to a high sensitivity to inhibition by FFA. Accordingly, insulin-induced hypoglycemia, which results in the decline of both FFA and glucose levels in blood, causes a high rise in GH level at the same time. This rise in GH level occurs chiefly because of the fall in the level of FFA but not glucose, because fat loading in conjunction with insulin hypoglycemia prevents a rise in blood GH concentration. These findings may be interpreted as an indication of the age-associated shift toward the predominance of the fat type of regulation.

Such opposite-directed, age-associated changes in the hypothalamic threshold of sensitivity to glucose and FFA are quite explainable from a biologic point of view. High levels of GH and FFA are indispensable in childhood for cholesterol synthesis and body growth. Therefore it is advisable to recall that cell division ceases when either cholesterol synthesis in the somatic cell or its transport from the blood into the cell is inhibited (Chen et al 1975). The simultaneous occurrence of the high levels of FFA and GH in children may be interpreted as a manifestation of the central type of homeostatic failure in the fat-regulated subsystem of the energy homeostat. This regulatory peculiarity is typical of a metabolic pattern that has been designated as "pre-prediabetes" (Dilman 1971, see Chapter 8). After the onset of sexual maturity, the hypothalamus becomes more sensitive to inhibition by FFA than to that by glucose. It is possible that metabolic suppression of GH secretion plays a certain role in the inhibition of the rate of body growth after onset of sexual maturity. It is not clear yet at what age the fat-regulated inhibition of GH secretion sets in. The data of Quabbe and coworkers (1977) demonstrate that lipolysis inhibition by nicotinic acid causes a sharp rise in GH concentration to occur in men as early as 20–21 years of age.

Some data confirming our findings on the elevation of the set point of hypothalamic sensitivity to homeostatic inhibition in the growth hormone-glucose system were published by Sandberg et al (1973). This study found that the growth hormone concentration after glucose loading was higher in older subjects than in younger ones despite a relatively high glucose level.

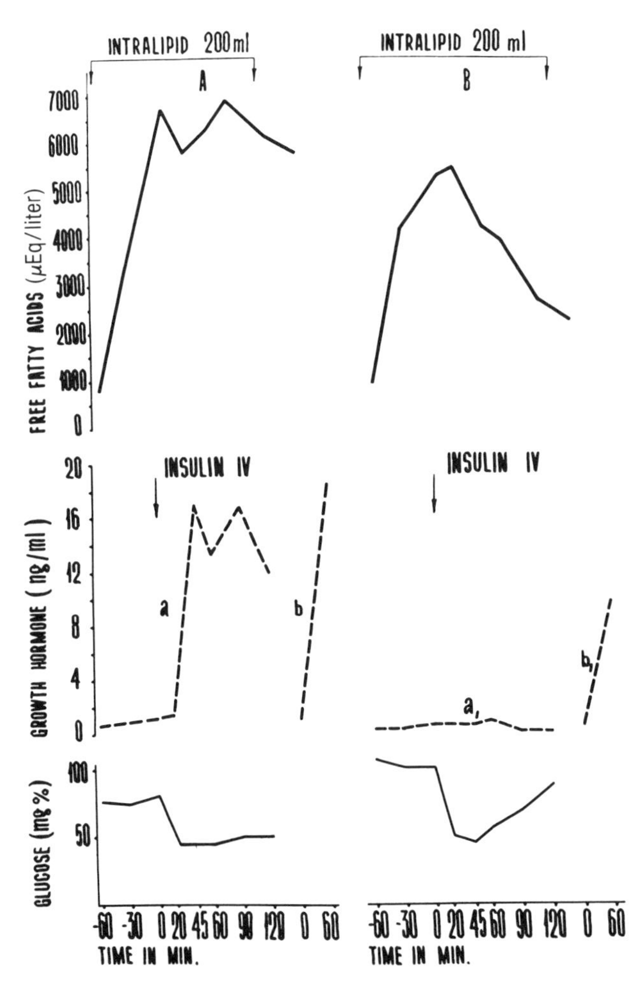

Figure 6-2 Dynamics of GH level during insulin test and intravenous injection of intralipid. A: A 29-year-old woman with normal body weight; B: A 45-year-old moderately obese woman; a and a_1: dynamics of blood growth hormone levels after insulin and intralipid; b and b_1: dynamics of blood growth hormone levels following insulin alone. Dynamics of blood glucose level were practically the same in both experiments.

Benjamin et al (1969) reported a paradoxical increase in growth hormone level after glucose loading in cases of endometrial carcinoma (see Chapter 17). However, they reported no fall in growth hormone level after glucose loading in healthy female controls over 50 years of age; this would indicate an elevation of the hypothalamic threshold.[1]

In another study (Dudl et al 1973), administration of a considerable intravenous load of glucose (20 gm over 20 seconds) showed no age-connected differences in the inhibition of growth hormone level. However, these data are open to criticism (Dilman 1974c). It is known that the blood GH level will change when the change in glucose concentration reaches 15–20 mg% (Luft and Cerasi 1968). The intravenous glucose load results in a very short rise in the blood glucose level, which rises as high as 260 mg%. Such a high level of hyperglycemia is never observed in healthy subjects following oral administration of glucose. Marked hyperglycemia may inhibit growth hormone secretion even when relevant hypothalamic centers are resistant to inhibition. In this connection it is interesting to point out that hyperglycemia produced by intravenous infusion of glucose has resulted in an approximately 58% decrease in growth hormone level in a case of acromegaly, whereas no decrease in growth hormone concentration has been observed after oral administration of glucose (Nakagawa and Mashimo 1973).

Such a situation is familiar to endocrinologists. Cases of obesity and Cushing's syndrome are generally distinguished by means of the dexamethasone test, in which 2 mg/24 hours of the drug is administered. In Cushing's syndrome a larger dose causes an inhibition of the hypothalamic-pituitary-adrenal cortex complex, although this syndrome is known to involve an elevated hypothalamic set point to inhibition by glucocorticoids. It should be pointed out that Danowski et al (1969) and Stephan et al (1973) used an unjustifiably large oral load (1.75 gm glucose per 1 kg body weight) in their comprehensive studies. Such a load may cause a reduction in growth hormone despite the increased hypothalamic threshold to inhibition. Hence, exorbitant loads should not be used for establishing the existence of an elevation of hypothalamic threshold. A similar situation seems to develop in growth hormone regulation when its level remains unchanged in postprandial hyperglycemia (Jung et al 1971). Normally in such a situation growth hormone secretion is inhibited even when the diet is isocaloric but rich in carbohydrates (Merimee and Fineberg 1973). Therefore age-associated rise in blood sugar should be interpreted as a sign of an excess of growth hormone caused by the resistance of relevant hypothalamic inhibitory

---

[1]Benjamin and Deutsch (Personal communication 1977) report that "if the response of the control women is compared to literature values or to our own clinical findings (unpublished), it can be seen that the suppression of growth hormone levels—often down to zero in younger women—is not obtained in older groups."

centers. Indeed, when the homeostatic system functions normally, postprandial hyperglycemia is followed by a decrease in growth hormone, and this creates optimal conditions for glucose utilization.

Another circumstance should be taken into consideration. The total 24-hour output of growth hormone cannot be assessed on the basis of its basal level. Numerous authors have reported cases of diabetes in which moderate physical exercise can induce overt hypersecretion of growth hormone (Hansen 1971, 1973b). And since age-associated metabolic shifts are similar to diabetic disturbances in many ways, we can obtain an adequate evaluation of age-connected changes in growth hormone by studying the results of examinations involving the use of physical exercise.

Elevation of the hypothalamic set point to inhibition by glucose is not an indication of aging alone. For instance in many cases of acromegaly no inhibition of growth hormone secretion by glucose has been observed (Lawrence et al 1970). This exemplifies the resistance of the hypothalamic centers to the inhibitory effect of glucose. The elevation of the hypothalamic threshold to inhibition occurs not only in acromegaly but in many other pathologic states as well. It has been found that glucose causes an increase rather than a decrease in growth hormone level in patients with endometrial carcinoma (Benjamin et al 1969). This paradoxical reaction also has been observed in cases of malnutrition (Alvarez et al 1972), in premature infants (Cornblath et al 1965), in patients with renal insufficiency, in Turner's syndrome, Wilson's disease, prediabetes (Sönksen et al 1973), breast cancer and endometrial carcinoma (Dilman 1970b, 1971; Samaan et al 1966), and in Huntington's chorea (Caraceni et al 1977). It is noteworthy that the paradoxical reaction observed in the thyrotoxicosis of Graves' disease subsides to euthyroidism (Cavagnini et al 1974).

The mechanism of paradoxical reactions remains obscure. All these syndromes share one feature in common: a diminished tolerance to glucose and, naturally, since there is no other alternative, an enhanced utilization of FFA for energy supply. Since such a situation is characterized by a predominant inhibitory effect of FFA on GH secretion, it is possible to advance the following hypothesis on the origin of a paradoxical response: as a result of the antagonism of the utilization of FFA and that of glucose, glucose loading leads to the hyperglycemia and reactive release of insulin seen in middle-aged subjects or in the above pathologies, which are much higher than normal. Since both factors cause a sharp fall in blood FFA level, the "fat brake" is rapidly eliminated, resulting in a rise in blood GH concentration despite hyperglycemia, ie, the "paradoxical reaction" occurs. The above hypothesis on the origin of paradoxical reaction is further supported by the data showing that patients with endometrial carcinoma often respond to glucose loading by a paradoxical rise in GH secretion (Benjamin et al 1969), and by data in these patients showing an excessive secretion of GH in response to insulin-induced hypoglycemia (Benjamin 1974). Thus, the very existence of the so-called paradoxical reactions, which are often observed in middle-aged subjects, in spite of their low basal levels of growth hormone, proves that the mechanism of the age-associated decline in growth hormone secretion is caused by functional shifts in the hypothalamus.

At present, there is no reliable evidence on the role of biogenic amines, hormonal receptors, and energy shifts in the mechanism of the age-associated changes in hypothalamic sensitivity to glucose and FFA. Therefore, it is expedient to summarize some preliminary conclusions on the problem.

It is known that there are metabolic, stressor, and diurnal types of GH secretion regulation, which are independent of each other (Martin 1973). While considering the age-associated changes in the metabolic regulation of GH it is necessary to mention that GH secretion is equally stimulated by serotonin and catecholamines (Müller 1973). In young age, the hypothalamic content of catecholamines and serotonin is at a maximum, and it is possible that it is the total effect of both factors that is responsible for a high level of GH secretion in young subjects. In this connection, the following data seem to be of interest. Endogenous mental depression is thought to be associated with lowered levels of catecholamines and serotonin in the brain. Since treatment of patients suffering from mental depression with 5-hydroxytryptophan does not result in a rise in GH secretion (Takahashi et al 1973), it means that an increase in serotonin level in the hypothalamus is not sufficient for stimulation of GH, unless the catecholamine level remains low. It is also probable that a high level of catecholamines is responsible for a high sensitivity of the hypothalamus to inhibition by glucose and, in addition, this may be associated with a glucose-induced decrease in the hypothalamic level of catecholamines. This hypothesis is corroborated by our experimental results showing that glucose loading lowers the dopamine level in the hypothalamus and boosts the rate of serotonin metabolism (Table 6-3). These data agree with results demonstrating that the decline in GH secretion, following glucose loading, may be prevented by treatment with L-dopa (Ajlouni et al 1975). This effect does not occur in diabetics, probably as a result of the diminished utilization of glucose by hypothalamic glucoreceptors.

It should be noted that two days' administration of a serotonin antagonist, cyproheptadine, decreased the plasma growth hormone concentration during oral tolerance test in four of six acromegalic patients (Feldman et al 1976).

Meanwhile, hypothalamic resistance to inhibition by FFA in young subjects seems to be determined by high levels of both catecholamines and serotonin. As can be seen from Table 6-3, fat loading increases the

Table 6-3
Effects of Glucose or Lipid Loading on Biogenic Amine Level in Rat Hypothalamus

Group	No. Animals	Noradrenaline (μg/g)	Dopamine (μg/g)	Serotonin (μg/g)	5-HIAA* (μg/g)
Control	13	1.12 ± 0.01	0.56 ± 0.13	0.59 ± 0.10	0.82 ± 0.10
Glucose†	17	1.06 ± 0.05	0.34 ± 0.04	0.88 ± 0.09§	0.92 ± 0.15
Control	10	1.80 ± 0.16	0.50 ± 0.07	1.25 ± 0.05	0.63 ± 0.07
Intralipid‡	10	1.73 ± 0.11	0.47 ± 0.05	1.21 ± 0.05	0.77 ± 0.05§

*5-Hydroxyindoleacetic acid, a metabolic product of serotonin.
†Solution of 40% glucose was injected intravenously, 1.5 mg/kg, 30 min before decapitation. Biogenic amine level was assayed in hypothalamic tissues, according to Anden and Magnusson (1967) and O'Hanlon et al (1970).
‡Intralipid was injected in the caudal vein of male rats, 1.5 ml, with 5 units of heparin, 30 min before decapitation. Biogenic amine level was assayed in tissues from four hypothalamuses, according to Ansell and Beeson (1968), Haubrich and Denzer (1973), and Cox and Perchuch (1973).
§Difference from controls is statistically significant.

rate of serotonin metabolism. Considering that aging involves a slow decline in the level of biogenic amines in the hypothalamus, it may be supposed that this factor raises hypothalamic sensitivity to inhibition by FFA. Hence, we suggest that high hypothalamic sensitivity to inhibition by glucose in young subjects is associated with an enhanced activity of the adrenergic system, while an elevated hypothalamic sensitivity to inhibition by FFA observed after onset of sexual maturity is caused by the age-associated decline in the hypothalamic levels of both serotonin and dopemine. It should be mentioned that metabolic shifts in the body influence the condition of hypothalamic systems. Apart from the known influence of glucose and insulin on the hypothalamic level of biogenic amines (Fernstrom and Wurtman 1971), Table 6-3 demonstrates the development of shifts as a result of fat loading. Moreover, it is well known that the blood FFA level rises with aging, leading to the elevation of the free tryptophan level, as a consequence of the competition between the latter substance and FFA for the protein carrier (Fernstrom 1974); thus, serotonin concentration in the brain increases. It should be interesting to discover whether the relatively predominant proportion of serotonin over catecholamines in the hypothalamus with increasing age is a consequence of the influence of this peripheral metabolic factor in terms of the cascade hypothesis of Finch (1976).

As far as the diurnal rhythm is concerned, the rise in the GH level is particularly frequent during slow-wave sleep, which is thought to be characterized by an intensification of serotonergic influences (Jouvet 1969, Laborit 1972). Therefore, the decay or complete absence of nocturnal peaks in subjects over 50 years of age (Finkelstein et al 1972) is likely to be caused by the age-associated decline in serotonin level in the hypothalamus. However, there are data that prove that a serotonin receptor-blocking drug, methysergide, exerts a moderate stimulatory effect on sleep-related growth hormone secretion (Mendelson et al 1978). It should be noted that the age-connected decrease in catecholamines is much greater than that in serotonin (Robinson 1975), which may result in a relative predominance of serotonergic influences. Moreover, metabolic shifts characteristic of aging (hyperinsulinemia and rise in blood FFA) may impede the age-associated decrease in hypothalamic concentration of serotonin. This factor, namely, the predominance of serotonergic influences, is responsible for a high nocturnal secretion of GH in some cancer patients who are middle-aged and overweight (see Chapter 17). This suggestion agrees with data on the stressor mechanism of GH regulation. Insulin-induced hypoglycemia, which reduces blood FFA and raises serotonin concentration in the hypothalamus (Bivens et al 1973), is known to bring about an almost identical elevation in GH level in young and old subjects (Pitis et al 1973, Kalk et al 1973) although basal (tonic) secretion of GH falls off with aging. Accordingly, the antagonists of serotonin reduce the reactive release of GH in response to insulin hypoglycemia (Bivens et al 1973).

I suppose that during aging the energy homeostat system undergoes opposite-directed changes in the hypothalamic threshold of sensitivity to the regulatory action of energy substrates. The high sensitivity of the hypothalamus to inhibition by glucose, inherent in the young body, is superseded by the rise in the hypothalamic threshold to inhibition by glucose. On the contrary, the hypothalamic threshold of sensitivity to inhibition by FFA declines. This leads to the age-associated decrease in the basal secretion of growth hormone. On the other hand, the dependence of the age-associated changes in GH secretion not only on specific hypothalamic alterations (eg, biogenic amine levels in the hypothalamus) but on the metabolic pattern in the body as well, lends some uncertainty and individual variability to the determined nature of the age-associated shifts in regulation. This deviation from the determination of the genetic program is caused by the multiplicity of factors that determine the extent and character of metabolic processes.

What disorders occur when the main elements of the four-component system of the energy homeostat are disturbed? Consider which disorders in the energy homeostat correspond to metabolic shifts intrinsic to normal aging.

At present there is a well-grounded point of view on hyperinsulinemia as a key factor in the formation of age-associated obesity, hypertriglyceridemia, and hypercholesterolemia. But hyperinsulinemia is a factor both promoting obesity and its consequence. What is the sequence of disorders that take place in the course of normal aging? Which is the first to occur, for instance, hyperinsulinemia or obesity? If it is hyperinsulinemia, then it is necessary to establish its cause. If obesity occurs first and produces hyperinsulinemia, then what are the causes of age-connected obesity?

It is obvious that there can be no answer to these questions if we limit the consideration of the problem to the two correlated parameters: hyperinsulinemia and obesity. Therefore, analysis should be made of disturbances taking place outside this pair of interrelated parameters. An analysis of a model of the energy homeostat shows that this syndrome of obesity and hyperinsulinemia may develop if the hypothalamic set point to the regulatory effect of glucose is raised. Elevation of the hypothalamic threshold to inhibition in the growth hormone-glucose subsystem is considered in our model to be a key factor of metabolic disorders in the energy homeostat in the course of aging. Further sequences of disturbances may be presented as follows (Figure 6-3).

When, after food intake, the growth hormone level decrease is not sufficient, postprandial glycemia arises because of the contrainsulin effect of growth hormone, thus lowering the muscle tissue sensitivity to insulin. This is followed by a rise in insulin secretion. Compensatory insulinemia, however, does not arrest the decline in glucose utilization completely. Therefore, tolerance to carbohydrates gradually diminishes as age advances (Figure 6-3, cycle I). At the same time, hyperinsulinemia

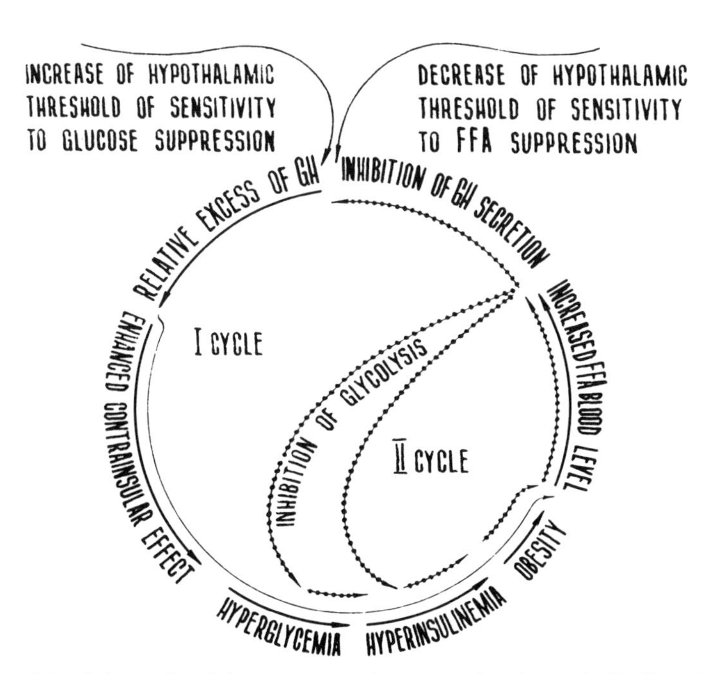

Figure 6-3 Schematic of the sequence of age-associated metabolic disturbances in the energy homeostat. See text for description.

in conjunction with an excessive glucose level stimulates triglyceride synthesis, leading to development of age-associated obesity. Subsequent hormonal-metabolic shifts are in positive correlation with the extent of overweight. Some data suggest that when the fat deposits exceed a certain critical level, a spontaneous lipolysis commences, which is manifested by an age-associated rise in blood FFA concentration. Consequently, growth hormone secretion is suppressed, thus switching off the primary mechanism of age-dependent metabolic disturbances. In the case of overweight, however, metabolic shifts persist (although, as a result of the diminished level of growth hormone, the pathogenic factor of cycle I of the metabolic disturbances is eliminated) because free fatty acid utilization inhibits the glucose uptake by the muscle tissue. This switches on cycle II of the disturbances, in which hyperglycemia is responsible for a secondary stimulation by hyperinsulinemia, while the latter leads to further accumulation of fat and intensification of lipolysis. This closed cycle can be denoted as the fat shunt, which does not need growth hormone for its reproduction. Under these conditions the routes of metabolism of energy-producing substrates change. Glucose taken with food is not fully used by muscle tissue and hyperinsulinemia converts further carbohydrate sources into depot fat. The deposits are drawn upon, and fatty acids, often in excess, are channeled to the target tissues. Thus the energy requirements of the organism are provided predominantly by fatty acid utilization, and metabolic conditions similar to those in maturity-onset diabetes mellitus develop (see Chapter 11).

Unfortunately, by the time the metabolic disturbances have been carried to this stage metabolism can no longer return to normal, even though the initial factor in their disturbance has been removed. Because of the well-advanced obesity that has developed by this point, the major pathogenic factors of the age-associated metabolic disturbances simply continue to operate. The main point is that obesity ensures a high level of lipolysis, which entails a decreased utilization of glucose by the mechanism of the so-called Randle effect, ie, through competition between the utilization of glucose and that of fatty acids. While fats burn in the flame of carbohydrates, carbohydrates do not burn in the flame of fats. Thus, as was shown earlier, a vicious circle of age-associated metabolic disturbances is formed. In the final analysis the human organism burns in the flame of fats, which means that the predominant utilization of fatty acids as a source of energy is inherent not only in normal aging but in such age-sepcific disorders as obesity, late-onset diabetes mellitus, atherosclerosis, metabolic immunodepression, and cancer (see Chapters 11–18). Hence the proposed model suggests a single pathogenic mechanism responsible for major metabolic disturbances inherent in aging. Moreover it suggests that the elevation of the hypothalamic set point to inhibition of the growth hormone-glucose system is sufficient to trigger a series of age-associated metabolic disorders. All subsequent metabolic disturbances occur according to the proposed model simply on the basis of relevant physiologic interrelations of the energy homeostat and other homeostatic systems. Now let us see to what extent this model complies with available factual data.

Age-Associated Hypersomatotropism

It is known that a glucose load reduces the growth hormone level in the blood by approximately 50% one hour after oral administration (Glick et al 1965). This decrease is characteristic of the normal functioning of the energy homeostat, but this shift is not observed in middle-aged subjects. However, judging from basal values the growth hormone level in the blood tends to decrease with advancing age. Such a decrease seems to be caused by the inhibition of growth hormone secretion, both as a consequence of an increased rate of FFA utilization and due to a lower concentration of biogenic amines in the hypothalamus. This raises the question as to whether or not it is possible to speak about age-associated hypersomatotropism at all.

Many hormones may exert an excessive influence on a target tissue as the result of a disturbance in their secretion cycle, even though there is no absolute increase in their level of concentration in the blood. This is observed, for example, when the diurnal rhythm of cortisol secretion is disturbed in prediabetic patients (Pfeiffer 1965). Based on this supposition, it cannot be excluded that a disturbance in the rhythm of growth hormone secretion, ie, lack of postprandial decrease of growth hormone level in the blood, can cause hypersomatotropism. It should be stressed that although the diabetogenic effect of growth hormone has been long established (Young 1968), there are still doubts about the fact that such effect may be caused by physiologic variations of the growth hormone level in the blood. It was shown recently that an increase of growth hormone within physiologic limits (up to about 6 ng/ml) promotes an increase of plasma β-hydroxybutyrate, glyceride and FFA (Gerich et al 1976). At the same time, little data can be produced now to illustrate the role of growth hormone in disturbing the energy homeostat. It has been shown that the rise of GH level which occurs four to five hours after oral glucose loading may be causally related to the relative glucose intolerance that ensues, possibly by delaying the early insulin response to hyperglycemia (Yalow et al 1969). Data obtained in our laboratory are consistent with this statement. As shown in Figure 6-4 the period of reactive hypersomatotropism is characterized by a decreased utilization of glucose, although the reactive insulinemia was more pronounced after the second glucose load than after the first. Thus, the hypoglycemic effect produced by the first load causes growth hormone to increase; therefore, physiologic variation in the growth hormone level may be directly responsible for the diminished utilization of glucose in subsequent loads. Bearing in mind that with advancing age postprandial hypoglycemia increases, hypersomatotropism may occur regularly owing to excessive food intake, although there are as yet no data on the age-associated dynamics of this reacton. Moreover the following data show that in patients with diabetes mellitus, administration of immune serum against an analog of growth hormone (capable of blocking the effect of native growth hormone) diminishes the requirement for insulin and reduces the level of blood sugar (Dilman et at 1971, Dilman 1974b) (Table 6-4).

Table 6-4
Decrease in Blood Sugar Level and Therapeutic Dose of Insulin as a Result of Administration of Immune Serum against an Analog of Growth Hormone*

	Duration of Observation (days)						
Assay	*1*	*4*	*5*	*6*	*8*	*11*	*13*
Blood sugar level* (mg%) at 8:30 AM	252	249	214	252	203	204	153
Blood sugar level* (mg%) at 12:30 PM	190	158	204	170	155	122	132
24-hour dose of insulin	140	140	120	112	112	112	112

*Immune serum administration completed on day 4.

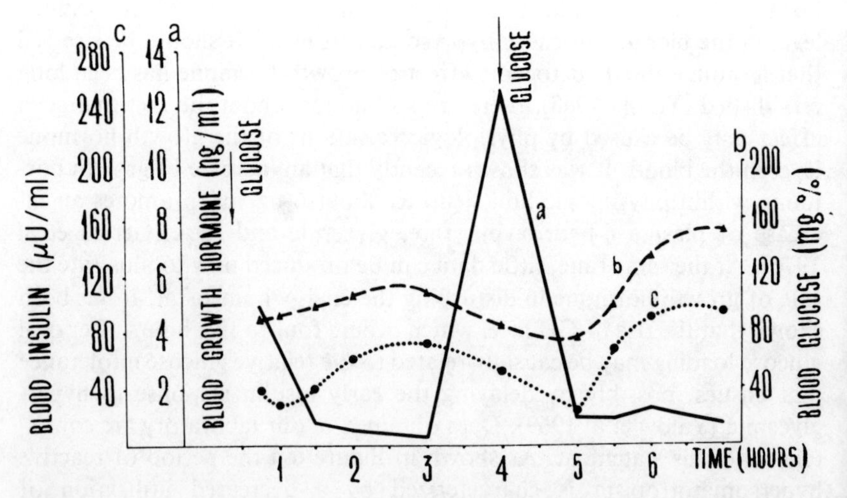

Figure 6-4 Decrease in glucose utilization following a double glucose load applied at four-hour intervals. Curve A: blood growth hormone level; Curve B: blood glucose level; Curve C: blood insulin level.

Of particular interest in this connection are the data on the improvement in glucose tolerance in diabetic patients with a carbohydrate-rich diet (Brunzell et al 1971), which may be considered to be a result of an inhibition of growth hormone secretion under such conditions (Merimee and Fineberg 1973). The data obtained in a study of prediabetes, which has many pathogenic features in common with the process of aging, should also be considered. Both states are characterized by compensatory hyperinsulinemia (see Chapter 11). Apart from manifesting a high level of growth hormone (Pfeiffer 1965, Hales et al 1968, Boden et al 1968), prediabetes reveals a paradoxical rise in growth hormone level after glucose load (Sönksen et al 1973). This disorder is also characterized by a "delayed" development of insulinemia following a glucose load, ie, a complex of hormonal and metabolic shifts typical of normal aging.

It should be noted that estrogen administration raises the sensitivity to insulin in patients with ischemic heart disease (Figure 6-5). Although estrogens increase growth hormone concentration (Frantz and Rabkin 1965), they simultaneously counteract the influence of growth hormone

[1]It should be noted that oral contraceptives containing modified estrogens affect the patient's tolerance to carbohydrates and promote hypertriglyceridemia, in contrast to the effect of natural estrogens (Dilman 1974a).

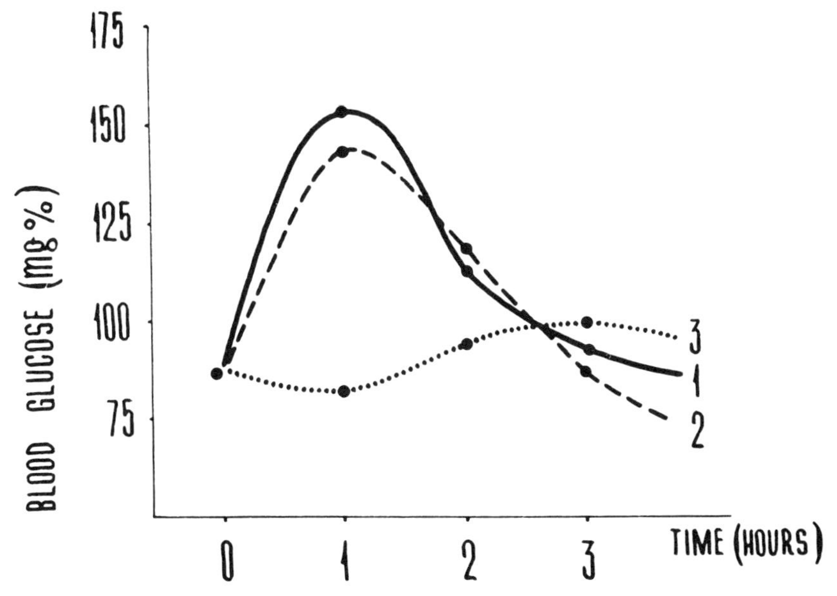

Figure 6-5 Effect of estrogen treatment on glucose tolerance in male patients with ischemic heart disease. Curve 1: Standard glucose load (100 gm orally); Curve 2: Glycemia after oral administration of glucose and intravenous injection of insulin (0.1 unit/kg body weight; Curve 3: Same parameters as in curve 2 following one month of treatment with estrogens.

on target tissues. For example it was shown earlier that estrogens considerably reduce the lipolytic effect of growth hormone (Kovaleva et al 1964, Wiedemann and Schwartz 1972).[1] Therefore the estrogen-induced increase in sensitivity to insulin may be regarded as an indirect indication of the importance of a relative hypersomatotropism in the development of this phenomenon. Thus, in spite of the limited amount of clinical data available, it can be supposed (bearing in mind all experimental data) that the disturbance in the rhythm of growth hormone secretion caused by an elevation of the hypothalamic set point to the inhibiting effect of glucose can result in physiologic hypersomatotropism (see Figure 6-3, cycle I). At the same time it is clear that cycle I operates until growth hormone secretion is decreased. However the same factor that causes this decrease, namely the intensified lipolysis and utilization of fatty acids, switches on cycle II (see Figure 6-3), which operates henceforth independently of the first cycle. A continuation of these disturbances is the age-associated reduction in glucose utilization.

Age-Associated Hyperglycemia

As age advances, tolerance to carbohydrates gradually declines (O'Sullivan et al 1971). Decrease in glucose tolerance may be observed in the elderly at two-year intervals (Hofstatter et al 1945). A diminished tolerance also continues into senescence after 80 years of age (Streeten et al 1965). Some authors believe that after 70 years of age practically all people develop diabetic features varying only in degree (Hofstatter et al 1945). According to the reports of several investigators, coefficient K, which describes the rate of glucose removal from the blood after intravenous injection, shows a gradual decline from 0.09 to 0.21 per decade (Andres 1971). Carbohydrate tolerance is decreased with advancing age regardless of body weight. This involves an enhancement of reactive insulinemia following a glucose load, an indication of diminished sensitivity to endogenous insulin (Hales et al 1968).

At the same time there is no evidence that long-term hyperglycemia-caused secondary insufficiency of insulin secretion is a factor responsible for the age-associated reduction in glucose utilization, since the insulin level two hours after glucose loading in subjects older than 85 is approximately 3½ times that at the age of 30 (Smith and Hall 1973). In addition, the metabolic clearance rate of native porcine insulin is identical in young and elderly subjects (Sherwin et al 1972). Thus the age-connected decrease in carbohydrate tolerance is caused by diminished effectiveness rather than a reduced level of insulin.

Age-Associated Decrease in the Sensitivity of Muscle Tissue to Insulin Action

One of the probable factors causing reduction of glucose utilization in muscle tissue is the decrease in the sensitivity of muscle tissue to insulin action. The phenomenon of age-associated decrease in the sensitivity of muscle tissue to insulin action has been reported by many authors. Our results are summarized in Table 6-5 and show again that sensitivity to insulin action diminishes with advancing age.

Table 6-5
Results of Insulin-Glucose Test (mg%) in Young and Middle-Aged Subjects

	Age Group	
	Young (n = 26)	*Middle-Aged (n = 54)*
0 minutes	85.1 ± 1.8	90.7 ± 1.7
60 minutes	82.6 ± 1.7	123.5 ± 3.9
120 minutes	77.6 ± 3.2	107.9 ± 3.0
180 minutes	76.4 ± 2.1	94.1 ± 5.4

The age-related decrease in sensitivity to insulin also is demonstrated by the fact that the age-connected increase in blood insulin concentration following a glucose load is accompanied by a rise in blood glucose (Welborn et al 1969). The causes for this are not clear. Growth hormone undoubtedly exerts an insulin antagonistic effect (Daughaday and Kipnis 1966). However, there may be other causes of the diminished hypoglycemic effect of insulin in such a complicated process as aging; therefore, it seems to be of considerable importance that a substantial reduction takes place in glucose tolerance after repeated glucose loading (with a four-hour interval between first and second loads). Some investigators had denied the idea of age-associated decrease in the sensitivity to insulin action. In particular, Shock (1977) wrote: "Dilman's arguments in support of his theory are often based on observations which are in error, as shown by more recent studies (for example, his presumptions that blood insulin levels increase with age and that 'muscular tissue becomes progressively less sensitive to the insulin' [Dilman 1971]). In the light of recent studies, neither of these assertions are true." In this connection he also claims that data on the age-associated rise in insulin level are inconclusive, and sensitivity to insulin does not decrease with aging (Shock 1977, Andres and Tobin 1977). The error made by Shock and certain gerontologists is realized after we have considered the following data on age-associated hyperinsulinemia.

Age-Associated Increase in Blood Insulin Level

Our data on the increase of the level of reactive insulinemia in response to glucose loading during aging have been presented (see Table 6-1). They are consistent with many other observations (Chlouverakis et al 1967, Welborn et al 1969). It is noteworthy that an age-associated hyperinsulinemia also develops in rats (Table 6-6), which supports the role of endogenous factors in the development of this phenomenon. However, arguments against this concept of the correlation between aging and blood insulin level are generally based on the assertion that obesity is the actual cause of hyperinsulinemia, because fat content increases with aging. However, such a conclusion gives no explanation for the causes of obesity, and it should be pointed out that age-associated hyperinsulinemia has been reported in a comparative study of groups of subjects varying in age but matched in the excess body weight (Hales et al 1968, Table 6-7).

Table 6-6
Age-Related Changes in Reactive Insulinemia in Rats

Age (months)	Insulin Level (μU/ml)	
	0 min	*5 min*
3	38.2 ± 1.6	82.3 ± 8.0
12	49.9 ± 2.8	199.2 ± 25.3
24	41.0 ± 4.0	144.0 ± 17.0

Source: Gommers and de Gasparo 1972.

Table 6-7
Correlation between Age and Reactive Insulinemia

Mean Age	Deviation of Body Weight from Mean (%)	Blood Insulin Level (μU/ml)				
		0 min	*30 min*	*60 min*	*90 min*	*120 min*
33	110	22 ± 2	69 ± 6	46 ± 6	31 ± 5	26 ± 4
54	111	25 ± 3	68 ± 12	67 ± 11	64 ± 13	40 ± 4

Source: Hales et al 1968.

The argument still holds that, for the same body weight, fat content in older subjects is higher. Nevertheless it would seem justified to attempt to dissociate these two processes. Fat does indeed accumulate in an organism in the course of normal aging. Hyperinsulinemia stimulates lipogenesis and seems to be a key factor in age-related obesity. Obesity in turn causes a rise in blood insulin level. Thus, irrespective of whether it is hyperinsulinemia that causes fat accumulation or whether the fat accumulation causes hyperinsulinemia, the latter, paralleling the increase of fat content in the course of aging, becomes a typical feature of aging. However, with the increase of insulin concentration in the blood, in particular, with elevation of the basal level of insulin, a situation develops where another irregularity comes into force, by which the insulin binding to membrane receptors is in negative correlation with the concentration of insulin in the blood (Kahn 1976). In particular, it has been shown that the insulin binding to membrane receptors of skeletal muscle was decreased 30% to 40% in older, fatter rats (Olefsky et al 1976). Many data indicate that the cell membrane hormone receptors decline in concentration during aging (Kahn 1976). As supposed by Roth and associates (1978b), "this phenomenon may be closely, if not causally, related to age-associated decreases in responsiveness to the same hormones." Thus, the critical remarks made by Shock (1977) appear to be obsolete in light of more recent data.

Some authors deny the phenomenon of age-related hyperinsulinemia (Gregerman and Bierman 1974) on the basis of observations that in nonobese elderly and young male subjects in whom blood sugar is controlled up to the same level, both the early and late phase of insulin secretion are clearly lower in the old subjects than in the young (Andres 1977, Sherwin et al 1972). These findings are open to argument, however, because under normal (not artificially controlled) conditions the postprandial blood glucose level in older subjects is higher than in the young; and therefore, blood insulin level is higher (O'Sullivan et al 1971). Thus in old mildly diabetic subjects, the same levels of hyperglycemia as in young mild diabetics can be maintained only by a much higher level of insulinemia. The comparison of subjects with identical glucose tolerance, when subjected to the same amount of oral or intravenous glucose, show that young people maintain the same blood glucose level with much smaller plasma insulin levels than their older counterparts (Johansen 1973a, 1973b). Some critics of the concept of age-related hyperinsulinemia also argue that blood insulin level in aged subjects is lower than in younger ones within the first three to five minutes after arginine or glucose infusion (Dudl and Ensinck 1972). This argument is fallacious, however, because both in age-associated reactive insulinemia and hyperinsulinemia in older diabetic patients an identical shift is observed toward a later-than-normal peak of blood insulin concentration ("delayed" curve of insulinemia). A similar shift in the curve of reactive hyperinsulinemia occurs in conjunction with carbohydrate metabolism disorders when growth hormone is administered to humans. And on the whole, insulin reserves in elderly subjects are not reduced (Joffe et al 1969).

As noted by Reaven and Olefsky (1978), "the delay in time of the peak insulin response in patients with chemical diabetes seems most reasonably attributed to the persistent hyperglycemia in such patients, and the persistence of hyperglycemia in the presence of hyperinsulinemia serves as evidence for the presence of insulin resistance in these patients." A similar pattern is typical of normal aging (see Table 6-1), ie, the difference between the age-associated decrease in glucose tolerance and chemical diabetes is based on quantitative (symbolic) criteria.

Some investigators deny age-associated hyperinsulinemia because, when insulin is assayed radioimmunologically, proinsulin is also determined, and the rise in proinsulin concentration may give a false impression of hyperinsulinemia (Duckworth et al 1972). Aging involves not only an increase in the level of so-called "immunoreactive" insulin, but also an elevation of the insulin-like activity of blood generally (Streeten et al 1965). Since biologic activity of proinsulin is low in these tests and has little influence on glucose uptake by tissues, the conclusion regarding an age-associated rise in insulin effect in the organism based on fat accumulation seems justified. Therefore, authors who deny the age-associated decrease in sensitivity to insulin action and the age-associated hyperinsulinemia appear to disregard the following:

1. Age-associated insulinemia cannot be evaluated on the basis of the basal level of insulin or a sharp release of insulin response to glucose loading (three to ten minutes), because aging is characterized by a delayed postprandial insulin secretion. If this is taken into account in the consideration of the data referred to by Andres and Tobin (1977), the phenomenon of age-associated hyperinsulinemia becomes apparent.
2. The observations of Andres and Tobin (1977) show nothing but the age-associated decline in the sensitivity of pancreatic β-cells to glucose stimulation. However, a relatively higher postprandial hyperglycemia in middle-aged individuals is responsible for an increased secretion of insulin, although the response of the pancreas to hyperglycemia is diminished.
3. Age-associated shifts in insulin sensitivity cannot be assessed by methods that are conceived on the principle of identity of basic conditions for young and middle-aged subjects, because this similarity does not exist due to the development of age-connected changes. For example, glucose loading is followed by a much higher hyperglycemia in middle-aged individuals than in younger ones. Accordingly, middle age is characterized by a pronounced reactive insulinemia that manifests a decreased sensitivity to endogenous insulin. Meanwhile a comparative study of subjects with identical tolerance to glucose showed that

younger individuals maintain the same level of glucose at a much lower blood level of insulin than do middle-aged subjects (Johansen 1973a).

4. It is erroneous to ignore the close relationship between age-associated hyperinsulinemia and age-connected insulin resistance, because it is hyperinsulinemia that is responsible for insensitivity to insulin action (Fineberg and Schneider 1975, Reaven and Olefsky 1978, De Meyts et al 1973). It is likely that the decline in the efficacy of insulin action during hyperinsulinemia is a result of decreasing hormone binding by specific receptors (Roth et al 1978a).
5. Finally, aging involves an increase in fat accumulation that predetermines hyperinsulinemia (Archer et al 1975).

Age-Associated Increase in the Somatomedin Activity of the Blood

Indirect evidence that may serve as an argument in favor of the existence of age-associated hyperinsulinemia is provided by the data obtained in our laboratory which indicate an increase in the somatomedin(s) activity of the blood both in older and in obese subjects, as well as in subjects with maturity-onset diabetes mellitus (Table 6-8). Concentration of somatomedins in the blood is controlled by growth hormone and insulin levels (Daughaday et al 1976) and probably by prolactin. Taking into account that in obesity the growth hormone level is decreased while the insulin level is increased, it may be supposed that the age-associated increase in somatomedin activity reflects the increased level of insulin in the body. Two additional arguments can be brought forward in

Table 6-8
Levels of Blood Somatomedin Activity in Healthy Controls of Various Ages and in Patients with Obesity, Diabetes Mellitus, and Atherosclerosis

Group	Age (years)	Deviation of Body Weight from Normal (%)	Somatomedin Activity (units)
Control subjects	21.0 ± 0.87	-13.8 ± 5.6	0.55 ± 0.09
	29.6 ± 0.67	-2.7 ± 2.7	0.79 ± 0.10
	39.2 ± 0.71	$+2.0 \pm 2.2$	0.91 ± 0.11
Obesity	42.1 ± 5.3	$+54.3 \pm 7.7$	1.87 ± 0.37
Diabetes mellitus	60.0 ± 2.5	$+13.3 \pm 6.2$	1.62 ± 0.32
Atherosclerosis	52.1 ± 2.4	$+16.6 \pm 9.5$	1.4 ± 0.35

favor of this supposition: 1) the highest level of somatomedin activity was observed in patients with Type IIb hyperlipoproteinemia, and 2) administration of phenformin decreases blood somatomedin activity (see Chapter 12).

Age-Associated Obesity

Fat content of an organism increases with aging even when body weight does not (Dudl and Ensinck 1977), because fat deposits are built up while the bone and muscle tissue mass is reduced (Novak 1972). Moreover, fat cells grow in size with age (Björntorp 1974). A gain in body weight occurs in normal subjects with advancing age. Some causes of this are age-connected hyperglycemia and hyperinsulinemia, diminished muscular activity, and excessive food intake, particularly of carbohydrates, as a result of the disturbed regulation of appetite. Aging features an increased intake of energy-producing substrates, a decreased consumption of energy, and stimulation of factors that tend to shift metabolism toward fat accumulation. The substantial rise in the insulin-like activity of blood should be emphasized in this respect (Pfeiffer 1970). It is remarkable that the fatty acid level also is raised (Rabinowitz 1970), and this points to an increase in lipolysis despite the intensified antilipolytic action of hyperinsulinemia.

Many authors believe that the rise in insulin level in obesity is a response to the accumulation of fat masses and the growth of adipose cells. This is thought to diminish the sensitivity of the adipose cells to insulin action and cause compensatory hyperinsulinemia. This conclusion is supported by studies that show a rise in the volume of adipose cells in obesity and a positive correlation between cell size and the increase of insulin and blood sugar levels (Björntorp et al 1970, 1971). Accordingly a loss of body weight is followed by a decrease in the blood insulin level. Such an approach to the mechanism of obesity inevitably implies that this disturbance is based primarily on hyperphagia resulting in alimentary obesity. This interpretation oversimplifies the problem, however (see Chapter 5).

It has been noted already that age-related hyperinsulinemia is actually a compensatory reaction to counteract the influence of factors that promote a decrease in glucose uptake by muscle tissue. It should be pointed out, however, that the compensatory influence of hyperinsulinemia has a wider range. For instance, when tolerance to carbohydrates diminishes, hyperinsulinemia-induced fat accumulation compensates for the loss of fatty acids through intensified lipolysis. Thus age-associated hyperinsulinemia is of great importance in the mechanism of age-connected gain in body weight. The accumulation of fat and the rise in FFA level occurring at a later stage provides additional, powerful stimuli for insulin secretion; this results eventually in basal hyperinsulinemia and obesity, a vicious circle wherein each factor reinforces the other. Eventually, age-associated obesity with hyperinsulinemia causes a reduction in the concentration of insulin receptors and thereby initiates or aggravates insulin resistance.

Antilipolytic Effect of Hyperinsulinemia

Insulin exerts a considerable antilipolytic effect, and this effect is retained by some derivatives that are devoid of the hypoglycemic effect. For example iodinated insulin, deprived of the property of stimulating glucose utilization, retains at least a partial antilipolytic effect (Dilman and Vasiljeva 1971). Dwarfs, who are characterized by a primary insufficiency of growth hormone and therefore diminished blood insulin, exhibit a high level of fatty acids. Thus the elevation of FFA level is caused largely by the reduced antilipolytic effect of insulin. It is probable that during aging the antilipolytic effect of hyperglycemia decreases, similar to the decrease that occurs in some patients with diabetes mellitus (Shafrir and Gutman 1965). This conclusion is supported by the results of the insulin-glucose test (Table 6-9), which shows that the antilipolytic effect is diminished in middle-aged subjects as compared with the young subjects, in spite of the more pronounced hyperglycemia in the former. This defect may cause a disturbance in the rhythm of utilizing the energy-producing substrates, ie, it may result in an excessive utilization of FFA, irrespective of the absence of any age-associated elevation of FFA basal level.

Table 6-9
Mean Free Fatty Acid and Sugar Levels in Blood in Cases of Ischemic Heart Disease and Controls in Insulin-Glucose Test

Group	Mean Age (years)	Parameter	Insulin-Glucose Test *0 min*	*60 min*	*120 min*
Young subjects	34	Sugar (mg%)	86.04 ± 4.4	84.0 ± 8.5	85.0 ± 35.0
		FFA (μEq/liter)	410.6 ± 21.0	197.3 ± 15.0	266.0 ± 19.3
Middle-aged subjects	56	Sugar (mg%)	96.5 ± 4.0	144.5 ± 6.6	119.0 ± 6.8
		FFA (μEq/liter)	518.5 ± 38.7	337.0 ± 24.1	306.0 ± 26.7

It should be noted that in many respects decrease in the sensitivity of peripheral tissues to the regulating action of hormones and metabolites resembles the elevation of the hypothalamic set point of sensitivity to the regulating stimuli. To illustrate, in both cases the mechanism of resistance may be connected with the decrease in the number of receptors to insulin or to catecholamines (Roth et al 1978b). However, an essential difference between these two phenomena may be pointed out. Hypothalamic disturbances are based on the genetic developmental program (see Chapter 1), while the variations in the sensitivity of the peripheral tissues seem to be caused by the regulatory shifts and consequent metabolic disturbances similar to the case of the induced synthesis of enzymes (Adelman 1976, 1978). The intensity of disturbances at the peripheral level may vary. Enlarged fat cells present in both obesity and hypertriglyceridemia, are probably insulin-resistant (Björntorp et al 1971). Accordingly, the sensitivity of the fat cell to the action of lipolytic factors, eg, adrenaline, can change in different directions (Ratzmann 1973), Di Girolano and Owens 1976).

Data on the influence of aging upon the intensity of lipolysis should be considered in light of these statements. Age-associated hyperglycemia and hyperinsulinemia (at certain stages of age-associated alterations) can have an inhibiting effect on lipolysis. For example, the antilipolytic effect of excessive insulin also may account for the well-known clinical observation that, although obese middle-aged subjects have considerable fat deposits, they often suffer from hunger even after a relatively short fast. However, many specific diseases of aging, like maturity-onset diabetes mellitus and atherosclerosis, whose metabolic pattern differs from the pattern of normal aging only quantitatively, are characterized by intensified lipolysis.

Age-Associated Changes in Rate of Lipolysis

We can state generally that aging features a decreased utilization of glucose as an energy substrate, with a simultaneous rise in fatty acid utilization. Put simply, the aged perish in the flames of fats. This age-associated intensification of lipolysis is caused, first of all, by obesity characterized by increased spontaneous lipolysis. At the same time, some investigators state that the level of plasma FFA does not appear to be influenced by increased age (Mitchell et al 1968), while others have observed an elevation of FFA level in elderly subjects (Metz et al 1966). Data obtained in our laboratory show that both in men and women there is a certain age-associated elevation of blood FFA level (Table 6-10). Elevated lipolysis also is typical of such age-specific pathologic disorders as diabetes mellitus, atherosclerosis, and cancer (see Chapters 11, 12, and

17). Available methods fail to detect this lipolysis intensification in its early states because a small excess of fatty acids is disposed of quickly. Therefore longitudinal data on the extent of FFA utilization are particularly important since individual blood levels may vary widely. It should be taken into account that at certain stages of aging the FFA level may decline as a result of inhibition of lipolysis by elevated glucose and insulin levels.

Table 6-10
Age-Associated Changes of Free Fatty Acid Levels in Healthy Subjects

	Men		Women	
Group	Mean Age (years)	FFA Levels (μEq/liter)	Mean age (years)	FFA Levels (μEq/liter)
1	35 ± 1	524 ± 30	34 ± 1	583 ± 22
2	53 ± 1	589 ± 28	51 ± 1	693 ± 26†
3	57 ± 1	654 ± 36*	53 ± 1	694 ± 50‡

*$p < 0.002$ for groups 1 and 3.
†$p < 0.01$ for groups 1 and 2.
‡$p < 0.05$ for groups 1 and 3.

Age-Associated Enhancement of Gluconeogenesis

Hormonal and metabolic shifts inherent in normal aging inevitably lead to enhanced gluconeogenesis for physiologic reasons, the main factor being the relative excess of cortisol intrinsic to normal senescence (see Chapter 3). This excess is known to stimulate the key reactions of gluconeogenesis (Exton 1972). Another factor is a metabolic shift toward intensified utilization of FFA as fuel. Increased FFA oxidation enhances gluconeogenesis and the production of glucose in the liver, because the increased FFA oxidation depresses the oxidation of pyruvate and leads to an accumulation of acetyl-CoA and of citrate, which in turn may reduce hepatic glycolysis and accelerate gluconeogenesis from pyruvate and lactate. Therefore it appears that in the course of normal aging an intensification of gluconeogenesis occurs regularly.

Age-Associated Hypertriglyceridemia

The synthesis of triglycerides in the liver is stimulated by insulin (Reaven et al 1967, Bagdade et al 1971). Triglyceride synthesis increases with relatively insignificant shifts in metabolism, and correlates primarily with the rise in blood insulin level (Bagdade et al 1971) and with the extent of fat accumulation. Plasma triglyceride levels also are known to correlate closely with free fatty acid turnover (Bortz 1973). Since both parameters increase in practically all humans after a certain age, it may be claimed that the triglyceride level rises even in relatively young subjects. For instance, an elevated blood triglyceride level is found in subjects who gain more than 4.5 kg after age 25, regardless of age at the time of weight gain (Albrink et al 1962). This accounts for the fact that blood triglyceride levels reach a plateau at an earlier age than blood cholesterol.

Hypertriglyceridemia also may depend on external environmental factors such as excess carbohydrates in the diet. In one study (Reaven et al 1967) where subjects were fed a diet rich in carbohydrates, 31 out of 33 males developed hypertriglyceridemia. Taking into consideration the metabolic relationships of all these factors, hyperinsulinemia often correlates with both obesity and hypertriglyceridemia (Bagdade et al 1971). However a correlation between hypertriglyceridemia and the degree of glucose tolerance may be lacking particularly in old age, since disturbances in carbohydrate utilization in older subjects may develop because of a relative insufficiency of insulin, despite a heightened output of this hormone.

There also are direct data on the rise in the blood triglyceride level following growth hormone administration, which is known to have an insulinogenic effect (Azizi et al 1973). However, the blood insulin level is not the sole factor regulating blood triglyceride levels (Bagdade et al 1971). Lipoprotein lipase, which regulates the removal from plasma of lipoproteins rich in triglycerides, also plays a role. Very low density lipoproteins (VLDL) are secreted mainly by the liver for transport of triglycerides to peripheral tissues such as muscle and heart. The hepatic synthesis of plasma VLDL correlates directly with FFA fluxes (Fredrickson et al 1967) as well as with FFA concentration in the plasma (Nestel and Whyte 1968).

In the periphery, VLDL are broken down to low density lipoproteins (LDL) by catabolic enzymes such as lipoprotein lipase and possibly lecithin: cholesterol acyltransferase. Correspondingly, cholesterol synthesis in subjects who had hypertriglyceridemia was almost three times

Table 6-11
Age-Associated Changes in Cholesterol and Triglyceride Levels in Rats

Age (months)	Blood Cholesterol (mg%)	Blood Triglycerides (mmole/liter)
1	69 ± 6	0.51 ± 0.06
4	94 ± 8	0.83 ± 0.07
9	218 ± 33	2.50 ± 10.38
18	307 ± 18	2.55 ± 0.34

Source: Carlson et al 1968.

greater than in those who had not (Sodhi and Kudchodkar 1973). As shown by Carlson et al (1968), cholesterol and triglyceride levels rise in rats during aging (Table 6-11).

Age-Associated Hypercholesterolemia

Many studies have shown an increase in serum cholesterol with age (Dilman 1958). Correspondingly, the fall of serum cholesterol levels after age 65 could be caused by natural selection by death (Schilling et al 1964).

The serum cholesterol level reflects a balance between absorption from the diet, biosynthesis, and degradation. Using isotope incorporation methods many investigators have concluded that with aging the synthesis of cholesterol in the liver decreases (Block et al 1946, Yamamoto and Yamamura 1971). Therefore, it is generally accepted that the age-associated increase of blood cholesterol level is connected with the slower degradation of cholesterol in the liver and the slower rate of its excretion. However, the latter statement is scarcely probable in light of the concepts discussed in this book, particularly if we take into consideration the fact that cholesterol synthesis is in positive correlation with adiposity (Bortz 1973), the blood level of insulin (Stout 1977), and the blood level of triglycerides (Sodhi and Kudchodkar 1973); ie, the values of all these parameters increase with age.

The level of cholesterol synthesis in the liver generally is agreed to be in positive correlation with plasma FFA concentration. These findings are consistent with the earlier data on the diminished synthesis of cholesterol in the liver of patients with hypercholesterolemia following nicotinic acid administration to inhibit lipolysis (Parsons 1961). The level of the utilization of FFA is of primary importance here. Accordingly, data on sterol balance in obese subjects shows an excess in daily cholesterol production, which is roughly equivalent to 20 mg/kg of adipose tissue (Miettinen 1971). Cholesterol synthesis is correlated with triglyceride synthesis in the liver, or to phrase it more precisely as suggested earlier by Sodhi and Kudchodkar (1973) "the plasma concentration of very low density lipoproteins (VLDL) reflected by hypertriglyceridemia is an important determinant of hepatic synthesis of cholesterol." This statement was later confirmed and expanded in several studies (Brunzell et al 1978). The source for cholesterol in the liver is acetyl-CoA. Excess acetyl-CoA is formed in the liver during intensive oxidation of fatty acids. Some of it may be resynthesized into fatty acids or used in the synthesis of cholesterol and ketone bodies. The balance between these metabolic pathways is probably determined, to a considerable degree, by the rate of glucose utilization in the organism. This is confirmed indirectly by data showing a decreased blood cholesterol concentration in diabetic patients following phenformin administration

(Grodsky et al 1963). This reduces compensatory hyperinsulinemia by improving glucose transport through the cell membrane and by inhibiting gluconeogenesis (Gordon and de Hartog 1973). The decrease in insulin level results in a diminished synthesis of triglyceride and cholesterol. It should be mentioned that cholesterol synthesis increases in obese subjects (Miettinen 1971), ie, when insulin output is enhanced. Hypercholesterolemia is therefore inherent in age-specific pathology (see Chapter 18). Some data assume that the increase in cholesterol synthesis occurs when there is a simultaneous increase both in triglyceride synthesis (hyperinsulinemia) and in FFA utilization. In this context it is noteworthy that serum cholesterol was observed to decrease significantly during high carbohydrate feeding, while the serum level of triglycerides increased (Sjöström 1973).

Aging may feature a delayed metabolism of cholesterol, particularly the reduction of bile acids following a fall-off in the level of thyroid hormones. The age-associated decline of thyroid gland function (see Chapter 7) can, therefore, promote a higher cholesterol concentration in the tissues by suppressing cholesterol degradation. This type of hypercholesterolemia is probably characteristic of Type IIa hyperlipoproteinemia, in which the triglyceride synthesis is not increased (Miettinen 1973). However, until now the classification of hyperlipoproteinemia worked out by Fredrickson et al (1967) has not been applied to studying the age-associated dynamics in the blood level of lipoproteins. Based on the regular age-associated increase in the insulin level, it may be supposed that the age-associated alterations correspond to Type IIb hyperlipoproteinemia, ie, a type with a more intense cholesterol synthesis. There is evidence of a negative feedback system in the liver that is controlled by the blood cholesterol level (Dietschy and Wilson 1970). It can be supposed that this mechanism seems to become ineffective in aged persons in a way similar to that in animals with aflatoxin-induced hepatomas (Siperstein 1967). In light of this assumption we can treat the data showing that in male Sprague-Dawley rats the cholesterol level increased in the liver steadily from 1 to 18 months, irrespective of the continuous increase in plasma cholesterol (Carlson et al 1968). Takenchi et al (1976) discovered the impairment of feedback control of cholesterol synthesis in aged rats. However, it should be taken into account that the feedback regulation of cholesterol synthesis by dietary cholesterol operates at the hepatic level, but it does not inhibit cholesterol synthesis in other tissues. In this context note that our data show an increase of cholesterol concentration in lymphocytes both in aging (see Chapter 18) and in cases of atherosclerosis (see Chapter 12), which indicates a disorder in the feedback mechanism.

At least two defects can be pointed out in the experimental data showing a decrease in cholesterol synthesis with aging. First, comparison of cholesterol synthesis values was made, as a rule, between younger (growing) rats and adult rats; however, only adult animals of different ages should be compared, since in younger rats, with their high rate of growth, cholesterol synthesis is naturally increased; this may reflect the high cholesterol requirement for cell membrane formation. Second, age-associated alterations in cholesterol synthesis were studied only in rats, without taking into consideration the diurnal activity pattern of these animals.

An analysis of our model of disturbances in the energy homeostat points to an intensification of physiologic interactions as the main cause of relevant pathologic age-associated metabolic shifts. These metabolic disturbances are, to a considerable degree, responsible for the fact that the normal process of aging is essentially a normal disease (see Chapter 18). Note however that the metabolic shifts accompanying the main diseases of man, namely, obesity, maturity-onset diabetes mellitus, atherosclerosis, metabolic immunodepression, and cancer, present an intensified variant of the normal age-associated disturbances (see Chapters 11–18), so that the metabolic pattern of aging, including decreased tolerance to carbohydrates, compensatory hyperinsulinemia, higher fat content in the body, intensification of lipolysis followed by the inhibition of glucose utilization, as well as increased synthesis of triglycerides, cholesterol, and VLDL, may be interpreted as a series of consequences of an intensification of physiologic functions normally performed within the energy homeostat.

Some Obscure Aspects of Age-Associated Changes in the Energy System

We have emphasized that a decline in the sensitivity of the peripheral tissues to insulin, resulting in a compensatory hyperinsulinemia, is one of the most typical age-associated changes. Though this phenomenon is no longer doubted, opinions vary as to its cause.

This chapter contains some arguments favoring the role of an elevation of the hypothalamic set point that upsets the normal secretion of growth hormone and therefore leads to the development of a resistance to insulin. This conclusion is based on an assumed lipolytic, insulin antagonistic, action of growth hormone in the four-component model of the energy homeostat. Such a phenomenon is indispensable for the regulation of energy influx, but it is possible that some other insulin antagonistic factors may exert a similar effect. For instance a diabetogenic factor was found in the animal pituitary (Louis and Conn 1972) that causes a much greater inhibition of the utilization of glucose than growth hormone does. ACTH also is a potent anti-insulin agent, as is prolactin. Prolactin secretion is known to change in the same direction as that of growth hormone. Thus the levels of both growth hormone and prolactin rise at a certain phase of sleep as well as in response to hypoglycemia and stress (Wilson et al 1972). However, in accordance with the proposed model of the energy homeostat, an insulin antagonistic effect may be exerted only by those lipolytic agents whose secretion is inhibited in hyperglycemia. This follows from the principle of energy homeostat functioning.

Therefore, prolactin cannot be an additional factor in the functioning of the energy homeostat (see Table 7-4). The age-associated rise in prolactin secretion (see Chapter 7) as well as disturbances in the cyclic functioning of the adaptive system, including the hypothalamic ACTH-glucocorticoid complex, may promote age-related metabolic shifts. It should be pointed out that children suffering from growth hormone deficiency were found to have a high level of prolactin (Aubert et al 1974). It is plausible therefore that a similar situation may develop in the age-associated decline in basal growth hormone level. All of this points to a more complex pattern of interaction rather than to a deviation from the general model of the energy homeostat. For instance, apart from growth hormone, the influence of ACTH, glucocorticoids, and adrenaline becomes very important in stress. However, their action obeys all the laws of the energy homeostat: intensifying the insulin antagonistic action of growth hormone, increasing the blood glucose pool, stimulating lipolysis, and raising fatty acid concentration.

Little is known about the role of lipotropin. It has a peculiar feature which has to be discussed. Figure 6-6 shows that bovine lipotropin administration is followed by a rise in tolerance to carbohydrates, although this hormone exerts a marked lipolytic effect. A similar phenomenon occurs in the case of administration of human lipotropin (Trygstad 1968). The cause of the lack of competition between the utilization of fatty acids and that of glucose in such a situation remains obscure however, and therefore the role of lipotropin in the development of age-associated metabolic changes is not clear. Lipotropin also seems to stimulate the secretion of glucagon, and the latter may play an important role in the pathogenesis of diabetic disorders (Unger and Orci 1975).

The interpretation of some data on growth hormone also presents difficulties. There are specific differences between the data for humans and those for animals, particularly rodents, and these differences seem to involve not only the structural features but also the properties, mechanisms of regulation, and ratios of isohormones of growth hormone. For instance, such factors as insulin-induced hypoglycemia, and stress, which stimulates growth hormone secretion in primates, reduce GH level in rats. And in guinea pigs and rabbits the growth hormone level does not rise in response to fasting and stress (Machlin et al 1968). Some data even show that glucose does not regulate growth hormone secretion in mice (Schindler et al 1972). All this suggests that the homeostatic regulation of growth hormone secretion by glucose is highly specific for primates; possibly this determines the characteristic features of age-related pathology in humans. To prove this hypothesis a more precise evaluation of the adequacy of the immunologic and biologic assays of growth hormone in animals is required. It also is necessary to study the role of other lipolytic hormones that seem to perform functions in animals similar to the functions of growth hormone in man. Should this be true, it may follow that the same factors also play a certain role in the energy homeostat system in man.

Note that hypophysectomy in rats is followed by hypercholesterolemia, which also is observed often in humans with growth hormone deficiency. In both humans and rats hypercholesterolemia can be eliminated by growth hormone administration. Such a metabolic pattern shows that cholesterol synthesis is intensified when fatty acid utilization is enhanced as a result of growth hormone deficiency, thus leading to a decrease in blood insulin and a rise in the rate of lipolysis (Merimee et al 1971). Therefore, somatostatin administration results in an appreciable rise in FFA level (Peracchi et al 1974). This occurs in dwarfs as a consequence of the decreased antilipolytic action of insulin (Merimee et al 1971). It also is noteworthy that growth hormone administration (5 mg twice a

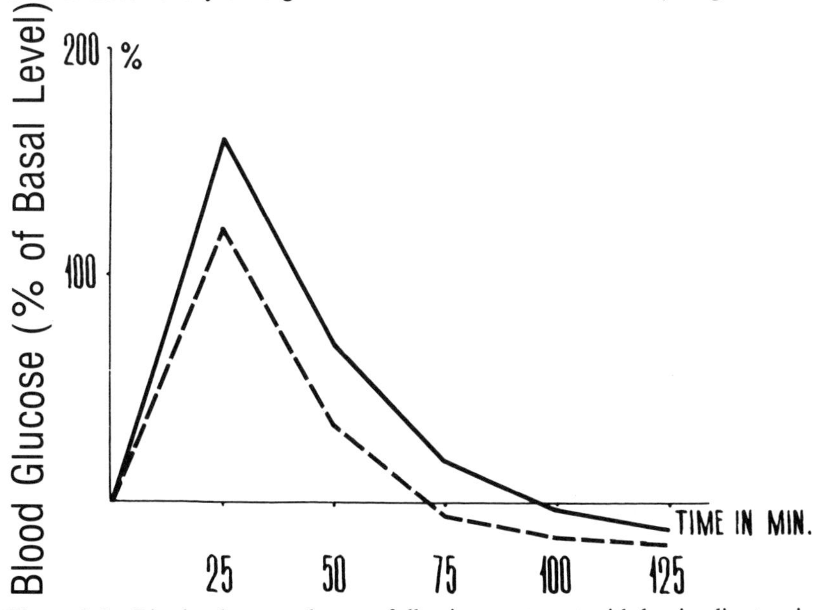

Figure 6-6 Rise in glucose tolerance following treatment with bovine lipotropic hormone. Solid line represents changes in curve following glucose (1.5 gm/kg body weight) and before lipotropin administration; (Y axis—Percent blood glucose change from basal level. X axis—Time [min]). Interrupted line represents changes after nine-day course of lipotropin (1 mg/day subcutaneously).

day for seven days) reduced blood cholesterol in four patients with hypercholesterolemia (Friedman et al 1972b), and in dwarfs with isolated deficiency of growth hormone. However, this was accompanied by a rise in pre-β- and β-lipoproteins and trigylcerides and a considerable fall in carbohydrate tolerance. We may suppose that the administration of large doses of growth hormone is followed by an immediate insulin antagonistic effect with a subsequent decline in glucose utilization and a compensatory rise in insulin level. This results in an intensified synthesis of triglycerides and a shift toward an increase in the pre-β-lipoprotein fraction. This sharp shift seems to cause a temporary decrease in cholesterol level, though the chronic administration of growth hormone produces some elevation of blood levels of cholesterol and triglycerides (Aloia et al 1975).

Hence, among the immediate tasks in the study of age-associated changes in the energy homeostat are the establishment of the role of a number of lipolytic hormones influencing this homeostat and a more detailed investigation of the importance of growth hormone, particularly its isohormones (Yadley et al 1973).[1]

---

[1] According to Ellis and Grindeland (1973) blood growth hormone level assayed by biologic tests is 200 times that in radioimmunologic testing, and the absolute level of growth hormone determined immunologically is nearly ten times that obtained in radioimmunologic assay.

7 Age-Associated Changes in the Thyroid Homeostat and in the Function of Other Hypothalmic-Hypophyseal Systems

Many problems of gerontology have been so insufficiently studied that difficulties arise even in attempting to find a monograph describing the problems.

While discussing the process of the age-related switching-on of reproductive function, logical arguments were summed up in favor of the concept that the key factor of the mechanism of sexual maturation is an elevation of the hypothalamic threshold of sensitivity to the inhibiting effect of sex hormones. This phenomenon provides both for the inhibition of the reproductive homeostat until body development has reached a certain critical level, and for the increase of capacity of the reproductive homeostat, which is an attribute of sexual maturity (see Chapter 4). Moreover, it is easy to show that the development and growth of an organism would not proceed, unless the capacity of the reproductive, adaptive, and energy homeostats were increased (see Chapter 1).

However, our studies show that the threshold of sensitivity to feedback suppression in the hypothalamic-pituitary-thyroid system decreases with age rather than increases. For instance the inhibitory effect of thyroxine (T_4) on the thyroid (enlargement) was less in young rats than in middle-aged ones (Berstein 1975, Table 7-1).[1]

[1] Similar data have been recently obtained in our laboratory, with thyroxine replaced by triiodothyronine (T_3).

Table 7-1
Age-Associated Changes in Compensatory Hypertrophy of Thyroid and Thyroxine Effect* in Rats

Age (months)	Compensatory Hypertrophy (%)	Compensatory Hypertrophy (%) with Thyroxine*
2.5–3	+20.6 ± 7.0 (n = 43)	+9.3 ± 7.0 (n = 28)
8–10	+33.2 ± 5.0 (n = 40)	−17.5 ± 8.0 (n = 40)
14–16	+40.4 ± 8.0 (n = 21)	−25.5 ± 5.0 (n = 22)

*Thyroxine was administered 2 μg/100 g body weight once daily for four days.

Similar results were obtained in experiments in which the functional status of the thyroid system was assessed on the basis of ^{131}I uptake by the gland. Hence, the age-associated changes in the sensitivity threshold of the hypothalamic-pituitary system controlling thyroid activity, are contrary to those that take place in the reproductive and adaptive homeostats with increasing age. It may, therefore, be suggested that a peculiarity such as the decrease in the sensitivity threshold of the hypothalamic-pituitary complex to inhibition by T_4 is associated with the requirements of the growing body for a high level of thyroid hormones. Should the hypothalamic-pituitary complex sensitivity to inhibition be maximum at the early stage of ontogenesis, thyroid hormones would cause, by negative feedback, a persistent inhibition of the central component of the complex, which governs thyroid function. Then, the requirements of the growing body for a high level of thyroid hormones would not be fulfilled. However, it would appear that the decline in the hypothalamic threshold in the thyroid system continues well after the completion of organismal development. This hypothesis may be supported by the following findings: although blood triiodothyronine (T_3) is lowered during ages 50–60 years approximately 25% to 40% from the initial value (Brunelle and Bohuon 1972), blood thyrotropin (TSH) concentration does not show such drastic changes (Lémarchand-Béraud et al 1969). On the basis of this discrepancy, Gregerman and Bierman (1974) suggested that aging involves an increase in the sensitivity of the hypothalamic-pituitary complex controlling TSH secretion, to inhibition by thyroid hormones. However, this hypothesis was not verified experimentally. On the other hand, evidence has been obtained proving that, because of the increase in the hypothalamic-pituitary complex sensitivity, the level of thyroid hormones remains sufficient to exert an inhibitory effect on the hypothalamic-pituitary system although their concentration is decreased.

Naturally, a question arises as to what determines the age-associated changes in hypothalamic sensitivity in the thyrostat. First of all, our experiments showed that the uptake of T_4 and T_3 by the pituitary does not decrease significantly in male rats with advancing age. However, aging reveals a trend of prevalent uptake of thyroxine by the anterior lobe of the pituitary at the expense of triiodothyronine (the ratio of uptake of T_4 to T_3 in young rats 2–2½ months old was 2.46 ± 0.20 and 3.40 ± 0.20 in adult rats aged 16–20 months; $p < 0.05$).

A special series of experiments with pharmacologic agents yielded results that throw light on the mechanism of age-associated regulatory changes in the thyroid system. Theophylline, cyclic AMP, tryptophan, disulfiram (which inhibits dopamine transformation to noradrenaline), and an antidiabetic biguanide, phenformin, (after a five-month administration) raise the threshold to inhibition by T_4. However, administration of γ-methyldopa led to a decrease in this threshold (Table 7-2).

Table 7-2
Effects of Drugs on Sensitivity of Hypothalamic-Pituitary Complex to Inhibitory Action of Thyroxine*

Treatment	Daily Dosage	Route of Admini-stration	Changes in Sensitivity to T_4 Inhibition (%)	
			T_4(2 μg/100 g)	*T_4 + drug*
Phenformin	5 mg	per os	−0.2±6	+26.4±8†
L-tryptophan	10 mg/100g	sc	+9.4±3	+26.7±6†
Reserpine	0.1 mg/100g	sc	+9.4±3	+5.9±4
L-dopa	10 mg/100g	ip	−9.6±3	−15.2±5
γ-methyldopa	10 mg/100g	per os	+11.1±5	+2.3±1.2
Disulfiram	10 mg/100g	per os	+0.7±5	+13.9±4†

*Drugs were administered to hemithyroidectomized male rats weighing 200–240 g beginning with the day of operation. Each experiment lasted five days.
†Statistically significant ($p < 0.05$)

The ability of tryptophan and disulfiram to change the sensitivity of the hypothalamic-pituitary-thyroid system is proof that the serotonergic and dopaminergic systems play a role not only in the regulation of activity of the hypothalamic-pituitary-thyroid system (Chen and Meites 1975, Grimm and Reichlin 1973), but in regulation of the hypothalamic threshold of sensitivity to homeostatic stimuli as well. It may be supposed that similar shifts in the hypothalamic level of biogenic amines, eg, a decrease in noradrenaline level and a relative increase in serotonin concentration, may cause a rise in the sensitivity threshold to estrogens and glucocorticoids (see Chapters 3, 4), simultaneous with a decrease in the sensitivity threshold to inhibition by T_3.

Systemic changes may affect the regulatory mechanism of a relevant homeostat. With regard to the hypothalamic-pituitary-thyroid system, it is necessary to consider the possibility of a thyroid hormone influence on the biogenic amine system in the brain. Interrelationships between metabolic processes and the functional state of the hypothalamic-pituitary-thyroid system are of considerable interest.

Many authors have shown that thyroid function decreases with aging in humans and in animals (Everitt 1972). However this is at variance with Keys' experiment to determine basal metabolic rates in the same subjects at 20-year intervals (Keys et al 1973). They found only about a 3% decrease in the basal metabolic rate of a group of subjects examined at age 22 and again at age 43. A second group examined at the ages of 49 and 71 showed a decrease only in cases with a gain in body weight, and elderly men whose weight had changed less than one kilogram did not show any change in basal metabolic rate. There now are indications that the age-associated decrease in metabolic rates may be explained best by an age-related decrease in metabolic mass, since oxygen consumption per unit of metabolic mass does not decrease with age (Gregerman 1967). These findings also throw light on the study by Keys et al (1973) regarding the negative correlation between the basal metabolic rate and body weight.

It is known that aging is characterized by an increased body content of fat (Björntorp 1974) and higher blood levels of cholesterol, triglycerides, and lipoproteins. Therefore, it is important to note that β-lipoproteins, like cholesterol in the experiments of other authors (Marquie et al 1973), inhibit the uptake of radioactive iodine by the rat's thyroid in vitro and in vivo (Table 7-3). Of particular interest is the fact that the inhibitory effect of blood lipoproteins on iodine uptake was more pronounced in adult rats (350 g body weight), than in those with a body weight of 250 g. It is possible that data (Keys et al 1973) concerning the relationship between body weight and thyroid function are related to this aspect of the problem.

Table 7-3
Inhibition of Thyroid ^{131}I Uptake by β-Lipoproteins in Rats*

	Number of Impulses (imp/10 sec)	
Treatment	*Over Thyroid*	*In 1 mg of Thyroid Tissue*
Control	35,526 ± 2760	2084 ± 112
Lipoproteins from serum of cancer patients	18,150 ± 1880	1138 ± 71
Lipoproteins from serum of pregnant women	24,059 ± 1580	1672 ± 153

Source: Berstein and Vasiljeva 1974.
*Lipoproteins were administered intraperitoneally during ten days in dosage equivalent to 0.5 ml of serum. In vitro, thyroid glands were incubated in Krebs-Ringer solution containing 3 to 5 μCi ^{131}I and the amount of lipoproteins contained in 0.5 ml of serum.

Thus, age-associated changes in the energy homeostat seem to promote the decline in thyroid function, although the central type of homeostatic failure does not develop in the hypothalamic-pituitary-thyroid system.[1] As far as the interaction with the energy system is concerned, it is interesting to note that administration of phenformin (which relieves many metabolic disturbances, eg, it decreases hyperlipidemia) raises the blood level of protein-bound iodine.

In summary, it would appear that the hypothalamic sensitivity threshold to thyroxine decreases, rather than increases, in rats with aging. I must admit, however, this conclusion is uncertain because it has been shown in our laboratory that in young women T_3 causes a greater decrease of blood thyrotropin level than it does in middle-aged women (Yevtushenko and Bobrov 1978). At present, the following explanation of the discrepancy between the experimental and the clinical data can be offered. The triiodothyronine inhibition test is made during a six-day period, with a total dose of 300 μg. It may be supposed that the persistent administration of T_3 decreases hormone binding by specific receptors in response to elevation of hormone levels, in accordance with the negative feedback mechanism between hormone binding and concentration of hormone. Consequently, it cannot be that the T_3 inhibition test itself affects the sensitivity of the hypothalamic-pituitary system. On the other hand, it cannot be excluded that the hemithyroidectomy-induced compensatory hypertrophy of the thyroid gland is able to alter the hormone balance in the thyroid homeostat. Favoring the validity of the experimental data is the fact that the γ-methyldopa was responsible for a decline of the threshold of sensitivity to the inhibiting stimulus in the thyrostat (see Table 7-2), while in the reproductive homeostat it caused an elevation of hypothalamic set point (see Chapter 4). In this context the opposite-directed changes in both homeostats are realized by the decrease in catecholamine concentration in the hypothalamus, ie, the hypothalamus reacts as a total system. This statement can be further considered as applicable to the age-associated changes in the levels of prolactin and melanocyte-stimulating hormone (MSH).

Age-Associated Changes in Regulation of Prolactin and Melanocyte-Stimulating Hormone

The data presented in previous chapters have made it possible to conclude that the three main homeostatic systems of the human organism undergo similar changes. The similarity of changes suggests the

[1] However, resistance to inhibition by thyroid hormones in thyroid cancer has been reported (Lémarchand-Béraud et al 1969).

possibility that the hypothalamus responds as a total system, not to each homeostat separately. Such total system changes have been recorded in experiments involving the use of continuous illumination (Taleisnik and Celis 1973), where the pineal gland is inhibited in frogs, causing an overall intensification of hypothalamic activity. This intensification results in enhanced secretion of pituitary hormones, specifically gonadotropins, thus accelerating the process of sexual maturation. On the other hand, intensifying hypothalamic activity also causes a decrease in the secretion of hormones that are inhibited by the hypothalamus. This is manifested in the discoloration of the frog's skin following illumination, and points to a decreased output of MSH. These observations show that the hypothalamus can indeed react as a single system.

Regulation of prolactin and MSH are similar. Normally, the secretion of both hormones seems to be inhibited by hypothalamic hormones (Kastin and Schally 1967), although there is evidence suggesting the existence of stimulating hypothalamic factors that control the secretion of prolactin and MSH. The prevalence of inhibitory hypothalamic factors is clearly discernible in that pituitary stalk section, as well as administration of chlorpromazine or reserpine, results in the intensification of prolactin and MSH secretion. Therefore, the administration of reserpine and chlorpromazine, which reduced the catecholamine level in the hypothalamus, results in the increased secretion of prolactin and probably MSH (Taleisnik and Celis 1973). On the contrary, L-dopa inhibits the secretion of these hormones (Kleinberg et al 1971). By virtue of regulation characteristics, the age-associated decrease in catecholamine concentration in the hypothalamus should lead to a rise in prolactin and MSH secretion. The blood prolactin level is reported to be high in older animals (Meites et al 1972). In humans, however, no age-associated increase has been found in the blood level of prolactin. To the contrary, Vekemans and Robyn (1975) showed that there is a progressive decline in serum prolactin concentration in women which they attribute to a decline in estrogen secretion.

It should be noted that serotonin increases prolactin secretion (Meites 1973), and it is suggested that this effect is produced by inhibition of prolactin-inhibiting factor secretion (Kamberi et al 1971b). Hence, it becomes clear why prolactin secretion rises in stress and during sleep, ie, when the influence of the serotonergic system prevails. Under these conditions, prolactin shows the same changes as growth hormone. Therefore, it would appear that the age-associated decline in serotonin level in the hypothalamus counteracts an increase in prolactin secretion that might occur because of the age-associated decline of dopamine level in the hypothalamus. In this connection, a hypothesis on the existence of a double system of control of prolactin secretion in which the prevalence of an adrenergic effect suppresses prolactin secretion, while the serotonergic system stimulates it (Lu and Meites 1973), seems convincing. There is, however, indication that serotonergic receptor antagonists produce a rapid and sustained increase in serum prolactin levels (Gala et al 1977). It may also be supposed that age-associated metabolic shifts suppress prolactin secretion, similar to their influence upon growth hormone (see Chapter 6). Data obtained in our laboratory show that glucose loading causes a decline in concentration of both growth hormone and prolactin in the blood (Table 7-4).

Table 7-4
Effect of Glucose Loading on Blood Prolactin and Growth Hormone Levels in Healthy Women Aged 20–29

	Concentration in the Blood			
Time (min)	*Prolactin (mU/ml)*	*Change (%)*	*Growth Hormone (ng/ml)*	*Change (%)*
0	610 ± 189		6.12 ± 1.97	
60	474 ± 151	−22	2.50 ± 0.66	−59
120	416 ± 109	−32	2.62 ± 0.91	−57
180	255 ± 133	−58	3.00 ± 0.60	−51
240	610 ± 162	0	9.00 ± 2.21	+47

Therefore, it may be supposed that prolactin is the additional element of the four-component energy homeostat and plays a role in metabolic regulation. Of interest are the data pointing to a possibility of the raising of blood prolactin level when growth hormone is deficient (Aubert et al 1974). The role of prolactin in metabolic regulation makes it necessary to study the question of probable association between the absence of age-associated increase in prolactin level and such factors as an increase with age of body fat content.

The possibility that there are common features in the development of the secretion of MSH and that of prolactin with advancing age is revealed by the continuous lighting model. However, as far as MSH is concerned, there are some peculiarities that are hard to interpret. Direct measurements have shown that stress raises MSH secretion (Francis and Peaslee 1974). Therefore, it is possible that serotonin stimulates MSH secretion in stress, similar to its effect on growth hormone and prolactin secretion. However, some differences in the regulation of secretion of prolactin and MSH cannot be ruled out. First, melatonin stimulates prolactin secretion (Kamberi et al 1971a, Lu and Meites 1973) and competes with MSH, at least at the peripheral level. Unlike other cancers, the incidence of melanoma decreases with age. If melanoma formation is dependent, to a degree, on the stimulating effect of MSH, the age-associated decrease in the rate of melanoma incidence, unlike other skin cancers, may be accounted for by the decline in MSH level. This also applies to the age-associated greying of hair, if the color of hair is controlled by MSH; however, it remains uncertain whether MSH secretion really declines with advancing age (Rust and Meyer 1968).

Although age-connected elevation of the hypothalamic threshold does occur in the three main homeostatic systems (energy, reproductive, and adaptational), and may explain the increased number of pathologic disturbances that occur in these systems with age, there are other vital homeostatic systems that do not undergo such age-connected changes, and the formation of age-specific pathology should not be established on the basis of the condition of these systems. For example, the aged human does not exhibit evidence of diabetes insipidus, although in humans two important antidiuretic hormone nuclei, the supraoptic and the paraventricular, both show striking age-specific changes without evidence of cell destruction. Adrenaline and noradrenaline excretion does not decrease with advancing age (Kärki 1956); to the contrary, plasma noradrenaline levels increase with age (Sever et al 1977). The decreased lipolytic effect of catecholamines during maturation and senescence actually may be caused by changes in other systems, a rise in blood insulin, for instance, because both lipolytic and antilipolytic effects of these hormones are exerted through the adenyl cyclase system.

The progressive decrease in bone density that accompanies aging most likely is associated with shifts in other hormonal systems, specifically the age-connected decline in classic estrogen output, although this factor is not the only one that contributes to bone resorption in osteoporosis. It is noteworthy that no age-related decrease in parathyroid hormone is seen in overtly osteoporotic subjects; and in fact, levels are significantly higher than in normal subjects of corresponding age.

Preliminary observations indicate that neither the basal level of plasma glucagon nor the glucagon response to arginine stimulation is impaired in older individuals (Dudl and Ensinck 1972). As to the secretion of aldosterone, urinary excretion of this corticosteroid hormone decreases with age as it does with other corticosteroids, particularly dehydroepiandrosterone, androsterone, and etiocholanolone. The biologic significance of these adrenal secretory products is not known, but on the whole they produce an anabolic action, and it should be emphasized that it is the decreased secretion of these corticosteroids that is responsible for the negative discriminant function of Bulbruck (1972) on which the increased incidence of aging pathology is dependent (see Chapter 3). Thus regular age-associated changes take place only in the systems that control the implementation of the Law of Deviation of Homeostasis (see Chapter 1).

8 Interaction of the Main Homeostatic Systems in Ontogenesis: The Four Metabolic Stages in Postnatal Development

The most obvious illustration of the relationship between the mechanism of development and that of aging seems to be the fact that both in old age and in childhood there is fat accumulation in the body, which determines the generally analogous metabolic pattern of the extreme ages of man. Indeed, old age is second childhood.

Data discussed in Chapters 3–7 demonstrate that changes in the main homeostatic systems that occur with age are independent of each other. However, the processes in these systems interact in a manner that determines many metabolic features of postnatal ontogenesis. The interrelation between the reproductive and energy homeostats is particularly important. Following the switching-on of the reproductive cycle many metabolic parameters show a decrease. For example, blood FFA and cholesterol levels are higher before puberty than after it (Heald et al 1967). Children also reveal increased fat content and cortisol output (Okuno et al 1972). During childhood, 95% of subjects have a glucose assimilation coefficient (K) between 1.7 and 3.9 (mean 2.8 ± 0.6), whereas 95% of adults have a coefficient between 1.1 and 2.4 (mean 1.7 ± 0.3) (Loeb 1966). During childhood fasting serum insulin levels appear to rise progressively with increasing age (Grant 1967). Cholesterol blood level is also higher during the period of intensive growth; it decreases during ages 13–17 and then starts increasing progressively (Adlersberg et al 1956).

All these metabolic shifts resemble the syndrome of prediabetes that occurs in middle age as a result of disorders in energy homeostat functioning (see Chapter 6). This metabolic pattern really corresponds to so-called prediabetes (Fajans and Conn 1965). Therefore, the metabolic pattern observed before puberty may be defined as "pre-prediabetes" (Dilman 1971, 1974a).[1] It appears most likely that the metabolic pattern of pre-prediabetes is a consequence of a relatively high growth hormone level. This leads to a metabolic shift that meets the energy requirements of the growing organism. For instance, young men show a gain in body weight and an accumulation of fat in certain parts of the body prior to the period of intensive growth. According to Tanner (1968), intensive growth in boys is associated with the mobilization of subcutaneous fat from stores in the shoulder and shoulder-blade areas. Similar developments follow the administration of growth hormone. In particular, all these metabolic shifts provide for an enhanced cholesterol synthesis in childhood, which in turn is necessary to provide the material for cell membrane formation.

A specific peculiarity of the prepubertal period is the existence of a high level of both growth hormone and FFA, despite the fact that FFA are known to suppress growth hormone secretion (Quabbe et al 1977). In Chapter 6 an assumption was discussed that the high levels of growth hormone and FFA are caused by an elevated hypothalamic set point toward the inhibiting effect of fatty acids in childhood, while the hypothalamus reveals a high sensitivity to the inhibiting effect of glucose during the same period. It may be supposed that a change in this relationship, namely, an elevation of sensitivity toward the inhibiting effect of FFA and, on the contrary, a decline of sensitivity to the inhibiting effect of glucose, will affect growth potential by suppressing growth hormone secretion.

The age-related switching-on of the reproductive function is characteristic of the next period in development, the period of postpubertal stabilization. Higher estrogen levels typical of the period of stabilization in the female organism may also counteract the metabolic shifts of the previous period of preprediabetes. An excess of body weight, which is typical of the growth period (or pre-prediabetes), is often seen in children whose sexual maturity is delayed.

---

[1]The term, pre-prediabetes, is not traditional. In most papers prediabetes is defined in terms of individuals who have two diabetic parents, or have an inherent condition begun at conception and extending to the onset of chemical diabetes. However, the term prediabetes may have another meaning, since in the course of normal aging there develop metabolic shifts typical of prediabetes. Therefore, in the context of my concept I regard prediabetes as a normal age-associated physiologic process manifested by a delayed and exaggerated insulin-secretory response to glucose loading, raised blood level of FFA, and age-related gain of body weight. Accordingly, the similar, though transient, metabolic pattern observed in the prepubertal period may be denoted as pre-prediabetes.

On the contrary, children with hyperplasia of the mammary glands, who have an increase of the total phenolsteroid excretion, show a decrease in blood FFA levels (Table 8-1). However, estrogens are thought to reduce rather than increase carbohydrate tolerance (Spellacy et al 1972). It would appear that this conception springs from the common application of contraceptive steroid preparations. These drugs, which often contain mestranol, do reduce utilization of glucose. However, the administration of natural estrogens or stilbestrol does not exert such an effect (Table 8-2). On the contrary, treatment with stilbestrol and progestins raises glucose tolerance (Vishnevsky and Dilman 1972). This effect seems to be due to an estrogen-induced increase in sensitivity to insulin (Chapter 6). On the other hand, castration results in increased body weight and an accelerated rate of atherosclerosis associated with a rise in blood insulin. These conclusions are further supported by observations of a decrease in blood cholesterol at the second phase of the menstrual cycle, when the estrogen output of the corpus luteum is marked. A steep rise in cholesterol after menopause (Weiss 1972) and a decrease in age-associated hypercholesterolemia following estrogen treatment (Boyd 1961) also have been reported.

The mechanism of these effects of estrogens is not yet clear. Estrogens raise the blood growth hormone level (Frantz and Rabkin 1965), which is supposed to cause relevant metabolic disturbances. Yet certain data indicate that estrogens counteract growth hormone effects on target tissue. We have observed that treating rats with a combination of growth hormone and estrogens suppresses the lipolytic effect of the growth hormone (Kovaleva et al 1964) (Figure 8-1). Estrogens also inhibit the influence of growth hormone on metabolism in cartilage (Henneman 1973), and the antisomatotropic effect of estrogens has been observed in humans (Schwartz et al 1969). Estrogens are capable of

Table 8-1
Blood FFA Levels and Excretion of Total Phenolsteroids in Females with Hyperplasia of Mammary Glands and in Normal Females

Age Range (years)	Group	Blood FFA Levels (μEq/liter)	Excretion of Total Phenolsteroids (μg/24 hrs)
4–7	Patients	494 ± 87	29.8 ± 11.9
	Controls	1031 ± 206*	1.0 ± 0.1*
12–16	Patients	577 ± 62	26.2 ± 8.2
	Controls	810 ± 120*	2.2 ± 0.8*

*$p < 0.001$

reducing the output of somatomedin (Wiedemann and Schwartz 1972). Hence it appears most likely that estrogens counteract many effects of growth hormone. Thus the switching-on of the reproductive system affects metabolic processes controlled by the energy homeostat, since it initiates the transition from the utilization of FFA as the predominant source of energy (suitable for the period of growth) to the prevalent utilization of glucose, leading to a phase of stabilization.

Table 8-2
Differences in Carbohydrate Tolerance (Glycemic Square) Following Treatment with Estrogens and Progestins, and Infecundin

Treatment	No. Patients	Glycemic Square*	*p*
1. Before treatment	12	920.5 ± 32.2	
2. Stilbestrol + Ethisterone	12	864.4 ± 41.1	< 0.05†
3. Infecundin (Enovid)	12	940.3 ± 58.0	< 0.05‡

*As determined according to Wynn and Doar 1969.
†Significance as determined after Wilcoxon between values 1 and 2.
‡Significance as determined after Wilcoxon between values 2 and 3.

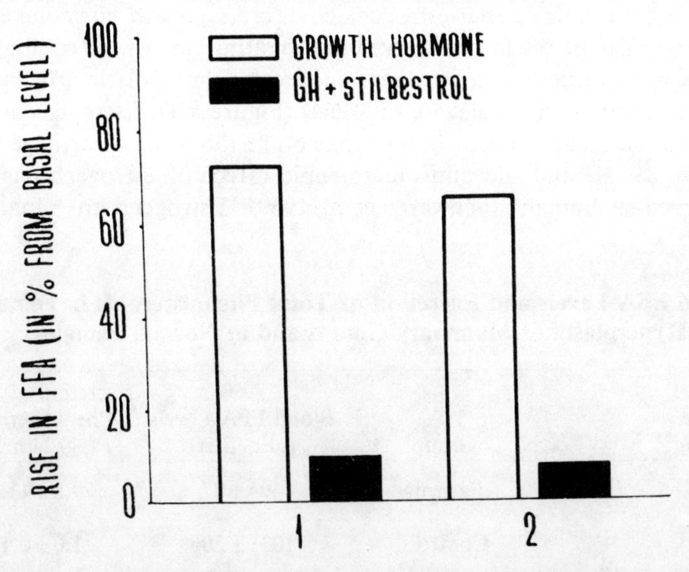

Figure 8-1 Diethylstilbestrol inhibition of lipolysis stimulated by treatment with human growth hormone. Blank Columns: percentage increase in FFA from basal level in control animals treated with growth hormone; Solid Columns: treatment with growth hormone in conjunction with diethylstilbestrol. 1 and 2 denote experimental series of rats.

Processes of the energy system influence the reproductive system. For example, the reproductive cycle is switched on when a critical body weight is reached (Frisch and Revelle 1970, Kennedy and Mitra 1963). This correlation between critical body weight and the switching-on of the reproductive cycle is of fundamental importance in the model of hypothalamic threshold elevation. If the age-associated switching-on of the reproductive function is in fact caused by this elevation of the hypothalamic threshold, it may be supposed that the elevation of the hypothalamic threshold is brought on by increased fat mass (see Chapter 5).

Is there such a correlation between the gain of body weight in ontogenesis and the elevation of the hypothalamic threshold of sensitivity? Of interest in this respect are findings that gonadotropin excretion decreases following treatment with the antidiabetic drug, phenformin (Dilman et al 1975). The improvement in the energy process that sometimes is observed as a result of phenformin administration reduces hypothalamic activity (see Chapter 18). Hence the reproductive and energy systems are subjected to reciprocal influences that determine the age at which the reproductive function is switched on and initiate the transition from the stage of growth or pre-prediabetes to that of stabilization. We designate this period following the completion of the growth of the organism as a period of stabilization because metabolic indices remain unchanged for a number of years. During this period metabolic conditions optimal for reproduction develop in the female organism.

Estrogens also have an appreciable immunodepressive effect; their main target is cellular immunity. In this respect the effect of estrogens is similar to that of glucocorticoids (Wyle and Kent 1977). The biologic significance of the immunodepressive action of estrogens seems to consist of the inhibition of response of cellular immunity during the reproductive period. It diminishes the likelihood of immunologic rejection of the fertilized ovum, which is genetically foreign to the maternal organism. It should be pointed out in this connection that pregnancy is characterized by a high level of estrogen output.

The adaptive-immunologic system also is subject to the influences of the energy homeostat (see Chapter 15). For example, the rise in growth hormone level in stress is a reaction directed at the restitution of function of the lymphoid system, impaired by an excess of cortisol (Chatterton et al 1973). Therefore it seems important to determine whether such a compensatory response is less striking when growth hormone secretion is inhibited by fatty acids in obese subjects. It should also be noted that insulin, and particularly somatomedin, are lymphocytotropic (Morell and Froesch 1973). Finally, it should be noted that the immune system in turn exerts an influence on the neuroendocrine functions in ontogeny (Pierpaoli et al 1976).

Thus optimal hormonal-metabolic interrelations develop at the phase of stabilization as a result of the interaction of the main homeostatic systems. It should be made clear that this phase of stabilization, so distinct in the development of the female organism, is practically nonexistent in men (see Chapter 9). However, in women, metabolic indices continue to change with age. Metabolic shifts are pronounced, particularly after reproductive function is switched off. Stabilization is transformed gradually into a stage of prediabetes that is characterized by disturbances in the constancy of the internal environment (see Chapters 3–7). The phase of prediabetes involves the formation of age-specific pathology, the so-called diseases of compensation (see Chapters 11–18). However, clinical studies show that some metabolic indices, eg, blood cholesterol, start to decrease in subjects older than 65 years of age. This phenomenon generally is accounted for by relatively higher death rates for cases with a high cholesterol level. However, an analysis of the data on age-associated changes in the hypothalamic threshold of sensitivity to inhibition by estrogens (see Figure 4-1) suggests the possibility of an actual decline in the hypothalamic threshold in old age. This may be attributed to the aging of the hypothalamic tissues, as is the case with the tissue of other organs. On the other hand, it may be accounted for by a diminished compensatory response to certain systems such as the decrease in blood insulin because of an exhaustion of the insulin secreting cells.

This evidence points to the existence of a fourth stage of ontogenesis: involution characterized by the decline in metabolic parameters. The stage of involution is sometimes accompanied by a loss of body weight. This statement is supported by the empiric observation that persons who have reached age 70 often continue to live without showing any dramatic advancement of age-specific pathology, and they may in all likelihood live for another eight to ten years. Considering the elevation of the hypothalamic threshold, and the interaction of the main homeostatic systems, the following four stages of postnatal ontogenesis may be distinguished: growth and maturation (the stage of pre-prediabetes); stabilization (in the female organism); the stage of prediabetes, ie, a period of profound deviation from the Law of Constancy of Internal Environment, which leads to the development of age-specific pathology; and the period of involution, or senescence (Figure 8-2). Taking into account the peculiar age-associated changes which occur in men, who do not pass through a stabilization phase, this conclusion seems to be still more convincing. These specific male-associated changes are the subject of Chapter 9.

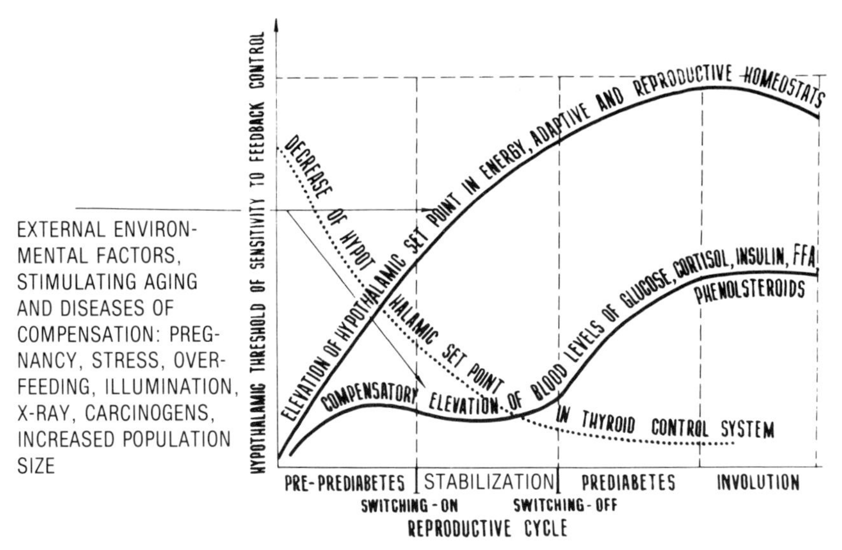

Figure 8-2 Program of development, aging, and age-specific pathology.

9 Peculiarities of the Neuroendocrine Program of Development and Aging in the Male Organism

The absence of the climacteric in the male, while being a biologically expedient phenomenon, is an advantage for which the male organism pays the price of a shorter life span, on the average, than is inherent in the female.

The postnatal ontogenesis of the male organism does not include a period similar to the phase of metabolic stabilization in women. This may be illustrated by the following comparison of the aging dynamics of blood cholesterol changes in men and women (Table 9-1).

It is clear that the blood cholesterol level in men rises by 67 mg% by the age of 37, whereas the rise in women is only 15 mg% during the same period. Cholesterol concentration eventually reaches the same level in both sexes, however. These differences may be accounted for on the basis of the concept described in Chapter 8 of a stabilization phase characteristic of the development of the female organism. Therefore the mechanisms operating at this stage have a normalizing effect on the levels of both reactive glycemia and insulinemia (Table 9-2).

It is evident that the age-associated increase of insulin level from age groups 21–29 to 40–49 is three times higher in men than in women (0.067 and 0.021). As previously mentioned, the higher the blood insulin level, the more active the formation of age-associated pathology, primarily atherosclerosis (see Chapters 6 and 12).

Table 9-1
Age-Associated Changes in Hypercholesterolemia in Males and Females

Age Group (years)	Blood Cholesterol (mg%)	
	Males	*Females*
3–7	179.8	209.0
8–12	180.4	196.4
13–17	175.5	182.9
18–22	185.2	192.6
23–27	194.5	201.9
28–32	243.1	200.1
33–37	246.9	224.5
38–42	246.9	224.5
43–47	237.2	238.9
48–52	238.8	249.5
53–57	239.7	285.8
58–62	236.2	263.8
63–67	249.7	259.9
68–72	242.5	241.8

Source: Adlersberg et al 1956.

Table 9-2
Age-Associated Changes in Insulin Level and Blood Sugar*

Age Group	Insulin Level (log units)		Blood Sugar (mg%)	
	Males	*Females*	*Males*	*Females*
21–29	1.51	1.60	86	95
30–39	1.53	1.59	92	91
40–49	1.57	1.62	97	102
50–59	1.62	1.68	107	106
60–69	1.73	1.77	114	121
70+	1.75	1.82	131	136

*Parameters were determined 1 hour after glucose load.
Source: Welborn et al 1969.

The data presented in Table 9-2 are of interest from still another point of view. Generally it is thought that there is a negative correlation between insulin level and blood sugar, ie, a high fasting blood sugar level is associated with a low level of insulin. However, Table 9-2 shows a simultaneous rise in blood sugar and insulin level in men. This points to the compensatory nature of hyperinsulinemia by mechanisms discussed in Chapter 6. This conclusion is in good agreement with the characteristics of the age-associated shift in these parameters in women. It is apparent that during ages 30–39 there is a decrease in both insulin and blood sugar levels in females, which indicates the diminished effect of those factors responsible for a compensatory hyperinsulinemia at this period. An appropriate decrease in blood sugar seems to result from a higher effectiveness of endogenous insulin action. In this connection it is noteworthy that the administration of estrogens improves tolerance to glucose in the prednisolone-glucose test in men (Table 9-3).

Table 9-3
Mean Blood Sugar Levels during Prednisolone-Glucose Test in Patients with Ischemic Heart Disease Before and After Estrogen Administration*

	Blood Sugar (mg%)		
Test Time	*Before Treatment*	*After Treatment*	p
One hour after glucose load	234.3 ± 8.3	192.1 ± 7.5	< 0.02
Two hours after glucose load	188.0 ± 7.1	146.3 ± 7.4	< 0.02

*0.5 to 1.0 mg of estradiol dipropionate or stilbestrol were administered 2–3 times a week during four weeks.

These findings suggest an explanation of a more delayed age-associated rise in cholesterol and insulin levels in women at the phase of stabilization. Some studies show that the phase of stabilization depends upon relationships at the level of the peripheral tissues, where estrogens counteract the growth hormone influence. Of similar importance is the fact that the female and male reproductive systems function differently; the female system is cyclic and the male system is continuous. These differences arise from relevant changes at the hypothalamic level. Neonatal administration of androgens is known to induce the male type of reproductive system functioning in genetically female individuals (Barraclough and Haller 1970). It has been found also that neonatal treatment with testosterone raises the hypothalamic threshold to feedback inhibition by sex hormones (Petrusz and Nagy 1967, Flerko 1974, Ullenbrock 1973).

However, elevation of both the threshold and noncyclic type of functioning constitutes specific features of aging and aging pathology. This is supported by data showing that neonatal administration of testosterone promotes the formation of diabetic disturbances in female rats (Foglia et al 1969) and results in a much higher frequency of tumors in animals with an androgenized hypothalamus (Vanha-Pertulla and Hapsu 1965). There is reason to suppose that sex-specific features of the hypothalamic function in the male organism are not limited to the reproductive system. For instance, the age-associated increase in the incidence of hypertension in men continues progressively, whereas this increase diminishes in women during the reproductive period (Hollingsworth et al 1965). The latter corresponds to the phase of stabilization in the female organism. It also is noteworthy that a glucose load results in a relatively smaller decrease in blood growth hormone in young men than in women, despite the fact that the absolute concentration of growth hormone is higher in women (Sandberg et al 1973).

Unlike estrogens, which are expected to ensure the cyclic functioning of the female reproductive homeostat, male hormones do not exert a distinct influence on hypothalamic function. This becomes evident particularly under clinical conditions when large doses of androgens, many times those of estrogens, are required to alleviate the symptoms of the climacteric, eg, menopausal hot flashes. It also is manifest in the absence of a cholesterol-lowering effect of testosterone. The differences in the patterns of reproductive homeostat functioning determine differences in the mechanisms of aging of this system, as well as account for the development of the central type of homeostatic failure, namely the switching-off of cyclic function (see Chapter 4).

The role of the male organism in reproduction is confined to the transfer of relevant genetic information. With increasing age this ability gradually declines because of a reduced potency caused by age-associated changes in the organism. Because of the permanent functioning of the reproductive homeostat and the absence of a stabilizing effect like the one provided by estrogens in the female system, the processes of compensation for age-associated changes in the energy homeostat start earlier in men than in women. Therefore age-associated pathology also occurs earlier in men.

Before such problems as the relationship between age-associated changes and age-specific pathology can be considered, however, it is necessary to establish the criteria for normal aging since, as shown in the preceding chapters, the norm recedes gradually in the course of natural physiologic aging.

10 The Definition of Norms in Aging

The idea of each age group having its own age-related norm of physiologic parameters proves to be a myth. It is not enough to be fit; it is necessary to be normal.

Aging is accompanied by numerous changes in physiologic parameters. In the three main homeostatic systems these changes actually are part of the organism's program of development, which would explain why the parameters of the norm should be different at different periods of childhood. These hormonal and metabolic parameters do not cease changing when growth is completed, however. For instance, gonadotropin excretion rises nearly sixfold between ages 20–29 and 40–49, even though this increase is no longer required, after reproductive function is switched on. Similar age-associated changes take place in the energy system; for example, blood concentrations of glucose, insulin, cholesterol, and triglycerides, rise steadily with advancing age.

Because of the universality of these age-associated changes, it is generally thought that a separate norm should be established for each age group. Thus Andres (1971) developed a special nomogram to establish the normal increase in blood glucose concentration for each age group (see also Pozefsky et al 1965). Similar age-related norms have been established for body weight and cholesterol levels. Such an approach has led to the formation of a concept of a "dynamic age-associated norm."

According to this concept, individual deviations from the norm are to be found by comparing the individual parameter with the available age distribution curve of that parameter in a population. The magnitude of the deviation is used to assess the difference between biologic and chronologic age of the individual, ie, to what extent the aging of the individual is accelerated or decelerated when compared with the average for his age group. That is how a myth appears of a "permissiveness" of the age-related changes in this or that physiologic parameter, eg, of the increase in the cholesterol blood level with age. However, the fact that age-related hypercholesterolemia develops in practically every individual must not delude us into believing that this phenomenon is normal or harmless.

On the contrary, the processes developing in everyone are dangerous for all. Cholesterol level rises by about 54 mg% in healthy men between ages 20–29 and 50–59, although the difference in cholesterol levels between healthy subjects and patients suffering from myocardial infarction is about 37 mg% (Gofman et al 1952). Statistics also show that between these two age groups the death rate from ischemic heart disease increases 140 times (WHO Manual 1967). Hence, any steady deviation of homeostasis is a disease. It is not enough to be fit—it is necessary to be normal. It also should be pointed out that these so-called normal parameters of the population as a whole are not reliable. Different countries, even different populations of the same country, show substantial differences. And since population make-up keeps changing, the norms must be re-evaluated at regular intervals.

Thus the current concept of the "dynamic norm" shows significant limitations. But there is an alternative to this in the concept of the "stable or ideal norm." According to this concept the parameters of the norm remain the same for all age groups and at all periods of ontogenesis after completion of growth (Dilman 1958, 1971). The norm is a constant established at age 20, ie, on completion of growth. Therefore, the norm is one and the same for all age groups. Parameters of the norm are ascertained for each individual at the age of 20–25 (Albrink et al 1962). All subsequent changes in these parameters are regarded as a departure from the norm, not as an age-associated change in the norm itself. Determining the norm on such a basis provides for specific reference points in individual cases, thus avoiding errors caused by individual uniqueness.

Traditional gerontology holds that the criteria of normal aging should be distinguished from those associated with specific diseases of senescence. This is based on the assumption that the mechanism of normal aging is separate from the mechanisms of age-specific pathology. However, there is now considerable evidence that pathologic processes such as diseases of compensation are direct consequences of normal aging, so that, as far as metabolic parameters are concerned, there should be no essential difference between normal aging and age-specific pathology (see Chapter 18).

There are difficulties involved in the selection of criteria, however. These difficulties arise from the fact that metabolic deviations identical to those inherent in normal aging and age-specific pathology also occur in diseases unrelated to aging. For example, the blood levels of total cholesterol, triglycerides, and LDL-cholesterol rise both with increasing age and in certain genetic diseases, eg, familial hyperlipoproteinemia. Therefore, in order to distinguish age-associated changes from pathologic ones, eg, atherosclerosis as an age-associated process from other types of atherosclerosis, it is necessary to develop both a battery of assay techniques (Comfort 1969), and a single system of criteria. Accordingly, it will be necessary to assess the origin of each metabolic disturbance.

Such an evaluation on the basis of isolated criteria, or even of a totality of parameters as in the case of lipid patterns, will not be feasible unless manifestations indicating the pathogenesis of the metabolic disturbances are included. One possibility is to determine the functional state of the main homeostatic systems along with the metabolic parameters. Norm recession is characterized by development of the central type of homeostatic failure, as shown in Chapters 3 through 7. Apart from disturbances in the rhythm of function of the homeostatic systems following hypothalamic threshold deviation, however, this state also involves a compensatory reaction from relevant peripheral endocrine glands. Table 10-1 shows the tests that determine the type of failure in the main homeostatic systems.

Such an evaluation should be complemented by the determination of secondary parameters that cover the hormonal and metabolic shifts caused by homeostatic disorders. This is important because, when compensation in the peripheral endocrine glands is sufficiently marked, the rhythmic functioning of the system may continue for a long time even though the hypothalamic threshold is elevated. An illustration of such a state is provided by the premenopausal period, when the rhythmic functioning of the ovaries is maintained at the same time that gonadotropic activity and ovarian function are enhanced. However, if secondary parameters (gonadotropin and phenolsteroid levels, in this case) are assayed, it becomes clear that the cyclic functioning of the system is maintained because of a much higher than normal level of the activity of both central and peripheral components of the reproductive homeostat. Therefore the state of normality should be assessed on the basis of two types of parameters: rhythmic function of homeostatic systems, and magnitude of secondary changes in hormonal-metabolic parameters.

Tests for the evaluation of age-associated changes may be simplified technically. It is, of course, impossible to assess in each individual all known or measurable physiologic parameters. Nor is it necessary to do so,

Table 10-1
Possible Tests for Elevation of Main Homeostatic Systems

Homeostatic System	Primary Test	Secondary Test
Energy System	Growth hormone level after glucose load and insulin-induced hypoglycemia; growth hormone level after fat loading	Two-hour blood sugar and insulin levels after glucose load; blood cholesterol, HDL-cholesterol and triglyceride levels; body weight; basal metabolic rate
Reproductive system	Inhibition of FSH and LH secretion by estrogens or pituitary inhibitors	Blood FSH and LH levels, or excretion of total gonadotropins and total phenolsteroids
Adaptive system	Inhibition of adrenal cortical function in dexamethasone test; response to insulin-induced hypo-; glycemia; diurnal rhythm of blood cortisol level	17-hydroxycorticosteroid/17-ketosteroid excretion ratio; tests for evaluation of cell-mediated immunity
Thyrostat	TSH blood levels after T_3 suppression test	Blood TSH, T_3 and T_4 levels
Regulation of MSH and prolactin secretion	L-dopa and chlorpromazine tests	Blood prolactin and MSH levels

since most physiologic parameters are protected by the Law of Constancy of Internal Environment and thus do not undergo any regular age-related changes. With advancing age, various accidental defects may appear in the organism, leading to the development of various diseases. It is not these accidental diseases but the so-called normal diseases that characterize the aging process. The battery of parameters necessary for determining the normal state of the organism is not immeasurable. Selection of a small battery of indices is determined by the fact that the Law of Deviation of Homeostasis manifests itself in uniform disturbances if aging develops in a normal way. Even without knowing about many intermediate links in the age-related disturbances, on the basis of several "final" indices determined by the main homeostatic systems, it is still possible to evaluate, with a certain degree of probability, the state of these systems as a whole. If the first examination is carried out between the ages of 20 and 25, the determination of the secondary parameters of aging alone may be sufficient for the appraisal of the organism's condition. They should include: body fat, cholesterol, triglyceride and HDL-cholesterol blood levels, sugar and insulin concentrations two hours after a glucose load, basal metabolic rate, 17-hydroxycorticosteroid/17-ketosteroid excretion ratio, and the level of total gonadotropin excretion (see Table 10-1). If these parameters are normal, it is not necessary to assay the condition of the homeostatic system; instead, determinations of the secondary parameters should be carried out approximately every two to three years. Theoretically, several phases of age-associated disorders may be distinguished according to the mechanism of normal recession resulting from the central type of homeostatic failure (Table 10-2).

Table 10-2
Phases of Development of Homeostatic Failure in Normal Aging

Phase	Homeostatic System Condition	Stage of Homeostatic Failure
I	Disturbed rhythmic activity	Dysrhythmic stage
II	No reaction or paradoxical reaction to inhibition test	Arrhythmic stage
III	Metabolic disturbance	Dysmetabolic stage (risk factor)
IV	Clinical signs of disease	Clinical stage

The application of primary and secondary tests offers an advantage in detecting deviations from the norm at an earlier stage than is possible based solely on risk factor determinations. It should be kept in mind, however, that the standard norm reached at ages 20–25 undergoes constant changes. These changes are brought about by numerous external stimuli, which alter the hypothalamic set point or intensify relevant compensatory reactions, and thus accelerate development and aging. Some of these factors include: different types of stress, obesity, decreased physical activity, influence of carcinogens and, primarily, the acceleration of development. So the establishment of the standard norm is an urgent task because the pattern of the norm changes under the influence of these factors. The patterns of the ideal norm also should be established for populations in different regions of each country, since differing physical and social environments promote unique patterns.

PART II
The Law of Deviation of Homeostasis and Diseases of Aging

It is not the disturbance of the Law of Constancy of Internal Environment of the organism, but the exact implementation of the Law of Deviation of Homeostasis, that determines the appearance of age-specific diseases. If these diseases do not develop during a certain period of life, this is an indication of an abnormality in the normal process of development and aging of the organism.

11 Diabetes Mellitus

Maturity-onset diabetes mellitus: the disease of diseases.

At present there are arguments in favor of the etiologic heterogeneity of idiopathic diabetes mellitus; maturity-onset type diabetes involves different types (Fajans et al 1978). Fajans and associates (1978) believe that "in maturity-onset diabetes the most important environmental factor appears to be a diet leading to obesity." It is my belief, however, that in this case, as in many similar cases, the importance of environmental factors is overestimated. As age advances, fat is accumulated in the organism while the overall mass of muscle and bone tissue is reduced (Dudl and Ensinck 1977). Thus elderly subjects contain more fat tissue than younger ones, despite comparable body weights. It has been calculated that a 20% rise in the body weight of a subject weighing 70 kg represents a twofold increase in adipose tissue (Keys and Brozek 1953). As age advances, carbohydrate tolerance is diminished (see Chapter 6). Furthermore, age-related hyperglycemia is so common as to be considered normal, and only when a conventional limit of glycemia is exceeded is it regarded as an indication of diabetes. The purely conventional character of these distinctions becomes still more apparent when one considers that not only does the level of glycemia increase with advancing age, but so do the levels of blood insulin and fatty acid. Changes inherent in prediabetes and maturity-onset diabetes make it impossible to draw a sharp distinction between age-associated hyperglycemia and these diabetic developments. Actually, each normal individual between 50 and 70 years of age suffers from a certain degree of chemical diabetes mellitus (Vinik and Jackson 1967). Meanwhile, many investigators are trying to solve a dilemma: which of the two phenomena develops first, obesity or decline of glucose tolerance? The problem is difficult. Since obesity is always accompanied by hyperinsulinemia (see Chapter 6), it is obscure whether hyperinsulinemia causes obesity or obesity leads to hyperinsulinemia.

Bagdade et al (1968) believe that hyperinsulinism is a metabolic consequence of obesity. According to this view, the following sequence of events may be surmised: obesity, hyperinsulinemia, decrease in insulin receptor concentration on the plasma membrane of target cells, insulin resistance, and decreased tolerance to carbohydrates.

On the other hand, there are arguments in favor of the concept that obesity is caused by the diabetic state, rather than it being a factor in the pathogenesis of diabetes. According to this viewpoint, the first phenomenon to develop is insulin resistance, which in turn causes both the development of obesity and a decreased carbohydrate tolerance. Woods and Porte (1978) believe that "although it is not clear whether insulin levels determine adiposity or whether adiposity determines insulin levels, it is clear that there is a close relationship between the two and that there is no a priori method for determining which is causative."

It seems, however, that a definite approach to the solution of this problem is possible. It is generally believed that there are two major types of obesity: metabolic and regulatory. According to Mayer (1965), "the general distinction can be made between regulatory obesities in which the impairment is in the central mechanism regulating food intake, and metabolic obesity in which the primary lesion is an inborn or acquired error in the metabolism of tissue per se."

The age-associated increase of fat accumulation should be referred to as a regulatory type of obesity, since this phenomenon is observed in practially every subject and is characterized by features of a central type of homeostatic failure in the mechanism of appetite regulation (see Chapter 5). However, as the deposition of body fat grows, tissue factors begin to play an important role in the pathogenesis of obesity regardless of the original causes. It is noteworthy that a 15% to 30% gain in weight by increased calorie intake in lean volunteers results in endocrine-metabolic changes similar to those observed in spontaneous obesity (Sims and Horton 1968). One of these tissue factors is an increase in fat cell size, which is associated with a diminished sensitivity of the adipose tissue to insulin action (Jahnke et al 1971, Olefsky 1977). The size of fat cells has a substantial influence on lipolysis (Östman et al 1973) and raises the level of free fatty acids in obese subjects with the result that glucose utilization deteriorates and hyperinsulinemia is induced (Jahnke et al 1971). Large fat cells have an increased sensitivity to the lipolytic effect of catecholamines (Bray et al 1977, Jacobsson et al 1976). In other words obesity brings about a metabolic situation in which normal regulation can be maintained only through hyperinsulinemia. Accordingly, fat cell size increases with age (Björntorp 1974), thus forming the total sum of metabolic disturbances that are connected with the behavior of the large fat cell. Thus, normal aging conditions promote the development of the metabolic type of obesity.

This mechanism includes two major components: a decreased uptake of glucose by muscle tissue, and a consequent compensatory hyperinsulinemia. These two components also are inherent in other types of obesity. Since glucose tolerance in obese subjects decreases significantly with age (Ditschuneit 1971), this in turn stimulates further development of obesity. Thus we can say that aging makes its contribution to the formation of two main types of obesity. Table 11-1 summarizes data on major metabolic disturbances occurring in normal aging as well as in regulatory and metabolic obesities. There are arguments supporting the concept of a simultaneous existence of two parallel processes: an elevation of the threshold of sensitivity in the hypothalamic centers controlling food intake, and the age-related disorders in the energy homeostat causing the development of obesity. Thus, aging leads to a simultaneous development of both regulatory and metabolic types of obesity (see Chapters 5, 6). In both cases hyperinsulinemia develops, since it is a key factor of the age-specific pathology. Therefore, I have long held that prediabetes and maturity-onset diabetes (to be more exact, in the light of the foregoing, diabetes of the obese) (Dilman 1961, 1968, 1971, 1974a) are each a disease of aging or, more precisely, a normal disease.

A number of papers published recently reflect the trend of research in this direction (Kent 1976, Shagan 1976). It should be of interest to discuss some data concerning the pathogenesis of prediabetes and maturity-onset diabetes, in order to document the statements in Table 11-1.

Table 11-1
Comparison of Data on Metabolic Disturbances in Normal Aging and in Regulatory and Metabolic Obesities

Characteristic	Normal Aging	Obesity
Sensitivity to insulin	Decreased	Decreased
Insulin binding	Decreased	Decreased
Blood insulin	Increased	Increased
Glucocorticoid output	Increased	Increased
Tolerance to glucose	Decreased	Normal, then decreased (depending on level of hyperinsulinemia and duration of disturbances)
Free fatty acids in blood	Increased	Increased
Synthesis and level of triglycerides in blood	Increased	Increased
Blood cholesterol levels	Increased	Increased
Growth hormone level	Decreased (in overt obesity)	Decreased

Prediabetes (the term was suggested by Fajans and Conn 1965) has much in common with the mechanism of age-associated hyperglycemia. It may last from conception to the period when first signs of a decrease in tolerance to carbohydrates appear (Marble 1970); although hyperglycemia is not yet developed at this stage, persons with prediabetes reveal such hyperglycemia-like symptoms as an increase in FFA, cholesterol, and β-lipoproteins, accompanied by a decrease in the antilipolytic effect of insulin (Mikhall et al 1972). Prediabetes also is characterized by diminished sensitivity to insulin, hyperinsulinemia (Ditschuneit 1964), and a propensity for birth of large babies. It is particularly noteworthy that prediabetics are apt to have an increased basal concentration of growth hormone (Pfeiffer 1965, Hales et al 1968, Boden et al 1968), as well as a paradoxical increase in growth hormone level one hour after a glucose load, coupled with a high reactive rise by the second or third hour (Sönksen et al 1973). Although the glycemic level in prediabetics is normal, subjects with prediabetes often suffer from vascular lesions of the kidneys, and hypophysectomy has been reported as effective in the treatment of angiopathy (Lundbaek 1973).

If we accept the role of hypersecretion of growth hormone in prediabetes, then a complete identity becomes evident between the mechanism of age-associated decline in carbohydrate tolerance and the mechanism of prediabetes. The same principle applies to the mechanism of maturity-onset diabetes mellitus. The role of growth hormone in the development of diabetes was suggested in connection with the concept of pituitary diabetes (Young 1968). It should be noted that, following growth hormone administration to humans, not only does the basal level of insulin rise, but the so-called delayed response is also observed (Yalow and Berson 1971). This response, typical of diabetes in its early stages, is considered to be an indication of the pathogenicity of growth hormone in diabetes (Sönksen et al 1972).

Some indirect evidence confirms the role of growth hormone in the reduction of the tolerance to glucose in humans. For example, it has been shown that when glucose is administered four hours after the standard glucose load, glycemic characteristics deteriorate in those patients with early-onset diabetes who reveal a considerable reactive increase in growth hormone concentration in response to the primary glucose load (rebound phase) (Yalow et al 1969). It should be noted that in diabetics the rebound phase of growth hormone secretion following a glucose load starts at a blood sugar level much higher than after fasting (Hunter et al 1966). Administration of growth hormone in humans shows a distinct diabetogenic effect potentiated by cortisone (Mitchell et al 1970).

The effect of hypophysectomy in diabetic retinopathy generally is accounted for by the elimination of the action of growth hormone. This conclusion seems to be fully justified, since diabetics with clinical signs of retinopathy or renal vascular disorders most often reveal an absolute rise in blood growth hormone level (Lundbaek 1973, Passa et al 1974).

Many investigators have reported increased concentrations of growth hormone in maturity-onset diabetes even without concomitant clinical manifestations of angiopathy (Hales et al 1968, Luft and Guillemin 1974). Of particular interest are the studies by a group of Danish researchers who showed that growth hormone output is strikingly high in both early- and late-onset diabetes if it is measured during the day or after physical exercise rather than at its basal level (Hansen 1970, 1973a, 1973b; Lundbaek 1973; Passa et al 1974). The possibility of a paradoxical increase in growth hormone after glucose load also should be noted (Hunter et al 1966, Sönksen et al 1972). Diabetic patients show a much smaller drop in FFA level following a glucose load than healthy subjects do (De Caro et al 1966). This decrease probably should be attributed to the influence of a relative excess of growth hormone. According to some reports, growth hormone clearance is reduced in diabetes. All these results point to the conclusion that the hypersecretion of growth hormone is inherent in diabetes mellitus. This phenomenon is more apparent at earlier stages when obesity is not advanced, or when diabetic patients are subjected to physical exercise or emotional stress (Lundbaek et al 1972). Some authors have failed to detect any increase in blood growth hormone level, however (Danowski et al 1969). Therefore the problem of what role this factor really plays remains unsolved. A confusing feature is that there are some factors that prevent an exact evaluation of growth hormone secretion in many cases of maturity-onset diabetes; for instance, a decreased level of growth hormone will appear in both maturity-onset diabetes and obesity (Tchobroutsky 1973). Taking into account the high sensitivity of hyperglycemic mechanisms regulating growth hormone secretion, a conclusion may be drawn that under the conditions of diabetic hyperglycemia, even a normal level of growth hormone should be interpreted as an indication either of increased output of this hormone or of resistance of suppression by glucose of the hypothalamic centers that regulate its secretion. This conclusion is consistent with observations that growth hormone secretion is inhibited markedly even in healthy persons who are on a high carbohydrate (but isocaloric) diet (Merimee et al 1973). This improvement in glucose tolerance was explained by the suppression of growth hormone output (Merimee et al 1973, Brunzell et al 1971).

A relative increase in cortisol level potentiates the insulin antagonistic effect of growth hormone (Pfeiffer 1965). A reactive excess of cortisol also may occur in diabetes mellitus (Goth and Gönczi 1972). Resistance to dexamethasone suppression has been reported in diabetics (Lentle and Thomas 1964), which corresponds to the central type of homeostatic failure in the adaptive system. All these factors contribute to hyperinsulinemia. In studying this problem, Reaven et al (1972) concluded that "the persistent hyperinsulinemia in patients with chemical diabetes in the response to the formula feeds, at a time when their plasma glucose levels were similar to those of normal subjects, suggests that the raised levels of plasma insulin must be a compensatory phenomenon designed to maintain glucose homeostasis." These data are in good agreement with the idea forming a basis for the concept of compensation diseases. On the basis of these findings I suggested that the elevation of insulin secretion is the key to maturity-onset diabetes development (Dilman 1967). This was also supported by the studies of Jackson et al (1972). It should be emphasized that this type of diabetes, particularly in its initial stages, involves hyperinsulinemia (Reaven et al 1972) and a delayed insulin reaction to stimuli, primarily glucose.

Insulin-like activity of blood also has been found to increase in patients with diabetes (Pfeiffer 1970, Streeten et al 1965). Moreover, Reaven and Olefsky (1978) stress that, although obesity is a determinant of the insulin response to oral glucose, "its impact should not be overestimated, and it is impossible to attribute the increased insulin response that is seen in many nonketotic diabetics to the coexistence of obesity." The presence of hyperinsulinemia can in turn cause insulin resistance typical of maturity-onset diabetes. As has been shown by De Fronzo et al (1978), in maturity-onset diabetes the rate of glucose metabolism stimulated by physiologic hyperinsulinemia was 30% lower than in healthy controls. Ginsberg et al (1974) showed that the resistance to insulin-mediated glucose uptake is a characteristic of nonobese patients with chemical diabetes. Recently, Reaven and Olefsky (1978) summarized a considerable amount of evidence that implicates resistance to the action of insulin as an important factor in the pathogenesis of chemical diabetes. If we exclude from this discussion the elevational model of the age-associated mechanism of insulin resistance, then in the light of modern knowledge this phenomenon may be connected with a number of various defects that are supposed to exist at the cell level (Fajans et al 1978). In this respect it is necessary to consider the relationship between hyperinsulinemia and insulin binding to target cells to be very important. At present the concept of receptor "down regulation," namely decreased hormone binding by specific receptors in response to the elevation of hormone level, has been well documented for insulin (Freychet 1976). With respect to insulin resistance in diabetes, reduced insulin binding to circulating mononuclear cells has been observed in maturity-onset diabetes, particularly when basal hyperinsulinemia is present (Olefsky and Reaven 1976). Moreover, the number of receptor sites directly correlates with insulin sensitivity in vivo, measured as the rate constant (K) for the fall in blood glucose after intravenous insulin administration (Harrison et al 1976). Taking into account the fact that, in at least 80% of all cases, maturity-onset diabetes coexists with adiposity, it should be of interest to consider the data showing that the calorie-restricted diet that ameliorates hyperinsulinemia produces an improvement in insulin binding in obese men (Archer et al 1975). These data allow one to suppose that the defect in insulin binding to receptors in maturity-onset diabetes is caused, at least partially, by hyperinsulinemia characteristic of this type of diabetes. There are data indicating that several cell membrane hormone receptors decrease in concentration during aging. As reported by Roth et al (1978b), "this phenomenon may be closely, if not causally, related to age associated decrease in responsiveness to their same hormones." In light of these data, an aspect of the relationship between normal aging, obesity, and maturity-onset diabetes, and other specific diseases of aging becomes more obvious.

In this respect, primary account should be taken of the fact that adiposity is associated with an increase in FFA mobilization while the plasma FFA turnover rate significantly correlates with the plasma FFA concentration (Nestel and Whyte 1968). It would be more precise to state that the shift toward a more intensified mobilization of FFA as an energy substrate takes place when adiposity is combined with a decline in carbohydrate tolerance, which is actually characteristic of chemical diabetes of the obese. At the same time, triglyceride turnover significantly correlates with FFA turnover (Nestel and Whyte 1968). It was noted, comparatively long ago, by Davidson and Albrink (1965) that "the resistance to exogenous insulin in hypertriglyceridemic obese, and elderly, persons is considered an evidence of some common etiologic factors in obesity, diabetes, and atherosclerosis." Many facts and arguments could be cited to support the idea that age-related hyperinsulinemia, maturity-onset prediabetes, and chemical diabetes are key factors in the formation of specific age-related pathology (see Chapters 12–18; Dilman 1968, 1974a). In particular, the diabetic state is associated with cellular characteristics of aging (Hamlin et al 1975). The activity of cellular immunity is decreased in diabetics (see Chapter 15), and the decreased activity of the suppressor T-cell function in diabetes mellitus (Horowitz et al 1977) seems to be one of the causes promoting the development of autoimmune disorders in diabetic subjects (see Chapter 16). Chemical diabetes is frequently observed in cancer patients (see Chapter 17), while administration of chemical carcinogens to experimental animals often causes hyperglycemia and hyperinsulinemia (see Chapter 20). Even in patients with essential hypertension one often observes a decreased carbohydrate tolerance combined with obesity (see Chapter 13). Finally, "diabetes of pregnancy" is a key factor in the acceleration of development and, accordingly, in the acceleration of age-related pathology (see Chapter 21).

It should be pointed out that long-term diabetic disturbances often result in a depletion of β-cell function. Therefore the blood insulin level drops lower as the diabetes becomes more overt and as hyperglycemia elevates. Hence the development of age-associated pathology also may be delayed. It is noteworthy that early-onset diabetes, which involves a low insulin level, is characterized by reduced incidence of cancer (Werner 1955) and atherosclerosis (Blagosklonnaya 1968), despite the increased growth hormone level as has been shown recently (Hansen 1970, 1973a).

The observations of Hansen (1973a, 1974) have shown that the blood of untreated male juvenile diabetics contains more immunoreactive growth hormone than the blood of controls. Hansen (1974) suggests that in diabetes mellitus defective glucose utilization in the hypothalamus caused by absolute insulin deficiency may account for the increased level of growth hormone. An increased growth hormone level is most frequent in brittle juvenile-onset diabetics. This is a fundamental feature of the distinction between late- and early-onset diabetes, since the increased level of growth hormone observed in juvenile-onset diabetes seems to be of secondary (compensatory) origin, and assures the utilization of fatty acids as the source of energy when insulin is deficient and glucose utilization is decreased. However, the insulin deficit in diabetic juveniles is a factor that somewhat decelerates atherosclerosis and, probably, cancer. It seems probable, however, that the hyperinsulinemia caused, not infrequently, by inadequate treatment leads to the loss of these advantages in the patients with juvenile-onset diabetes mellitus.

12 Atherosclerosis

Atherosclerosis is an ancient disease, nearly as old as the world, since it originates for man and the spawning Pacific salmon alike, in the regulatory mechanism which secures both the reproduction and growth of the organism.

Atherosclerosis is the pathologic phenomenon most frequently associated with aging. Nevertheless, it is generally believed that the development of atherosclerosis is dependent chiefly on external environmental factors, primarily excessive food intake and stress. It is true that there is a rather stable correlation between the caloric content of the diet (and the relative content of carbohydrates) and the frequency of atherosclerosis. There also is a correlation between atherosclerosis and the influence of stress, the level of muscular activity, and tobacco smoking. Atherosclerosis has been one of the most often cited of the so-called diseases of civilization. If we examine the pathogenic mechanisms of atherosclerosis, however, it becomes obvious that the effect of these external factors is superimposed on preexisting, age-related internal factors, which accounts for the increased frequency of this disease with age. Before this relationship is considered, it is necessary to discuss briefly the data available on the pathogenesis of atherosclerosis.

Atherosclerosis is caused by the accumulation of lipid, mainly cholesterol, in the arterial wall. This process is determined by several factors: 1) the condition of the vascular tissue, 2) the level of cholesterol synthesis in the arterial wall, and 3) the level and properties of lipoproteins in the blood, as well as by some other factors.

Alterations in the arterial wall are essential for the development of atherosclerosis. Response of the arterial wall to injury is a factor, as are changes in the level of activity of enzymatic systems that contribute to the degradation of lipoproteins during their passage through the arterial wall (Niehans et al 1977). Still another factor is blood pressure.

The tissue factor in the genesis of atherosclerosis still is underestimated, largely because an adequate methodologic approach to the problem is lacking. For example, Kuo (1969) believes that the damage in small venules and capillary changes that promote atherosclerosis in Types III and IV of essential hyperlipidemia seem to be associated with carbohydrate metabolism disturbances at the stage of prediabetes. It also has been observed that, apart from insulin, cholesterol synthesis in the arterial wall is affected by the glucose level, by fatty acids, and by catecholamines.

Cholesterol synthesis in the arterial wall, which seems to be another important source of atherosclerosis, is regulated by the same factors as cholesterol synthesis in the liver. The insulin level is particularly important (Stout 1968). The exposure of arterial tissue to insulin results in the proliferation of smooth muscle cells and synthesis of cholesterol and triglycerides (Stout 1977). Cholesterol synthesis in the arterial wall is independent of the negative feedback mechanism controlling cholesterol synthesis in the liver (Dietschy and Wilson 1970).

However, synthesis of cholesterol in the tissues is regulated by a mechanism controlling the flux of lipoproteins into the tissues. The major function of plasma low density lipoproteins (LDL) may be to transport cholesterol from its site of synthesis in the liver and intestine to its site of utilization in the peripheral tissues. LDL delivers cholesterol to peripheral tissues for the renewal of cell membranes and also inhibits the cellular synthesis of cholesterol. Elevation of LDL level in the blood causes a reduction of the synthesis of the LDL receptor, thus preventing excessive accumulation of cholesterol within the cell (Brown et al 1975). Circulating LDL-cholesterol thus regulates, by feedback inhibition of cholesterol synthesis, the cellular content of cholesterol. However, the net flux of LDL into the arterial intima appears to increase with age (Niehans et al 1977). This may account in part for the association between hypercholesterolemia and the development of atherosclerosis. It has been found that in the normal intima the concentration of intimal lipoproteins is significantly correlated with serum cholesterol. For every 100 mg% increase in blood cholesterol the lipoprotein cholesterol increases by 1.8 mg per 100 mg of dry tissue, and this represents an increase of nearly 50% in total intimal cholesterol (Smith and Slater 1972).

The level of high density lipoproteins (HDL) does not increase with age, though the level of HDL is known to play a significant role in the removal of cholesterol from tissue (Miller et al 1977b). HDL is formed in the liver and, perhaps, in the gut. The interest in human HDL recently has grown, largely because of the finding that plasma HDL-cholesterol is negatively associated with the incidence of coronary artery disease in man (Williams et al 1979) and longevity of individuals (Glueck et al 1977).

There is some evidence for a monoclonal origin of human atherosclerotic plaques developing from smooth muscle cells (Benditt and Benditt 1973). At the same time, it has been shown that some lipoproteins promote hyperplasia of arterial smooth muscle cells. In this context some data obtained in our laboratory are of interest, since they show that patients with ischemic heart disease reveal an increase of cholesterol concentration in the lymphocytes, which can be considered as a model of interaction between the cell and the internal environment of the organism (Table 12-1). It is not yet clear, however, why the mechanisms controlling the constant level of cholesterol concentration in the cell lose their capability to maintain a balance. This failure may be caused by alterations within the internal environment of the organism since phenformin, along with the improvement of blood lipid indices, was responsible for a decrease of cholesterol content in the lymphocytes of atherosclerotic patients. It seems, therefore, that the level of LDL and the composition of the internal environment of the organism are key factors in the development of atherosclerosis.

Table 12-1
Cholesterol Content of Lymphocytes in Control Subjects (mean age 43 ± 2.0 years) and in Patients with Ischemic Heart Disease (mean age 43 ± 2.0 years)

	Control	Patients	Significance (*p*)
Content of cholesterol in lymphocytes (μg/mg protein)			
Total cholesterol	34.3 ± 2.7	54.3 ± 3.0	< 0.001
Free cholesterol	31.4 ± 2.9	43.4 ± 3.0	< 0.01
Cholesterol ether	8.8 ± 2.34	18.7 ± 4.26	> 0.05
Blood parameters (mg%)			
Total cholesterol	236 ± 11.9	313 ± 18.7	< 0.01
β-Lipoproteins	461 ± 49.2	753 ± 42.6	< 0.001
Triglycerides	110 ± 21.1	304 ± 87.5	< 0.05

The level and properties of the blood lipoproteins are determined by many factors and, above all, by the synthesis in the liver of VLDL. In its turn, the intensity of VLDL synthesis is determined by the intensity of triglyceride synthesis (Eisenberg and Levy 1975).

Plamsa LDL are derived from the plasma VLDL (Schafer et al 1978a). Arterial cells can also degrade lipoproteins. VLDL is metabolized in endothelial cells by the enzyme lipoprotein lipase, and the product particle, LDL, can filter through the endothelial barrier to be taken up by smooth muscle cells in the subintimal space. Under normal conditions all these processes are controlled homeostatically. Hence, in order to understand the causes that may induce an increase in the rate of synthesis and, accordingly, an elevation of cholesterol blood level, which occurs in atherosclerosis, it is essential to analyze the processes during which such an increase develops physiologically.

Pregnancy is one of the states in question. It may be supposed that enhanced cell division in the pregnant organism calls for a high level of synthesis of cholesterol which is vital for the "synthesis" of new cells as a building material for cell membrane formation. Intensification of cholesterol synthesis during pregnancy is achieved in the following way (see Chapter 21). The output of chorionic somatomammotropin, which has the properties of growth hormone, as well as the production of some other hormones, reduces the level of glucose utilization by muscle tissue in the pregnant organism. This is followed by compensatory hyperinsulinemia, which leads to body fat accumulation and results in intensified lipolysis in the second half of pregnancy (Felig 1977). With a high level of FFA utilization, a secondary decrease in the muscle uptake of glucose occurs (Randle 1965). As a consequence, an intensified utilization of FFA becomes the chief source of energy supply, which eventually results in a more intensive synthesis of both triglycerides and cholesterol (see Chapter 6). This thesis is supported by our data demonstrating that administration of phenformin to pregnant rats reduces the blood cholesterol level (see Chapter 21).

Thus, a higher rate of cholesterol synthesis takes place in the cases of combined glucose intolerance and adiposity. Accordingly, in repeatedly bred female rats, with each succeeding reproductive cycle the arterial lesions grow in complexity; in many aspects these correspond to atherosclerotic lesions in humans (Wexler and Lutmer 1975, Lewis and Wexler 1975).

The Pacific salmon (see Chapter 1), within one to two months, builds up vast stores of sperm and eggs. During this short time their sera becomes milky, containing as much as 1000 mg% cholesterol (Wexler 1976). In spawning Pacific salmon, generalized atherosclerosis and myocardial infarction may develop (Wexler 1976). This mechanism provides conditions for intensive cell division during pregnancy. However, the existence of this physiologic mechanism results in an intensification of atherosclerosis development in all situations where similar metabolic shifts are brought about by other factors, even though there is no physiologic need to create conditions providing for intensive cell division. In this sense the age-associated development of atherosclerosis is determined by the inappropriate hyperfunctioning of the mechanism that is needed to provide for the requirements of reproduction and development of the organism.

Some data show that patients with atherosclerosis may develop antibodies to lipoproteins (Beaumont 1970, Klimov 1973). However, the induction of antibodies to normal lipoproteins is theoretically impossible because of natural immune tolerance. As an explanation of this discrepancy I would suggest that the presence of such antibodies points indirectly to changes in the composition of lipoprotein compounds that result in the breakdown of natural tolerance, and that it is the increased need for the synthesis of triglycerides and cholesterol in the liver that brings about these changes (Dilman 1974a). Indeed, the enhanced synthesis of cholesterol and triglycerides should be accompanied by a relevant increase in the synthesis of apoproteins in the liver. It cannot be excluded that the overstimulated synthesis of apoproteins may result in changes in their structure, and consequently in the breakdown of natural tolerance to lipoproteins. Recently, significant modifications of the lipid and apoprotein composition of VLDL in rabbits made hypercholesterolemic by cholesterol feeding were described by Rodriguez and associates (1976).

The following aspect connected with the problem of atherosclerosis appears to be of interest. Data given in Chapter 15 indicate that the metabolic shifts typical of atherosclerosis are responsible for the development of the syndrome of metabolic immunodepression. Suppression of phagocytic activity, characteristic of the syndrome, can probably decrease the lipid resorption in the atheromatous plaque. Metabolic immunodepression stimulates the development of autoimmune disorders (see Chapter 16), which can intensify the autoimmune component of atherosclerosis. The hypothalamic mechanism of age-associated hypercholesterolemia presented in my earlier hypothesis (Dilman, unpublished data, 1958, 1960) suggests (with the support of numerous subsequent studies) an integrated network of atherosclerosis pathogenesis.[1] The basic element of this network is an elevation of the hypothalamic threshold of sensitivity to homeostatic stimuli, which in turn leads to an excessive effect of growth hormone, ACTH, and cortisol. This results in the following sequence of events: 1) a reduction in glucose tolerance; 2) hyperinsulinemia and fat accumulation; 3) an increased utilization of

[1]There is no doubt about the existence of age-associated hypercholesterolemia. However, cholesterol synthesis is generally considered to decrease with age (see Chapter 6). A number of considerations and data, such as the age-associated elevation of FFA levels and the age-associated intensification of the synthesis of triglycerides in the liver, as well as an intensified cholesterol synthesis in obesity and in stress, is not consistent with the statement that cholesterol synthesis decreases in man with advancing age.

FFA as energy-producing substrates; 4) an intensification of the synthesis of triglycerides, cholesterol, and VLDL, and probably of the modifications of the lipid and apoprotein composition of VLDL; 5) an increase in the blood level of LDL; 6) disturbances in the mechanism controlling the lipid content in the cell; 7) the intensified proliferation of arterial smooth muscle cells; 8) a decrease of HDL blood level; 9) metabolic immunodepression (decreasing in particular the activity of macrophages); 10) intensification of autoimmune disorders; and 11) an enrichment of cholesterol concentration in platelets, which alters their function in a manner that may promote aggregation and thrombosis (Colman 1978).

In the context of the above suggestions, let us compare some major stages of the elevating mechanism, which renders atherosclerosis a disease of aging, to the mechanisms of some internal and external environmental factors that promote atherosclerosis development. Of major importance are: 1) obesity, 2) maturity-onset diabetes mellitus, 3) decreased physical activity, 4) stress and depression, 5) tobacco smoking, 6) hypothyroidism, 7) hypertension, 8) ovariectomy before the age of 40; and 9) essential hyperlipoproteinemia. Let us consider some data showing that all factors that contribute to atherosclerosis induce metabolic changes similar to those inherent in normal aging, which accounts for their influence in the development of atherosclerosis.

The role of obesity in the development of atherosclerosis is determined by relevant metabolic shifts. For instance, obesity is characterized by hyperinsulinemia (see Chapter 11), a key factor in the development of subsequent pathogenic changes promoting atherogenesis. Also, in obesity both the synthesis of cholesterol and its blood level are increased. Of interest here are data correlating the quantity of fat cells with plasma glycerol; glycerol level with the rate of free fatty acid metabolism; size of fat cells with blood insulin level; triglyceride concentration with insulin level and carbohydrate tolerance; and finally, data showing that hyperinsulinemia increases the synthesis of very low density lipoproteins in the liver (Björntorp et al 1970).

The atherogenic role of late-onset diabetes mellitus and the high incidence of minimal signs of decreased glucose tolerance in patients suffering from atherosclerosis, are well known (Berns et al 1967, Wahlberg 1962). Moreover it has been shown that atherosclerosis incidence does not rise in familial Type I hyperlipoproteinemia, which does not involve disturbances in glucose tolerance (Kuo, 1969). Atherosclerosis is promoted by prediabetes and late-onset diabetes mellitus (Blagosklonnaya 1968), ie, in states characterized by excessive insulin levels (Kuo 1969). On the other hand, after analysis of the causes of death of 1500 patients with juvenile-onset diabetes mellitus, Bell (1952) found that atherosclerotic lesions were not solely responsible for the death of these patients. Therefore it may be inferred that atherosclerosis development is associated with hyperinsulinemia, which is typical of prediabetes, chemical late-onset diabetes, and aging.

Statistically it appears that treatment of diabetics with tolbutamide, which stimulates insulin secretion, results in an increased mortality from vascular diseases (Knatterud et al 1971).

Physical activity has been found to decrease blood insulin levels and to improve glucose tolerance (Björntorp et al 1972), as well as to increase HDL-cholesterol levels (Wood et al 1976). Accordingly, the sera from runners inhibits the incorporation of thymidine in the arterial cells (Rönnemaa et al 1978).

The role of stress in atherosclerosis is related to the fact that metabolic shifts inherent in stress and normal aging have much in common (see Chapter 21), particularly when lipolysis is intensified. The absence of hyperinsulinemia in stress does not improve the atherogenic situation because the loss of the insulin-suppressing effect on the adipose tissue leads to the enhancement of FFA levels. Stress does seem to raise the level of serum cholesterol, although no intensification of triglyceride synthesis is observed (Rothfeld et al 1974). Moreover thrombogenesis is increased in stress (because of a high concentration of free fatty acids [O'Brien et al 1976]), and platelet behavior is altered as a result of hyperadrenalinemia (Carvalho et al 1974) and hyperbetalipoproteinemia (Colman 1978). A negative correlation between blood oxysteroid level and fibrinolytic activity also plays some role (Menon et al 1967).

The effect of psychogenic factors and constitution on metabolic processes must also be considered. Noteworthy are data showing high blood levels of cholesterol, triglycerides, insulin, oxysteroids, and ACTH in coronary-prone (Type A) individuals (Friedman et al 1970, 1972a). This type of person also risks atherosclerosis.

The effect of tobacco smoking is similar to that of stress. Nicotine seems to intensify adrenaline secretion and lipolysis (Kershbaum et al 1963). It also has been shown that coronary blood flow is changed, which may affect the filtration mechanism. The intensified development of metabolic alterations inherent in atherosclerosis in dwarfs with isolated deficiency of growth hormone (Merimee et al 1972) may be explained by an increased lipolysis that is determined by an insufficient secretion of insulin.

In hypothyroidism there is a delayed conversion of cholesterol to bile acids, which leads to the development of hypercholesterolemia (Fowler and Swale 1967). The activity of lipoprotein lipase also is reduced (Bierman et al 1970). It was observed that a rise in the frequency of hidden autoimmune thyroiditis may start with hypercholesterolemia, revealing the syndrome of pre-myxedema (Fowler and Swale 1967, Vanhaelst et al 1977).

The role of arterial hypertension in atherosclerosis cannot be determined primarily by filtration mechanisms. Elevated blood insulin levels (Welborn et al 1966), gain of body fat content, and metabolic shifts—a complex of changes typical of hypothalamic pathology—often occur in essential hypertension (Lang 1950), and these may be the main factors determining the association of atherosclerosis with essential hypertension.

The influence of ovariectomy on atherosclerosis is determined by the estrogen effect on the energy homeostat according to the mechanism discussed in Chapters 6 and 8. The rate of development of atherosclerosis is greatly intensified in young women after castration. In addition to the influence of the estrogen deficit on metabolic pathways, these hormones also seem to exert an antiatherogenic effect on the vessels (Pick et al 1952). The administration of estrogens reduces age-associated hypercholesterolemia both in men and women (Barr 1955, Blagosklonnaya 1959, 1968). Administration of contraceptive steroid preparations reduces tolerance to carbohydrates and raises the level of insulin and triglycerides in the blood, which may contribute to the development of atherosclerosis.

There are several types of essential hyperlipidemia (Fredrickson et al 1967). Unlike Type I and Type V, which are characterized by a high blood chylomicron level but involve no simultaneous decrease in carbohydrate tolerance, the other types of essential hyperlipidemia, particularly Types IIa, IIb, and IV, provide metabolic factors conducive to atherosclerosis. These factors include increased blood levels of LDL, VLDL, triglycerides, and cholesterol (Jones 1973), as well as decreased HDL-cholesterol levels (Schafer et al 1978b). Hyperinsulinemia becomes a factor when the disturbances are carbohydrate-dependent (Reaven et al 1967, Tzagournis et al 1972). When they are fat-dependent, mechanisms responsible for triglyceride transport regulation, particularly that of lipoprotein lipase, are deranged, resulting in a rise in blood chylomicrons and a very low density of lipoproteins.

Thus the intensification of atherosclerosis as a result of certain provocative states appears to be caused by the same mechanisms that are responsible for this process in normal aging. Therefore, when atherosclerosis develops in young individuals, a higher cholesterol blood level is observed in these patients as compared with the control subjects, since the latter usually develop atherosclerosis because of inherent or acquired disorders, eg, hypothyroidism. On the contrary, no essential differences in the level of hyperlipidemia are found in the age group of 50–59, since the regulatory disorders typical of normal aging provide conditions for the development of atherosclerosis in each individual. When the factors accelerating the development of atherosclerosis come into play, their influence contributes to the different stages of a process already well under way.

Accordingly, symptomatic syndromes of atherosclerosis should be distinguished from atherosclerosis as a disease of compensation developing by a uniform mechanism. Like other diseases of compensation, the rate of atherosclerosis development is determined by a number of external environmental factors, thus creating the impression that atherosclerosis is a disease of civilization.

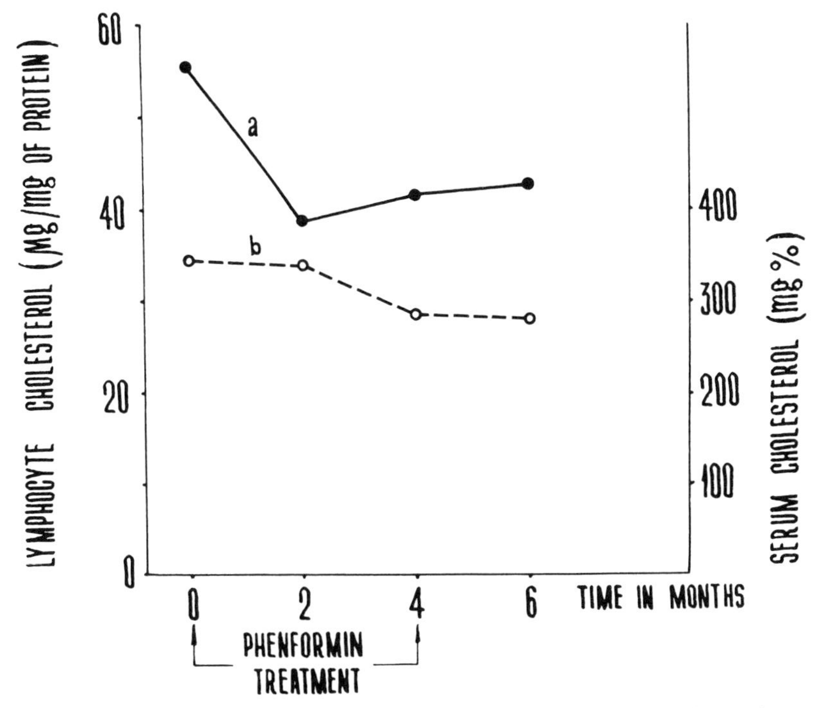

Figure 12-1 Effect of phenformin treatment (100 mg/day) on cholesterol concentrations in lymphocytes and in blood of patients with ischemic heart disease. Curve a: Concentration of cholesterol in lymphocytes. Curve b: Concentration of cholesterol in blood.

13 Essential Hypertension

When V.F. Lang in 1950 put forward a theory that hypothalamic disturbances provide the main pathogenic factor of essential hypertension, no one could have predicted that this concept could be tested by means of measurements of the blood level of prolactin, a hormone that stimulates lactation.

There are reports that blood sugar level, particularly after glucose loading, is higher in hypertensive patients than in normal (Berglund et al 1976). However, instead of useless probing into the influences of glucose on blood pressure, it is advisable to seek clues to the solution of this problem in the mechanisms of the hypothalamus.

An evaluation of the significance of external and internal factors for the development of arterial hypertension is complicated. On the basis of some parameters this disease would be regarded as a disease of adaptation, because the main etiopathogenic source of essential hypertension is provided by continuous, pent-up, negative emotions (Lang 1950), or by chronic stress. The influence of internal environmental factors undoubtedly is essential as well, with the elevation of hypothalamic activity of primary importance. The latter offers an explanation as to why the frequency of arterial hypertension increases with advancing age (Lang 1950). It would appear that in aged subjects even a relatively insignificant stress is sufficient to account for a rise in blood pressure. In young subjects, whose hypothalamic activity is not raised, arterial hypertension occurs rarely but assumes a more serious form, which points to considerable shifts taking place in the hypothalamus as yet undisturbed by aging.

It should be noted that the existing concepts of the etiopathogenesis of essential hypertension have undergone considerable cyclic changes. In the past the renal factor was considered to be of primary importance. Lang and his followers drew attention to the role of the hypothalamus, specifically its intensified activity in the course of development of arterial hypertension (Lang 1950), thus offering an explanation for the concomitant decrease in tolerance to carbohydrates, body weight gain, and hypercholesterolemia, as well as the increased blood insulin level (Welborn et al 1966). The frequent co-occurrence of these hypothalamic disturbances is a specific manifestation of the pathogenic role of the hypothalamus in the development of essential hypertension (Dilman 1958). The slowly rising incidence of hypertension in women at the stage of stabilization (Hollingsworth et al 1965) is in agreement with the concept of the hypothalamic-dependent genesis of this disease.

As the pathogenesis of systemic arterial hypertension was studied further, however, primary importance again was attached to the renal factor. The following sequence was suggested: renal ischemia-increased secretion of renin, rise in angiotensin I and II levels, and increased output of aldosterone (Crane 1978). This hypothesis was based on evidence showing that derangements in renal function take place even at early neurogenic stages of essential hypertension. At the same time it was established that the renal pressor mechanism of hypertension is implemented by a variant in which the main pathogenic factor is an augmented cardiac output rather than an increased peripheral vasoconstriction. Since cardiac output depends chiefly on the condition of some homeostatic systems, further investigations led ultimately to the interpretation of hypertension as a disease of homeostasis (Shapiro 1973), ie, dependent to a considerable degree on hypothalamic function. This approach was supported by the findings of Postnov (1973), which pointed to an enhanced neurosecretory function of the hypothalamus in different types of arterial hypertension.

This signifies a return to the hypothalamic-dependent genesis of hypertension where the age-associated increase in hypertension is caused by the elevating mechanism of aging. The disturbances of a homeostat regulating arterial blood pressure should be caused by a certain mechanism, for instance, a decline in biogenic amines in the hypothalamus. Of interest are the observations that some hypertensive patients reveal increased plasma prolactin concentration. This is a manifestation of the decline in dopamine level in the hypothalamus, as bromcriptine, agonist of dopamine, lowers both blood pressure and blood prolactin level (Stumpe et al 1977).[1] Essentially, if these findings are supported by other results, increased blood prolactin level will probably be considered a criterion for the differentiation of essential hypertension of hypothalamic origin from many types of symptomatic arterial hypertension. Moreover, if homeostatic disturbances responsible for arterial hypertension are caused by inevitable age-connected processes, eg, the drop of biogenic amines in the hypothalamus or some other areas of the CNS, essential hypertension may be regarded as a normal disease rather than one brought about by external environmental factors like chronic stress. Such an interpretation is supported by Boyle (1970), indicating that not only does the prevalence of hypertension increase with increasing age, but so does the mean blood pressure. It also provides an explanation of the co-occurence of hypertension and disturbed tolerance to carbohydrates, hypercholesterolemia, hyperinsulinemia, obesity, and cancer. It should be pointed out that although the development of systemic arterial hypertension is independent of other diseases of compensation, its development also is promoted by aging (Table 13-1).

Table 13-1
Frequency of Elevated Arterial Blood Pressure as Function of Body Weight and Age

Deviation of Body Weight from Ideal	Frequency of Elevated Arterial Blood Pressure (%)	
	25 to 35 years old	*40 to 45 years old*
− 15 and less	6	7
from − 14 to + 14	8	28
+ 15 and more	15	44

It is seen from Table 13-1 that obesity does not significantly influence the incidence of hypertension in younger subjects (25–35 years); however, this rate is lower in middle-aged subjects (40–45 years) with a relatively low body weight than in those who are overweight. This shows that the delayed, age-associated hypothalamic changes (manifested by a relatively small gain of body weight) are consonant with a reduced predisposition to hypertension, linking hypertension to diseases of compensation. It is interesting from an historical perspective that Way (1951)

[1]On the contrary, Holland and Gomez-Sanchez (1977) reported that plasma prolactin is decreased in essential hypertension. It should be mentioned that the mean age of the patients examined by the latter investigators was 51 ± 3 years, while in the study of Stumpe et al (1977), it was 21–27 years. It is possible that the accumulation of fat stores causes a drop in the secretion of both growth hormone and prolactin (see Chapter 6).

referred to arterial hypertension, obesity, and diabetes mellitus as the triad of symptoms most frequently found in patients with endometrial carcinoma. It should also be mentioned that elevated blood pressure is a risk factor for cancer (Dyer et al 1975). From the regulatory viewpoint, hypertension is a disease that involves an elevated excitability (or activity) of several hypothalamic centers. Such hyperactivity could not be maintained unless the hypothalamic threshold of sensitivity to regulatory stimuli were elevated. This thesis, however, has not been tested experimentally in essential hypertension.

14 Mental Depression

Low spirits in old age are a byproduct of the implementation of the program of organism development.

It is known that the rate of mental depression increases with age, particularly in postmenopausal women (Robinson 1975). Many aged persons regularly suffer from depression after an exposure to stress. At present, two groups of facts may be used to account for this relationship.

There is substantial evidence showing that depressions are associated with an absolute or relative decrease in catecholamines, particularly in noradrenaline, available at central adrenergic receptor sites (Schildkraut 1965). At the same time, insufficiency of the central serotonergic processes may be one of the reasons for the high rate of anxiety and tension in depressed elderly people (Averbukh and Lapin 1969). Thus, both adrenergic and serotonergic functional depletion of the brain is important to the mechanism of depression (Mass 1965).

Normal aging is accompanied by a decrease in the level of biogenic amines in the hypothalamus (Robinson et al 1972, Robinson 1975). The drop in biogenic amine level in the hypothalamus seems to be of particular importance for age-associated changes in the hypothalamic threshold of sensitivity to homeostatic regulation (see Chapter 18). If a shift in the hypothalamic threshold is a key factor in the implementation of the neuroendocrine program of the organism in development and aging, shifts in concentration of biogenic amines and the resultant age-associated depression that accompany this process may be interpreted as normal disease. From this point of view the occurrence of age-associated depression is an inevitable outcome of the organism's genetic program for development and aging.

There is a plausible explanation for the stress-induced development of depression. The rise in ACTH secretion is a component of stress reactions. Meanwhile, there is considerable neuropharmacologic evidence that a brain noradrenergic system exerts tonic inhibition of ACTH secretion (Ganong 1974, Scapagnini et al 1973, Gruen 1978). Therefore, increased ACTH secretion is caused by a decrease in the hypothalamic level of noradrenaline. Stress may cause depression, particularly in middle-aged persons, who are characterized by the age-associated drop in catecholamine level in the hypothalamus. This interpretation of the depression mechanism is consistent with the hypothesis of Lapin and Oxenkrug (1969) on the self-reproduction of the depressive cycle in stress. According to this hypothesis, supported by the findings of Curzon (1969), stress stimulates hypothalamic activity, which leads to a rise in blood cortisol. The latter activates tryptophan pyrrolase, leading to reduced synthesis of serotonin, inhibition of the amygdala, and activation of the hypothalamus. As a result, a vicious circle is formed which aggravates depression (Dilman et al 1979b).

Regardless of the influence of stressor factors, the age-associated disturbances in biogenic amine metabolism affect the hormonal secretory pattern in a depressed individual, particularly that of cortisol. According to Gruen (1978), in depressed individuals there are more secretion spikes with a higher absolute plasma level of cortisol. Hence, stress may contribute to mental depression development, while mental depression proper leads to an elevation of cortisol, characteristic of stress. In turn, the fall in brain monamines may also be a consequence of increased adrenocortical activation (Nisticò et al 1969). Although there is a large body of convincing evidence on the role of the fall in biogenic amines in the hypothalamus in the pathogenesis of mental depression, the determinations of biogenic amine excretion level do not provide conclusive data on their concentration in the hypothalamus because they are also produced by other systems.

However, application of the dexamethasone suppression test offers a means for estimating the biogenic pattern of the hypothalamus, since there is a correlation between the sensitivity of CNS structures to inhibition by dexamethasone and the level of biogenic amines in the brain (see Chapters 3 and 18). Carroll and coworkers (1976) used a short-term dexamethasone test to show that the steroid-sensitive neurons of the hypothalamus in depressive patients are subjected to an abnormal drive from another limbic area. These findings agree with our results. For example, Table 14-1 shows that 0.5 mg of dexamethasone administrated at 11 PM in the depressive phase in patients with endogenous depression did not affect blood cortisol level in the blood sampled at 9 AM the following morning. However, in the intermission phase, the same dose of dexamethasone was followed by a decrease in blood cortisol similar to that in healthy subjects. Since this type of dexamethasone test gives an evaluation of the impulse mechanism of ACTH secretion (see Chapter 3), it is desirable to study sensitivity of the hypothalamic-pituitary complex to dexamethasone in depressive patients by means of a long-term dexamethasone test. The latter technique is preferable because it assesses the hypothalamic basal feedback mechanisms rather than the impulsive extrahypothalamic mechanism that governs adaptive homeostat func-

Table 14-1
Short-Term Dexamethasone Test
in Normal Subjects and in Depressive Patients

		11-Hydroxycorticosteroids (μg%)		
	No. Cases	*Basal Level*	*After Dexamethasone*	Inhibition (%)
Normal subjects	17	13.2 ± 1.4	4.3 ± 1.4	−65 ± 1
Depressive Patients				
Depressive stage	24	20.2 ± 1.1	18.0 ± 1.4	−9 ± 7
Remission stage	24	19.5 ± 1.5	7.8 ± 1.0*	−63 ± 3*
L-Dopa†				
Before treatment	14	20.6 ± 1.8	11.5 ± 1.3	−38 ± 7
After treatment	14	19.3 ± 1.9	6.1 ± 0.9*	−52 ± 10
L-Tryptophan‡				
Before treatment	20	20.1 ± 1.5	12.0 ± 1.5	−40 ± 7
After treatment	20	20.0 ± 1.9	8.2 ± 1.4*	−59 ± 4*

Short-term dexamethasone test performed as in Table 3-4.
*Difference is statistically significant ($p < 0.05$).
†L-Dopa (1 to 3 g daily) was administered during one week to depressive patients or patients with parkinsonism.
‡L-Tryptophan (3 to 6 g daily) was administered during one week to depressive or neurotic patients.

tion. It is likely that a long-term dexamethasone test will be able to establish whether there is a biogenic amine deficiency in the hypothalamus of depressive patients in the intermission phase. Such data are desirable both for evaluating the role of stress in the pathogenesis of mental depression and for establishing a tendency to mental depression whenever such predisposition has been caused by metabolic disorders or the decline in biogenic amine level in the brain.

Table 14-1 shows that administration of L-tryptophan, 3 to 6 g daily for seven days, improves sensitivity of the hypothalamic-pituitary complex to suppression by dexamethasone in patients with mental depression. It is also known that 5-hydroxytryptophan treatment, particularly in combination with nicotinic acid administration, mitigates mental depression. This serves to indicate that the dexamethasone test can be used to evaluate the condition of the serotonergic system of the brain, which is one of the factors of mental depression pathogenesis.

The effect of L-dopa treatment on the dexamethasone test in depressive patients has not been studied yet, although there are data available on the influences of this drug on the secretion of growth hormone and prolactin (Gold and Goodwin 1977). It should be pointed out that the results of determination of the action of neurotransmitters or their precursors on pituitary hormone secretion are not sufficient for establishing the threshold of hypothalamic-pituitary complex sensitivity to various homeostatic stimuli. Unless stress is considered to be the main etiopathogenic factor of mental depression, it seems desirable to study changes in the threshold of sensitivity of the hypothalamic-pituitary complex not only in the adaptive homeostat but in other main homeostatic systems as well. Such studies are indispensable both for better understanding the etiopathogenesis of mental depression and elucidating the relationships between this syndrome and specific diseases of aging.

15 Metabolic Immunodepression

It is likely that, when assessing the age-associated decline in the blastogenic response of lymphocytes to the tuberculin skin test, we actually study a certain metabolic syndrome rather than intrinsic changes in the function of the immune system.

The efficiency of cell-mediated immunity decreases with advancing age. In particular, elderly individuals have a depressed delayed skin reaction (Waldorf et al 1968), and lymphocytes from aged subjects show decreased blastogenesis in response to mitogens (Pisciotta et al 1967). Some reports show a progressive decline in the number of circulating T cells in humans (Smith et al 1974, Teasdale et al 1976), but others show no change (Davey and Huntington 1977).

To some extent, these discrepancies may be accounted for by the reports that aging involves an increased incidence of certain diseases that are characterized by the rise in T-lymphocytes (Ferguson et al 1977). However, it is important to point out that although no significant alteration in the absolute number of total T and B cells and unmarked cells occurs among various age groups, many reports indicate a reduction in cellular immune response in the aged. Thus, the age-associated reduction in cellular immune response may relate rather to T-cell dysfunction than to the reduction in thymic cell population (Davey and Huntington 1977). In this respect, it is necessary to stress that in an immune response the antigen (mitogen) triggers T cells to proliferate and transform into effector cells. Therefore. the diminution of the proliferative capacity of T cells may lead to a diminished intensity of specific immune reactions, which are realized or controlled by T-dependent lymphocytes.

In contrast, the capacity for autoantibody synthesis does not appear depressed with aging. Older humans exhibit a rise in the incidence of autoantibodies. It may be stressed that the incidence of autoantibodies increases significantly among subjects with low levels of phytohemagglutinin response (Hallgren et al 1973). Consequently, aging individuals can become prime targets of T-cell-susceptible microbes and other naturally occurring intrinsic and extrinsic agents (eg, mutated cancer cells and drugs), and these attacks can lead to various types of debilitating diseases (Makinodan 1977, 1978).

There are different hypotheses on the cause of age-dependent immunodepression. There is a consensus that the involution and atrophy of the thymus is the key to aging of the immune system (Makinodan 1978). Burnet (1969, 1976) suggested the role of clonal exhaustion, where thymic cells with a genetically programmed clock mechanism for self-destruction die, having undergone a fixed number of divisions.

Recently, I adduced some arguments suggesting the functional nature of age-related immunodepression (Dilman 1977, 1978a; Dilman et al 1976). This concept is based on both experimental results and theoretical considerations. Regarding experimental data, it should be mentioned first of all that present-day investigations on the problem are being conducted in two directions.

Mertin and colleagues (Field and Shenton 1974, Mertin and Hughes 1975, Meade and Mertin 1978) described the inhibitory effects of polyunsaturated fatty acids on immune cells in vitro and in vivo and suggested an immunoregulatory role of unsaturated fatty acids.

Our laboratory reported some evidence demonstrating that the age-associated decline in the effectiveness of cellular immunity is, to a considerable degree, caused by metabolic changes involved in normal aging. For example, the administration of an antidiabetic drug, phenformin, and an antiatherosclerotic preparation, clofibrate, improved metabolic parameters and the indices of the blastogenic response of lymphocytes to PHA and raised the phagocytic index and lysosomal activity of monocytes in patients with ischemic heart disease (Dilman et al 1976, 1978; Nemirovsky et al 1978).[1] Hence, both phenformin and clofibrate appeared to improve cellular immunity indices, which results suggest an interrelation between metabolic and immunologic parameters.

---

[1]The choice of ischemic heart disease as a model of an aging process was determined by the fact that it involves metabolic shifts, similar to those of normal aging, yet more pronounced (see Chapter 12).

The above data made it possible to suggest a phenomenon of metabolic immunodepression, ie, immunodepression caused by a set of metabolic shifts.[1] Three points should be emphasized in this connection. First, the increase in the number of T cells caused by phenformin treatment supports the hypothesis of a metabolically regulated affinity of the receptors on the surface of T cells (Wybran and Fudenberg 1975). Extrinsic modulation of T lymphocyte E-rosette function in many respects appears to be similar to the changes in insulin receptors in accordance with the blood level of insulin (Archer et al 1975). Second, metabolic immunodepression may be mitigated and even eliminated by a pharmacologic correction of the metabolic pattern. Third, if metabolic immunodepression involves the suppressor T cells, then their disturbance should be accompanied by an increase in the response of B-lymphocytes. It follows that the elimination of metabolic immunodepression can contribute to normalizing B-lymphocyte function, thus improving the trend toward some autoimmune processes (Dilman 1977, 1978a). This aspect of the metabolic immunodepression mechanism is also related to the mechanism of immunization and may be used to improve the effectiveness of immunization in middle-aged patients with a metabolic immunodepression syndrome (see Chapter 16). Initially, I thought that the immunoregulatory action of polyunsaturated fatty acids (PUFA) proposed by Mertin and coworkers and the syndrome of metabolic immunodepression were two manifestations of the same phenomenon. This approach seems to be supported by Meade and Mertin (1978). PUFA are dietary essential fatty acids. Therefore, though these acids play a key role, particularly as membrane components and prostaglandin precursors, they should be regarded rather as the extrinsic factors of immunoregulation. For instance, Mertin and Hughes (1975) reported that linoleic acid and, to an even greater extent, arachidonic acid, suppressed the PHA-induced blastogenic response of lymphocytes, while saturated fatty acids and even oleic acid had very little specific activity.

An enhanced lipolysis, concomitant with pathologic states involving metabolic immunodepression, is not accompanied by a predominant rise of PUFA in the blood. Moreover, diets rich in PUFA produce immunosuppression (Mertin and Hughes 1975), although PUFA are known to lower the blood levels of cholesterol, β-lipoprotein, and possibly insulin, ie, the major factors of metabolic immunodepression.

Therefore, it is desirable to consider the data available on the possible role of separate metabolic and hormonal factors in the mechanism of metabolic immunodepression.

---

[1] The suggestion that "there is a strong correlation between metabolic shifts and the condition of immunologic defenses" was made earlier (Dilman 1974a, p 371).

Free Fatty Acids (FFA)

It is known that some prostaglandins inhibit lymphocyte activity. The influence of prostaglandin precursors, PUFAs, on cellular immunity was studied and they were found to markedly suppress the blastogenic reaction of lymphocytes (Meade and Mertin 1978). FFA inhibit the activity of the reticuloendothelial system (Berken and Benacerraf 1968). The high level of FFA produces a cytotoxic effect in lymphoid cells (Kigoshi and Ito 1973). It is also possible that FFA participates in lymphocyte lysis caused by glucocorticoids (Turnell et al 1973). This serves to indicate that the deterioration of cellular immunity may occur when FFA, rather than glucose, becomes the main source of energy supply. Lipids suppress the activity of macrophages, too (Smith and Stuart 1975).

A correlation between a fat-rich diet and longer survival of a skin allograft was observed, and a diet poor in linoleic acid accelerates allograft rejection (Mertin and Hunt 1976). Thus, Mertin and colleagues point to the importance of the specific effects of polyunsaturated fatty acids, whereas the mechanism of lymphocytosis caused by long chain free fatty acids does not seem to be associated with the peculiarities of fatty acids. Moreover, there is evidence that starvation suppresses and overfeeding activates certain diseases (Newsholme 1977). Meanwhile, blood FFA level rises considerably during fasting (see Chapter 6).[1] Therefore, the rise in blood fatty acid level is not likely to be the key factor responsible for the syndrome of metabolic immunodepression.[2]

Cholesterol and Lipoproteins

The immune response of cells is elicited by the reception by lymphocytes of an stimulus that causes the latter to proliferate. Cell membranes play a key role in this process. Therefore, among metabolic factors capable of producing metabolic immunodepression, of particular importance is the rise in the level of cholesterol, an indispensable component of cell membrane structure.

One of the immediate consequences of mitogenic action on lymphocytes is the reduced microviscosity of their cell membranes (Toyoshima and Osawa 1975, Barnett et al 1974). It is known that saturation of membranes with cholesterol increases their microviscosity (Schinitzky and Inbar 1976). It was reported that the increased cholesterol concentration

[1]A long period of nutritional deprivation, particularly protein deprivation, produces a "nutritional thymectomy," ie, a decrease in immunologic vigor (Jose et al 1972), although moderate dietary restriction improves cellular immunity (Jose and Good 1972, Fernandes et al 1978).

[2]It was shown at our laboratory that an intravenous injection of fat emulsion (intralipid) into normal subjects is followed by a fall in the rate of the lymphoblast transformation reaction induced in humans by PHA.

in lymphocytes inhibits the mitogen-induced microviscosity of lymphocyte membranes and the subsequent incorporation of thymidine in the DNA of cells (Toyoshima and Osawa 1976). Membrane saturation with cholesterol leads to an elevated activity of adenylcyclase (Sinha et al 1977), while lymphoblast transformation involves a decrease in adenylcyclase activity. Hence, excessive cholesterol inhibits a number of processes indispensable for carrying out the reaction of lymphoblast transformation.[1]

At the same time, however, cholesterol is required for the proliferation of cells, inducing lymphocytes. It was demonstrated that dividing cells are characterized by an increased endogenous synthesis of cholesterol and a higher concentration of receptors of low density lipoproteins that ensure the cell supply of exogenous cholesterol (Brown et al 1975, Goldstein and Brown 1975). Inhibition of cholesterol synthesis in lymphocytes blocks the mitogen-induced incorporation of thymidine in DNA (Chen et al 1975), whereas the supply of exogenous cholesterol restores this process (Kandutsch and Chen 1977).

Since cholesterol exerts opposite effects on the processes taking place during lymphocyte stimulation, there should be some optimal level of this substance in cells and a shift toward either direction should impair function. Therefore, it is not surprising that reduced blast transformation was observed in in vitro experiments with liposome-induced changes in the cholesterol level of lymphocytes, both at an increased (Alderson and Green 1975) and decreased (Chen and Keenan 1977) level of this substance. In both cases, differences in cholesterol levels were approximately 15% of control concentration.

Concerning situations in vivo, it should be mentioned that blood cholesterol is a component of different classes of lipoproteins, which interact with cells, including lymphocytes. The chief source of exogenous cholesterol supply to cells are low density lipoproteins (LDL), which are produced from very low density lipoproteins (VLDL) secreted by the liver (Eisenberg and Levy 1975, Schafer et al 1978a). LDLs are absorbed by the special receptors of cells (Brown et al 1975; Rechless et al 1978; Ho et al 1976a, 1976b, 1977). Cholesterol may penetrate into cells in the course of nonspecific pinocytosis and the immediate exchange of lipids between cell membranes and lipoproteins (Brown et al 1975). Some cholesterol is excreted from cells when they interact with high density lipoproteins (HDL) (Stein and Stein 1976). The regulation of the endogenous synthesis and exogenous supply of cholesterol is provided to maintain its concentration in cells at a constant level (Nervi and Dietschy

[1] Kandutsch et al (1978) stressed that the biologic activity of some oxygenated derivatives of cholesterol are more potent than cholesterol itself. In particular, Humphries and McConnell (1979) showed that oxidized cholesterol, 25-hydroxycholesterol, exerts an immunosuppressive effect.

1978) and is effected by changing LDL receptor concentration. It is particularly important as far as lymphocytes are concerned, because the maintenance of the optimal concentration of cholesterol for their function must be assured. The rate of endogenous cholesterol synthesis increases as exogenous cholesterol supply decreases (Fogelman et al 1975, 1977; Ho et al 1977; Laporte et al 1978) and cholesterol excretion from cells is intensified (Ho et al 1977). Cholesterol synthesis is enhanced when it is increasingly used for the build-up of cell membranes during lymphocyte division (Chen et al 1975, 1978).

It may be supposed that the mechanisms of maintenance of cholesterol concentration in lymphocytes in vivo at an optimal level continue to function properly even in some inborn diseases. The lymphocytes from patients with such extreme disorders as familial hypercholesterolemia and abetalipoproteinemia were reported to show the same level of cholesterol as those from healthy subjects (Ho et al 1977). Waddell et al (1976) showed that plasma from patients with primary type IV and V hyperlipoproteinemia inhibited ^{3}H-thymidine incorporation into lymphocytes. The inhibiting effect was identified with the chylomicron and VLDL fraction isolated from the plasma and was concentration dependent. These data suggest that the effect of lipoproteins on lymphocytes is determined by some other factors which act upon the feedback mechanism responsible for the control of the plasma cell traffic of lipoproteins.

Curtiss and Edgington (1978) identified two subsets of low density lipoproteins that possess bioregulatory properties, namely: rosette-inhibitor factor and LDL-inhibitor. Subsequently, a lymphocyte surface receptor for low density lipoprotein inhibitor was found (Curtiss and Edgington 1978). It is possible that immunoregulatory lipoproteins can influence the uptake or synthesis of cholesterol by lymphocytes.

Our investigations show that the cholesterol level in lymphocytes increases in men and women with advancing age (Table 15-1).

Table 15-1
Relationship of Cholesterol Level in Lymphocytes to Age

Age (years)	Cholesterol Level (μg/mg protein)			
	Total		*Free*	
	Men	Women	Men	Women
20–29	25.0 ± 1.5	33.8 ± 2.0	20.8 ± 1.0	30.4 ± 2.2
30–49	34.3 ± 2.6	47.5 ± 5.0	31.4 ± 2.0	42.0 ± 3.8
Significance *(p)*	< 0.01	< 0.02	< 0.01	< 0.02

These changes are probably part of the decline in cellular immunity activity with aging. This conclusion is also supported by the results showing that administration of phenformin, a drug capable of mitigating metabolic immunodepression, lowers lymphocyte cholesterol level (see Figure 12-1). It may be suggested that this effect of phenformin is realized through its influence on the levels of certain hormones which may influence the function of the immune system.

Insulin

Reactive insulinemia is a typical manifestation of aging (see Chapter 6). Consider the possible role of hyperinsulinemia in the mechanism of metabolic immunodepression. It is doubtless that insulin deficiency can cause metabolic immunodepression. This may be inferred from the data demonstrating that insulin-induced palliation of metabolic disturbances in patients with insulin-dependent diabetes mellitus results in an improvement in some indices of cell-mediated immunity (Table 15-2). Similar results have been reported by other authors (MacCuish et al 1974, Bagdade et al 1974).

Insulin and other ligands (which increase intracellular level of cyclic GMP) augment thymus-derived lymphocyte effector activity, and the elimination of insulin deficit may improve the indices of cellular immunity by itself. Delespesse et al (1974) reported that addition of insulin to lymphocyte culture did not improve the PHA-induced blastogenic response in patients with diabetes mellitus. At the same time, normalization of metabolism induced by insulin, and particularly the antilipolytic effect of insulin, lowers the blood levels of many factors, to which I assign the pathogenic role in the mechanism of metabolic immunodepression. I suggest that improvement in glucose utilization leads to a drop in the blood FFA level, which lowers the cortisol level in the blood; consequently, insulin binding to lymphocytes is increased. Insulin-induced augmentation of lymphocyte-mediated cytotoxicity was observed by Strom and Bear 1975).

On the other hand, I suppose that hyperinsulinemia is a factor in the development of metabolic immunodepression. An increase in blood insulin reduced the concentration of insulin receptors of the plasma membrane of lymphocytes (monocytes) (Gavin et al 1974), which may result in a deterioration of glucose transport to these cells. This factor promotes the toxic effect of FFA on lymphocytes. The emergence of insulin receptors of lymphocytes during blastogenic response (Krug et al 1972) may be mitigated by hyperinsulinemia. It is possible that hyperinsulinemia also inhibits the phagocytic activity of macrophages (Bar et al 1976). Hence, the influence of insulin on the immune system is determined, to a considerable degree, by the blood insulin level, with both hypo- and hyperinsulinemia as possible sources of metabolic immunodepression.

Table 15-2
Comparison of Metabolic and Immunologic Parameters in Healthy Subjects and in Patients with Uncompensated and Compensated Juvenile Diabetes Mellitus

Parameter	Healthy Controls (20–29 years)	Diabetes Mellitus (n = 14)		
		Uncompensated	*Compensated*	*p*
Blood glucose (mg%)	80 ± 3	270 ± 11	145 ± 8	< 0.001
Blood cholesterol (mg%)	188 ± 8	248 ± 20	236 ± 8	< 0.05
Blood triglycerides (mg%)	108 ± 10	224 ± 39	181 ± 22	< 0.05
Free Fatty Acids (μEq/liter)	452 ± 35	890 ± 70	455 ± 43	< 0.001
11-Hydroxycorticosteroids (μg%)	12.1 ± 1.0	20.6 ± 0.7	15.0 ± 0.7	< 0.001
T-lymphocytes (%)	70 ± 1	64 ± 1	72 ± 1	< 0.01
B-lymphocytes (%)	15.5 ± 1.2	31 ± 2	30 ± 2	< 0.05
PHA-induced blast transformation (imp/min)*	67,927 ± 7018	32,077 ± 6473	87,997 ± 7782	< 0.01
Phagocytosis index (%)†	43 ± 3	16 ± 3	30 ± 5	< 0.05
Phagocytic activity (%)‡	135 ± 14	48 ± 14	107 ± 20	< 0.05
Lysosomal activity of monocytes (units per 100 cells)	388 ± 24	208 ± 21	240 ± 24	< 0.05

*Imp/min – impulses per minute.
†Phagocytosis index: percentage of phagocytes with intracellular latex particles.
‡Phagocytic activity: mean number of "ingested" latex particles per 100 phagocytes.

Growth Hormone and Prolactin

Some experimental data show that growth hormone (GH) deficit lowers immunologic activity (Pierpaoli et al 1970, Fabris et al 1972, Astaldi et al 1972). But some findings indicate that prolactin is the hormone most likely to play a major role in the thymus-regulated immune function (Pierpaoli et al 1976). It should be mentioned that obesity typical of the elderly is responsible for the decline in the basal level of GH (see Chapter 5). This factor may be conducive to metabolic immunodepression. It cannot be ruled out that, with obesity, secretion of prolactin is inhibited, too, since its level should rise with advancing age as a result of the decrease in dopamine level in the hypothalamus. However, the fact that patients with uncompensated diabetes mellitus reveal metabolic immunodepression (see Table 15-2) (although such cases are characterized by an elevated GH level) indicates that the age-related decrease in GH concentration cannot be regarded as a key factor of metabolic immunodepression.

Thyroid Hormones

These hormones stimulate the efficiency of immunity (Pierpaoli et al 1970). Meanwhile, a rise in blood cholesterol (β-lipoproteins) level reduces the iodine uptake by the thyroid (see Chapter 7). Therefore, it is possible an improved metabolism caused by administration of phenformin may stimulate thyroid function, thus leading to an improvement of cell-mediated immunity.

Glucocorticoids

The immunosuppressive action of glucocorticoids is well known. It is important to point out that even physiologic variations in cortisol level probably influence the immune system (Tavadia et al 1975). Apart from the direct action of glucocorticoids on lymphocytes, excessive cortisol causes metabolic shifts which lead to the predominant utilization of FFA for energy supply, thus intensifying gluconeogenesis (see Chapter 3). Phenformin treatment, on the other hand, reduces blood cortisol level (Dilman et al 1975), probably as a result of improved glucose utilization. It is impossible at present to adequately distinguish the direct immunosuppressive action of glucocorticoids and immunodepression caused by glucocorticoid-induced metabolic shifts.

The Thymus and Its Hormones

It may be supposed that metabolic immunodepression is brought about, at least partially, through changes in thymic function. There is some evidence that the pituitary gland produces a certain effect on the thymus (Fabris et al 1972), while the thymus influences the hormonal profile of the organism (Pierpaoli et al 1976). Moreover, recent studies strongly suggest that the thymus can actively modify the internal environment (Fabris and Piantanelli 1978).

However, the effect of the pattern inherent in metabolic immunodepression on thymic function has not yet received sufficient attention. Injection of free fatty acids is followed by a reduction in the weight of the thymus (Meade and Mertin 1978). Therefore, none of these factors can be considered solely responsible for metabolic immunodepression.

A review of our data points to several metabolic factors in the suppression of cell-mediated immunity: increased free fatty acid blood levels, hypercholesterolemia (or more precisely the increased blood level of β-lipoproteins), hypertriglyceridemia, and hyperinsulinemia. This metabolic pattern occurs in such different processes as normal aging, obesity, maturity-onset diabetes mellitus, atherosclerosis, mental depression, and various types of cancer (see Chapters 11–17). Correspondingly, immunodepression is observed in all these states. A similar metabolic pattern and immunodepression are induced by pregnancy as well as by chemical carcinogens (see Chapter 20). Thus, it seems that metabolic factors do contribute to the immunodepression development inherent in all these states.

However, the suggested correlation between a definite metabolic syndrome and the decrease in the efficiency of cell-mediated immunity does not explain the relationship between these two syndromes. Hypercholesterolemia caused by the rise in the blood levels of VLDL and LDL is most likely the key factor in metabolic immunodepression development, because hypercholesterolemia as well as the elevated FFA level in the blood inevitably occur in the states exhibiting the syndrome of metabolic immunodepression. Of these two factors, the raised blood levels of FFA and cholesterol, the latter is of greater importance. For example, a reduced calorie diet improves immune vigor, which may be partially caused by the decrease in blood corticosterone level (Pierpaoli 1977). However, calorie restriction lowers the cholesterol level in blood and raises that of FFA. An elevation of blood levels of insulin and triglycerides is not an indispensable component of metabolic immunodepression because stress simultaneously reduces these indices and immune vigor. On the other hand, age-associated hyperinsulinemia is a key factor in the formation of the metabolic pattern inherent in normal aging (see Chapter 6).

It is evident that there are no conclusive data on the role of separate metabolic and hormonal factors in the metabolic immunodepression mechanism. Conversely, certain states involving the metabolic immunodepression syndrome are characterized by a set of metabolic shifts that probably disturb homeostatic mechanisms in lymphocytes, resulting, for instance, in an increased level of cholesterol. In this context, it is possible to explain the fact that the cholesterol level in lymphocytes is not elevated, as compared with considerable shifts in blood cholesterol concentration observed in patients with familial hypercholesterolemia (Ho et al 1977). The age-connected rise in cholesterol level in lymphocytes is concomitant with relatively insignificant increases in blood cholesterol. Therefore, to elucidate the mechanism of metabolic immunodepression, it seems justified to adduce some highly hypothetical considerations based on the analysis of physiologic interrelations which probably underlie this syndrome.

Most T lymphocytes circulate in peripheral blood as differentiated cells. Like all differentiated cells of higher organisms, they possess a definite life span. But once they come into contact with a new antigen, T cells undergo a sequence of changes that eventually culminate in the blastogenic response of lymphocytes and T cell division.

There is still another consequence of blast transformation which distinguishes T cells from somatic cells. This is the ability of a T lymphocyte to deviate from the course of natural development of a common mature somatic cell, ie, to avoid age-associated death. In this respect, T lymphocytes may be rightfully likened to unicellular organisms that are virtually immortal because of cell division. It seems reasonable to suppose that the internal environment of the animal organism, which constitutes the external environment for T cells, should determine the destiny of the latter, like the external environment does for unicellular organisms. Figuratively speaking, the body of a higher organism is an ocean in which unicellular-like lymphocytes float, engage all extraneous matter in their habitat, and multiply and eliminate foreign bodies by means of immunologic defenses.

Using this metaphor, one cannot fail to see still more profound interrelationships between the higher organism and T cells: while the organism serves as a habitat for T cells, the latter are used by the former as a peculiar source of energy-producing substances. A stable homeostasis in any organism would be impossible unless the stores of the main energy substrates, glycogen, FFA, and amino acids, were provided. Glucose is stored in glycogen, FFA in adipose tissue, and amino acids, probably, in T lymphocytes. The lymphatic system has a considerable mass which is easily destroyed, releasing protein and amino acids into blood. Moroz and Kendych (1975) cite experimental findings showing that the chief mobile source of free amino acids mobilized by glucocorticoids is lymphoid rather than muscle tissue. The lysis of lymphocytes is, in this respect, similar to the lipolysis in adipose tissue and to glycogen degradation in the liver. In many cases, eg, in stress, all these processes occur simultaneously and are induced at initial stages by the same stressor hormone, adrenaline. Let us consider the interaction between energy-producing and immune processes underlying the phenomenon of metabolic immunodepression, from this point of view, using the instance of stress reaction.

The animal organism uses two substrates for energy supply, glucose and FFA. During fasting, eg, at night, when food is not taken, FFA supplied from fat depots is used as a source of energy. FFA are mobilized from fat depots by mediation of lipolytic hormones, ie, chiefly, by GH. At the same time, FFA is capable of inhibiting the glucose uptake by muscle tissue. As a result, glucose reserves are kept for energy supply of the neurons. However, the intake of such energy substrates as carbohydrates and fats makes the utilization of glucose stores unnecessary and, therefore, both the secretion of GH and lipolysis become inhibited.

Hence, there exist two separate and antagonistic rhythms of energy substrate utilization (see Chapter 6). For example, in stress this antagonism is distinct. It is natural that the defense from stressor factors should call for an increased consumption of energy. Stress involves a predominant utilization of FFA. Therefore, stress switches on a mechanism that ensures the uptake of FFA rather than glucose by target tissues. One of the features of this mechanism is the elevation of hypothalamic activity followed by a rise in the levels of secretion of such lipolytic and contra-insulin hormones as growth hormone, ACTH, and prolactin (see Chapter 19). As a result, lipolysis is enhanced. An increased utilization of FFA leads in turn to a decrease in glucose uptake by muscle tissue. As a result, when FFA become the main source of energy supply a compensatory synthesis of glucose from noncarbohydrate substances, eg, amino acids, is intensified. FFA stimulate gluconeogenesis and causes the lysis of lymphocytes, thus contributing to the pool of glycogenic amino acids. The same effect is exerted by cortisol, the level of which rises in stress.

These changes cause a shift in the energy supply system indispensable for the defense from stress. At the same time, the death of some T-lymphocytes results in a decline in the efficacy of cellular immunity. This indicates that the deterioration of cellular immunity may occur, when FFA, but not glucose, becomes the main source of energy supply.

Therefore, the deterioration of cellular immunity as a result of a shift toward the predominant utilization of FFA for energy supply was designated as "metabolic immunodepression." Metabolic immunodepression caused by the participation of the immune system in energy homeostasis may be designated as an acute type, or type I of metabolic immunodepression. This condition may transform to type II, a more stable metabolic immunodepression related to cell division.

An enhanced cell division calls for a certain set of metabolic conditions. These include a high blood level of cholesterol or an enhanced rate of cholesterol synthesis in the cell for the production of the additional plasma membrane required to enclose two daughter cells. Cholesterol synthesis, however, will not increase unless a metabolic shift toward the predominant utilization of FFA for energy supply takes place. Such a metabolic shift naturally occurs during pregnancy, when a rapid increase in the cell mass of the fetus is required (see Chapter 21). The efficiency of cellular immunity is reduced during pregnancy; otherwise the fetus would be rejected by cellular (transplantation) immunity. Numerous hormonal factors which are at work during pregnancy, as well as fetal proteins, produce an immunosuppressive effect, particularly in incipient pregnancy (Contractor and Davies 1973) when the lipid metabolic shift has not occurred. However, as pregnancy progresses, the output of chorionic somatomammotropin, which has the properties of growth hormone, reduces the level of glucose utilization. This is followed by a compensatory hyperinsulinemia which leads to fat accumulation, resulting in intensified lipolysis in the second half of pregnancy.

FFA does not pass through the placental barrier (Felig 1977). Therefore, with the high level of FFA utilization in the maternal organism, a secondary decrease in muscle uptake of glucose occurs. As a consequence, an intensified utilization of FFA becomes the chief source of energy supply. This shift leads to an intensified synthesis of cholesterol in the maternal organism. Cholesterol is transported to the fetoplacental unit where it is utilized for cell formation and steroid hormone synthesis. Simultaneously, in the maternal organism, hypercholesterolemia or the increased blood level of specific low density lipoproteins causes the suppression of T cell division, since it increases cholesterol accumulation in the plasma membranes of T lymphocytes, thus bringing about metabolic immunodepression of type II.

Both types of metabolic immunodepression often occur in succession under the same conditions because the development of hypercholesterolemia results, in most cases, from the increased utilization of FFA for energy supply. Thus, disturbances in carbohydrate metabolism induce hypercholesterolemia, indispensable for an intensified "synthesis of cells" during pregnancy, as well as for maintaining metabolic immunodepression. This thesis is supported by the data obtained in our laboratory showing that administration of phenformin to pregnant rats lowers blood cholesterol level (see Chapter 21) and may reduce metabolic immunodepression in humans (Dilman 1978a). In other words, the suppression of cell-mediated immunity and development of metabolic conditions for cell mass build-up are achieved by the same pathway.

At the same time, the process of aging involves a complex of metabolic shifts similar to the changes inherent in normal pregnancy. A decreased uptake of glucose by muscles, build-up of adipose tissue, intensification of FFA utilization, a rise in the blood levels of insulin, VLDL, LDL, triglycerides, and cholesterol, a slight increase in blood cortisol level, and some other signs are typical of the metabolic patterns of pregnancy and aging (see Chapter 18).

Evidence of the two physiologic mechanisms (demonstrable in stress and in pregnancy) which are probably responsible for the metabolic immunodepression syndrome, makes it clear why it is impossible to identify the key factor of its development on the basis of present data. The administration of phenformin, clofibrate, and sometimes insulin reduces metabolic immunodepression and affects the different pathogenic components of the general network. It should be noted that, under certain conditions, the same effect is produced both by raising blood insulin level (in the treatment of uncompensated insulin-dependent diabetes mellitus, as in Table 15-2) and lowering the same, as in phenformin treatment. Table 15-3 presents our observations of certain hormonal, metabolic, and immunologic shifts caused by administration of phenformin to patients with ischemic heart disease and mammary cancer.

Table 15-3
Effect of Phenformin Treatment on Endocrine, Metabolic, and Immunologic Parameters in Patients with Breast Cancer or Ischemic Heart Disease

Parameter	Before Treatment (mean ± SE)	After Treatment (mean ± SE)	Significance*
Breast Cancer:			
Body weight (kg)	80.4 ± 2.7	77.3 ± 2.4	S
Body fat content (%)	44.0 ± 0.8	41.6 ± 0.6	S
Glucose tolerance (mg%)			
60 min	163 ± 10	128.4 ± 7.6	S
120 min	148.0 ± 9.8	114.7 ± 8.7	S
Insulin (μg/ml)			
60 min	68.1 ± 12.0	42.8 ± 10.2	W
120 min	78.7 ± 16.2	34.8 ± 8.9	W
Growth hormone (ng/ml)			
0 min	2.3 ± 0.6	1.6 ± 0.7	NS
60 min	3.7 ± 0.5	2.0 ± 0.6	W
120 min	0.7 ± 0.4	0.5 ± 0.2	NS
Somatomedin (unit/ml)	1.80 ± 0.42	0.80 ± 0.24	W
FFA (μEq/liter)	811 ± 56	639 ± 24	S
Cholesterol (mg%)	282.5 ± 9.5	243.2 ± 12.0	S

Table 15-3
Effect of Phenformin Treatment on Endocrine, Metabolic, and Immunologic Parameters in Patients with Breast Cancer or Ischemic Heart Disease

Parameter	Before Treatment (mean ± SE)	After Treatment (mean ± SE)	Significance*
Triglycerdie (mg%)	205.4 ± 23.1	188.1 ± 27.2	W
PBI (mg%)	4.5 ± 0.2	5.3 ± 0.3	S
AMP (μM/g creatinine)	3.18 ± 0.26		S
PHA-induced blast transformation of lymphocytes (imp/min)	14,541 ± 3820	38,221 ± 5130	S
Rosette-forming cells (T cells) (%)	55.6 ± 2.4		NS
Lymphocytes (%)	31.8 ± 2.7	37.6 ± 3.2	W
DNCB†	3.5 ± 2.0	8.5 ± 1.2	S
PPD†	3.2 ± 3.3	15.5 ± 5.0	W
Candidin†	3.2 ± 2.0	12.4 ± 1.8	S
Schemic Heart Disease:			
Rosette-forming cells (%)	64 ± 2	73 ± 1	S
PHA-induced blast transformation of lymphocytes (imp/min)	3554 ± 111	36,599 ± 9560	S

*S: significantly different as determined by Student t-test ($p < 0.05$); W: significantly different as determined by non-parametric method after Wilcoxon ($p < 0.05$).
†Skin test results are expressed in mm and show the maximum diameter of papule.

It is obvious that these drugs act on the factors that may be conventionally referred to as the key factors of metabolic immunodepression (blood level of cholesterol or LDL, to be more precise), as well as auxiliary factors that contribute to hypercholesterolemia development. This fact makes it difficult at present to adequately identify the key contributing factors to metabolic immunodepression development. However, the same fact distinguishes this syndrome from that of cellular immunity suppression by polyunsaturated fatty acids.[1]

[1]Recently Mertin and Stackpoole (1978) showed that immunosuppression induced by polyunsaturated fatty acids is abolished by indomethacin.

Undoubtedly, one of the most intriguing problems is the mechanism by which an antigen switches on the neuroendocrine-metabolic component of immunologic response. Besedovsky and Sorkin (1977) suggest that endocrine responses occur as a consequence of antigenic stimulation of the hypothalamus. This viewpoint is consistent with the data that supported the existence of hypothalamic centers controlling the immune system (Filipp and Szentivenyi 1958, Lupparello et al 1964, Korneva et al 1978). Furthermore, if the hypothalamus is a target organ for an antigen, analysis of this problem should consider the shift in the set point of hypothalamic sensitivity with aging. Moreover, if Basedovsky and Sorkin (1977) are right in proposing a network of immunoneuroendocrine interactions, the latter should include not only hormonal but metabolic factors as well. Finally, interrelationships between cellular and humoral immunity provide another argument in support of the existence of physiologic mechanisms underlying the metabolic immunodepression syndrome (see Chapter 16). It should be mentioned that the phenomenon of metabolic immunodepression poses the question of whether the immune system itself becomes less efficient with increasing age, or whether metabolic shifts are the main causative factor of age-associated immune system suppression.

It was mentioned in the beginning of this chapter that the proliferative capacity of T cells in response to mitogens (phytohemagglutinin and concanavalin A) declines with age. However, it is precisely this proliferative capacity of T cells that is a function of the properties of blood plasma and, primarily, lipoprotein profile (Waddell et al 1976). Therefore, when the reaction of lymphoblast transformation is tested, it is the metabolic pattern of the internal environment of the organism rather than the immune system proper that is actually evaluated. In this case, we assess changes in body metabolism by means of indirect immunologic tests, eg, by suppression of the mitogen-induced lymphoblast transformation. It is possible that other tests for assessing the efficiency of cellular immunity have the same limitation, if the results of these tests depend on the condition of the internal environment. For instance, it cannot be ruled out that a negative DNCB or tuberculin skin test, which immunologically corresponds to the decline in cellular immunity, will directly correlate with death rates, for example, for traffic accidents because of the disorientation of patients suffering from cerebral atherosclerosis. This suggestion, no matter how inconsistent it may seem at first, is supported by the data showing that phenformin treatment lowers the blood levels of factors promoting atherosclerosis development (see Chapter 12) and raises the sensitivity of DNCB and tuberculin. Even if the processes influencing involution and atrophy of the thymus are thought to be the key to aging of the immune system (Makinodan 1978), it is necessary to consider the data indicating that fatty acids cause the suppression of the thymus (Meade and Mertin 1978). Therefore, it is possible that body fat tissue build-up, which suppresses the secretion of GH and probably prolactin as well as fat accumulation in the thymus, also causes thymic involution as a consequence of suppression of secretion of some hormones, eg, GH, and the direct action of fatty acids on thymocytes. Investigations of this problem may elucidate the contribution of changes in the cellular environment (ie, metabolic immunodepression syndrome), and age-connected changes in immune competent cells, to the decline in the vigor of cellular immunity with aging.

16 Autoimmune Disease

If someone thinks that to refer to climacteric, dysadaptosis, and obesity as a group of "normal diseases" is a far-fetched concept, then a question arises: Aren't normal antibodies a manifestation of the "normal disease" of the immune system?

Aging brings about an unusual immunologic situation that has not yet been properly explained: with the apparent decline in cellular immunity older humans exhibit a rise in the incidence of autoantibodies (Blumenthal 1967). Serum levels of IgG and IgA increase with age. According to Hallgren et al (1973), "these observations suggest that hyperglobulinemia, impaired lymphocyte phytohemagglutinin responsiveness, and increased frequency of autoantibodies are characteristic of surviving older humans and represent associated events in the natural history of human life."

Since aging involves an increased frequency of somatic mutations, some investigators including Burnet (1970) and Comfort (1972) are searching for a relationship between mutations, cancer, autoimmunity, and aging. Thus, the primary age-related effect of normal aging on the immune system is a decrease in T cell functional capacity. This decreased function is associated with the development of autoimmune phenomena, malignancy, and shortened life span (Greenberg and Yunis 1968).

However, Allison (1977) points out that if autoantibodies to the thyroid antigens may be induced by a simple procedure like immunization by saline extract of thyroid tissue, mutations cannot be the cause of autoimmunity. On the basis of the analysis of his own results, Allison (1977) concluded that T lymphocytes might provide a general mechanism for preventing or delaying autoimmune responses. This hypothesis is based on numerous data showing that T and B immune systems are connected by a reciprocal relationship (Stutman 1972, Hallgren and Wood 1972). Taking into consideration the physiologic role of the subpopulations of T suppressor cells, it may be supposed that as the activity of cell-mediated immunity decreases with advancing age, the T suppressor inhibition of B lymphocytes is relieved. This may contribute to the development of age-associated hyperglobulinemia and to the increase in the so-called normal autoantibody titer (Irvine et al 1970, Naor et al 1976). Therefore if metabolic immunodepression involves T suppressor cells, their disturbance might be accompanied by an increase in functional response of B lymphocytes (Dilman et al 1977a, 1977b; Dilman 1978a). In this context, metabolic shifts responsible for the suppression of cellular immunity (see Chapter 15) may stimulate the hyperactivity of humoral immunity. This point is in full agreement with the results of Fernandes and coworkers (1976, 1978). These investigators showed that calorie restriction in kdkd mice with genetically determined renal disease and autoimmunity produces suppression of autoimmune disorders and prolongs their life span. Taking into account the possibility of overactivation of the system of humoral immunity in metabolic immunodepression, it is possible to explain some well-known phenomena.

The above data on metabolic immunodepression are in agreement with the results that, in general, thymus-dependent responses to antigens and mitogens decline earlier and at a faster rate than thymus-independent responses, whereas the mitogenic response to the precursor B cell mitogen, dextran sulfate, does not decline until much later in life (Singhal et al 1978).

The incidence of autoantibodies and their titer are increased in diabetes mellitus (Irvine et al 1970, Whittingham et al 1977, Hann et al 1976, MacKay et al 1977) and atherosclerosis (Jezkova and Pokorny 1967). At the same time, obese subjects show a reduced immune capacity.

Autoimmune disturbances often occur concomitantly with hyperlipidemia, and these observations serve as the basis for identification of the syndrome of autoimmune hyperlipidemia (Beaumont 1970). It is possible, however, to suppose that it is primarily hyperlipidemia that promotes the development of the autoimmune processes. Taking into consideration the suggestion by Besedovsky and Sorkin (1977) that the rise in glucocorticoid levels in the course of immunization may suppress the generalization of the immune response, it may be supposed that, conversely, hyperlipidemia contributes to the development of immune reactions associated with T dependent B lymphocytes by inhibiting T suppressors. In this context, the effect of the administration of polyunsaturated fatty acids as immunosuppressors for treatment of autoimmune disorders (Meade and Mertin 1978) may be determined by the contribution of the T and B systems to these disorders. If one proceeds from the concept of metabolic immunodepression and its effect on humoral immunity, it is easier to understand why one factor, calorie restriction, should inhibit the development of experimental tumors (Fernandes et al 1976) and autoimmune lesions (Fernandes et al 1978).

Cancer patients, particularly those with breast cancer, exhibit a tendency for intensification of autoimmune processes (Mittra et al 1976). This fact cannot be explained.

If metabolic immunodepresion involves T suppressor cells, this syndrome might be accompanied by an increase in B lymphocytes (Dilman 1977, 1978a). It was found in our laboratory that the T lymphocyte/B lymphocyte ratio (T/B) was 3.76 ± 0.24 in younger healthy subjects (mean age 25.4 ± 1.2 years), and 3.55 ± 0.67 in mastectomized breast cancer patients (mean age 58.1 ± 1.6 years). Subsequently, a subgroup of the breast cancer patients was distinguished, in which the T/B ratio was low (2.1 ± 0.1). The members of this subgroup exhibited a significant negative correlation of immunologic indices and metabolic parameters ($r = -0.68$; $p < 0.01$). This means that the disturbances caused by metabolic immunodepression lead to a rise in B lymphocyte count. This increase seems to manifest disturbances in humoral immunity because of a decline in T suppressor activity as a result of metabolic immunodepression development. In turn, the reduced T/B ratio may probably contribute to the development of autoimmune disorders.

An analysis of the relationship of metabolic immunodepression and autoimmune processes suggests that it stems from the physiologic mechanism of the interaction of the immune and endocrine systems in the course of forming an immune response. This hypothesis may be supported by certain findings, although some links are missing. For instance, data show that immunization by thyroglobulin is accompanied by the development of hyperinsulinemia (Premachandra 1971). This phenomenon is interpreted as a particular case of autoimmune thyroiditis. At the same time, considering that antigenic challenge should stimulate T lymphocytes, the rise in blood insulin level may play the role of an endogenous mitogen which promotes the division of T-dependent lymphocytes.[1]

[1] Both antigens and mitogens stimulate an increased utilization of glucose by cells. This is an insulin-dependent process, and is an indispensable factor of the cell mitotic cycle. Persistent hyperinsulinemia involved, for instance, in obesity, may block the mitogenic effect of insulin on lymphocytes because hyperinsulinemia reduces insulin receptor concentration by negative feedback.

In support of this role of hyperinsulinemia it may be recalled that immunization results in a rise in blood cholesterol level (Di Perri 1975, Beaumont 1970). Since hyperinsulinemia intensifies the synthesis of triglycerides in the liver, and triglycerides enter the circulation as very low density lipoproteins, hyperinsulinemia and hypertriglyceridemia inevitably lead to a rise in blood cholesterol level (see Chapter 6). Concurrently, immunization causes the blood cortisol level to rise (Besedovsky and Sorkin 1977), thus intensifying the utilization of free fatty acids for energy supply (see Chapter 6).

How can the biologic significance of all these changes be interpreted? In antigen challenge, T lymphocytes and monocyte-macrophages are liable to be activated at a faster rate than the system of humoral immunity. The emergence of an insulin receptor on the plasma membrane of T lymphocytes indicates such activation (Helderman and Strom 1977). It is also possible that antigens trigger both insulin secretion and emergence of the insulin receptors on T lymphocytes. Thus, hyperinsulinemia is probably a factor stimulating T immunity activity.[1] Meanwhile, subsequent hormonal-metabolic shifts, eg, rises in the blood levels of cortisol, free fatty acids, triglycerides, and cholesterol, may inhibit the activity of T suppressors, thus causing B lymphocyte activation, ie, the activation of humoral immunity. Therefore, according to my hypothesis, the hormonal-metabolic shifts, occurring in the course of immunization, provide an artificially intensified mechanism, which normally assures the activation of T-dependent and, subsequently, B-dependent immunity in response to antigen challenge. I suggest that this physiologic mechanism is responsible for the metabolic immunodepression when metabolic disturbances pertinent to aging arise.

Whenever this physiologic mechanism is boosted by metabolic disturbances, eg, obesity, it may in turn become an important factor of the interrelationship of metabolic immunodepression and autoimmune processes.[2]

This hypothesis may be tested experimentally. For instance, administration of an insulin antiserum is supposed to reduce immune response. Elimination of age-associated hypercholesterolemia should result in reduced autoimmune disorders. Perhaps, the slowing-down of the autoimmune process by a calorie restricted diet (Fernandes et al 1978) illustrates such a relationship (Dilman 1977, 1978a).

---

[1]Until the present time, there was no plausible explanation of the origin of postprandial lymphocytosis. In the light of my hypothesis it may be suggested that the intake of food, particularly protein, causes hyperinsulinemia, which produces postprandial lymphocytosis as a nonspecific immunologic response.

[2]The metabolic shifts can cause (or promote) the autoimmune disturbances inherent in aging. It is precisely this situation that justifies referring to autoimmune processes as a group of normal diseases, which are largely caused by the regulatory-metabolic shifts characteristic of normal aging.

It follows from the above that annulment of metabolic immunodepression can contribute to normalizing B lymphocyte function, thus improving the trend of some autoimmune processes. Along with this, it is possible that the increase in T suppressor cell activity with aging (Singhal et al 1978) is caused by metabolic immunodepression. Therefore, it may be suggested that application of some means of pharmacologic correction of metabolism, eg, lowering or raising cholesterol concentration in lymphocytes, may be used for control of the induction of antibodies to viral or microbial antigens. In this connection, it is noteworthy that immunization was found to be followed by a significant increase in the mean level of total cholesterol and by a decrease in the mean level of HDL-cholesterol in man (Mathews and Freery 1978).

17 Cancer Susceptibility

If a human population as homogeneous as an inbred strain of cancer-prone mice had existed and had lived under such strictly controlled conditions as do experimental mice, the date of the age-associated increase in cancer incidence might have been pushed outside the life span of modern man. One of the most striking features of cancer is that carcinogenesis can be controlled, although the nature of malignant transformation is not understood.

Most types of cancer show a pronounced increase in incidence with aging (Doll 1962). However, it is not clear yet why cancer rates increase sharply with age. Summing up the analysis of this problem, Peto et al (1975) concluded that "the observed approximate power-law increase of most human adult cancer incidence rates with age could exist merely because age equals duration of exposure to background and spontaneous carcinogenic stimuli."

There are certain pathophysiologic conditions under which the risk of cancer is increased, such as overweight (Tannenbaum 1959, Wynder 1976). Therefore, carcinogenesis involves changes in both the cells and in the organism as a whole. But in what manner may obesity promote the development of cancer? If we accept the present hypothesis that chemical carcinogens are responsible for most cases of cancer and that the carcinogenicity of aging is a function of duration of exposure to carcinogens (Peto et al 1975), we should conclude that time flies "quicker" for obese people.

Moreover, if we take into account that normal aging is concomitant with the increase of body fat content, it may be suggested that obesity-stimulated carcinogenesis is related to an intensified aging. Our findings show that body fat content is the same in fibroadenomatosis and breast cancer patients, aged 50–59 years, but higher than in healthy females (41.0 ± 0.4, 41 ± 1.0, and 38.7 ± 0.5 kg, respectively). As compared with healthy females, patients suffering from fibroadenomatosis or breast cancer reveal the signs of intensified aging, if body fat stores are assumed to be a criterion of aging. Moreover, similar levels of body fat content in patients with fibroadenomatosis and cancer suggest that overweight only provides certain conditions that promote tumorigenesis, whereas malignant transformation of cells is induced by other factors. It would appear that an intensified aging contributes to cancer development. However, obesity is merely a component of the pattern of aging, which, according to my concept, is characterized by the development of a central type of homeostatic failure (see Chapters 1 and 18). Data on the symptoms of the central type of feedback failure in the main homeostatic systems in cancer patients will be discussed in this chapter. A hypothesis on the manner in which the syndrome of cancer susceptibility, ie, the confluence of metabolic factors promoting carcinogenesis, is formed in the course of normal aging, will be explored. Finally, evidence demonstrating the possibility of reducing the incidence of cancer induced by chemicals or some viruses by means of annulment of cancer susceptibility will be considered.

Changes in the Energy Homeostat in Cancer Patients

The data presented in Table 17-1 show that the standard glucose load fails to suppress growth hormone level in patients with breast cancer and endometrial carcinoma. This points to an elevated hypothalamic threshold to homeostatic inhibition typical of the central type of homeostatic failure.

Figure 17-1 shows the results of a six-hour observation of a patient with endometrial carcinoma. Glucose load is followed by a paradoxical rise in growth hormone level and by a high compensatory hyperinsulinemia. In other words, two major symptoms of the central type of homeostatic failure are present. This paradoxical reaction to glucose load was also observed in breast cancer patients by Samaan et al (1966) and in cases of endometrial carcinoma by Benjamin et al (1969).

It should be noted that there is nothing paradoxical about this reaction if it is examined on the basis of the elevating mechanism concept. Indeed, any system resistant to inhibition can (or should) respond to stimuli by an increased activity (Dilman 1971; see also Chapter 6). This point is confirmed by the data of Benjamin (1974) showing a relatively high rise of the blood growth hormone level produced by the insulin tolerance test in patients with endometrial carcinoma. Similar results may be found in the reports of Carter and colleagues (1967, 1975) on

Table 17-1
Levels of Serum Growth Hormone during Oral Glucose Tolerance Tests in Patients with Breast, Endometrial, and Colon Carcinoma

			Serum Growth Hormone (ng/ml)	
Tumor	No. Patients	Mean Age (years)	*Before Glucose Load*	*One Hour after Glucose Load*
Healthy controls	13	42.5 ± 0.3	1.01 ± 0.20	0.35 ± 0.66
Endometrial carcinoma	11	56.4 ± 1.6	1.4 ± 0.3	1.4 ± 0.3
Breast cancer	12	52.8 ± 1.86	2.2 ± 0.4	2.3 ± 0.4
Cancer of the colon	11	57.6 ± 1.8	1.57 ± 0.79	0.82 ± 0.22

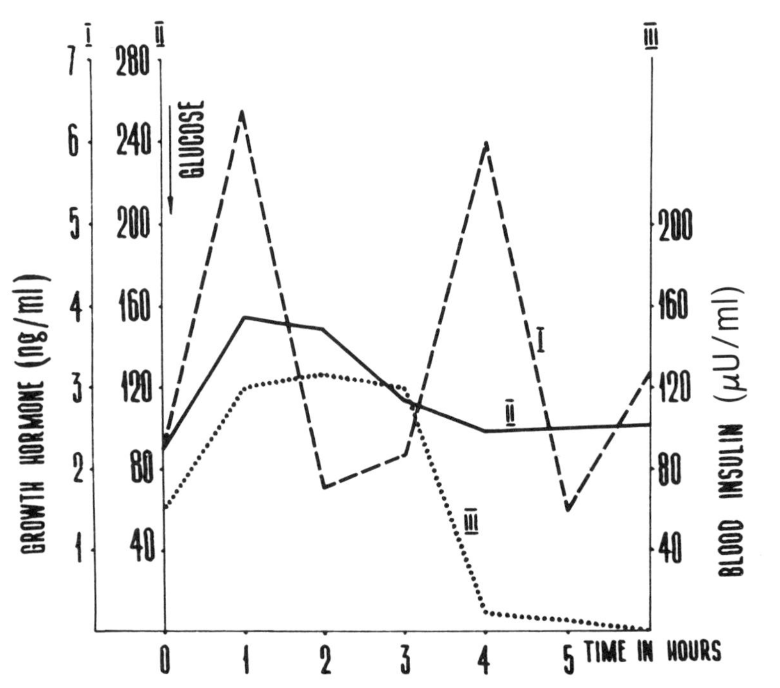

Figure 17-1 Effect of glucose load on blood growth hormone and insulin levels in endometrial carcinoma patient (100 g glucose per os). Curve I: Blood growth hormone; Curve II: Blood glucose; Curve III: Blood insulin.

breast cancer, and in the study of Spellacy et al (1972) on uterine fibromyoma. In observations made in our laboratory a high level of nocturnal growth hormone secretion was found in some cancer patients even though they were old and obese (Figure 17-2). This shows that the effect of inhibition of growth hormone secretion by free fatty acids is obviated, possibly by the influence of the tumor itself. Disorders in growth hormone secretion in lung cancer also have been reported (Glass et al 1972, Claeys-DeClerg et al 1975). Some experiments demonstrate that growth hormone may induce cell proliferation in lung cancer (Brody and Buhain 1972). The findings obtained in our laboratory show that a glucose load fails to lower blood growth hormone level in many cases of lung cancer, which indicates a central type of homeostatic failure. Abundant experimental data also point to a possible role of growth hormone in the processes of carcinogenesis, particularly in tissues characterized by rapid cellular turnover (Pierpaoli and Sorkin 1972).

The data obtained in our laboratory on the increased level of growth hormone and insulin in some types of tumors in children also are of interest (Table 17-2). Goodman et al (1978) revealed an abnormal glucose tolerance, hyperinsulinemia, and elevated levels of blood GH and somatomedin in five out of seven patients aged 6 to 25 years with primary osteosarcoma. Although these authors think that these hormonal shifts represent a new "paraneoplastic syndrome," this conclusion, contradicts their other data showing that glucose loading produced an inhibition of GH level. Such a response points to hypothalamic-pituitary disturbances in patients with primary osteosarcoma.

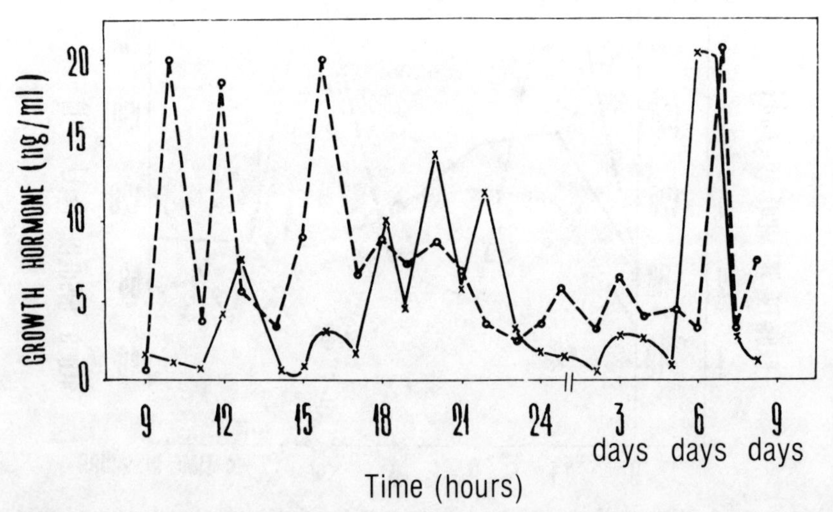

Figure 17-2 Diurnal rhythm of blood growth hormone level in patients with endometrial carcinoma. o—o—o—o—: 82-year-old patient; x—x—x—x—: 65-year-old patient weighing 102 kg.

Table 17-2
Basal Growth Hormone and Insulin Levels in Healthy Children and Children with Cancer

Group	Mean Age	Growth Hormone (ng/ml)	Insulin (μU/ml)
Healthy children (n = 14)	9.0 ± 1.0	2.40 ± 0.5	14.0 ± 2.4
Hodgkin's disease (n = 22)	7.50 ± 0.7	6.46 ± 1.28	25.9 ± 4.2
Lymphosarcoma (n = 10)	6.85 ± 1.80	4.89 ± 1.07	20.9 ± 4.5
Dysembryonal tumors (n = 28)	6.80 ± 1.8	7.63 ± 1.59	28.7 ± 3.4
Osteosarcoma (n = 10)	11.2 ± 1.3	basal: 4.11 ± 0.59	15.0 ± 2.1
		60 min after glucose load: 3.76 ± 0.40	33.8 ± 2.9

Many cancer patients reveal metabolic disorders typical of aging, such as obesity, decreased glucose tolerance, a rise of free fatty acid level in the blood, and hypercholesterolemia. It should be stressed that metabolic shifts often observed in cancer conform to the pattern typical of diseases of compensation. Reduced sensitivity to insulin has been reported for different tumors (Bishop and Marks 1959), particularly cancer of the rectum (Vasiljeva and Dilman 1973). Decreased glucose tolerance is frequent in tumor patients (Glicksman and Rawson 1956). Such changes are observed particularly in cases of endometrial carcinoma (Way 1951, Lucas 1974, Dilman 1974a, Dilman et al 1968). In cases with very large tumors, gluconeogenesis also is enhanced (Carey et al 1966; Shapot 1972, 1973).

Many cases of cancer are also characterized by a relatively high level of blood free fatty acids (Mueller and Watkin 1961, Dilman et al 1968). A glucose load is followed by a lower than normal concentration of FFA in such patients, and the lipid content in the tumor itself is found to be high (Haven et al 1949).

One of the most detailed studies of metabolic parameters in patients with metastatic breast cancer was carried out by Carter et al (1975), who found an elevated GH level and reduced glucose tolerance. Simultaneously, insulin secretion was delayed and prolonged in those patients. Table 17-3 contains our data on certain metabolic disturbances in patients with different sites of cancer. It is evident that blood cholesterol levels in females with cancer of the rectum, stomach and mammary gland do not differ significantly from those in the age-matched control group. However, different chapters of this book cite evidence in support of the concept that any deviation from the ideal norm, ie, the indices typically observed in the age group 20–29 years, is an indication of disturbed homeostasis, a disease (see Chapter 10). Hence, a cholesterol level typical of young healthy subjects is assumed to be the norm; cancer patients should be considered to be suffering from hypercholesterolemia. Since the pathogenicity of hypercholesterolemia is much the same as for atherosclerosis and cancer, particular mention should be made of the data indicating that a man with a blood cholesterol level of 250 mg% or more has about three times the risk of heart attack as a man with a cholesterol level below 194 mg% (Walker 1976). These values are identical to those observed by us (Table 17-3). The cases of lung cancer revealed a normal blood cholesterol level and, yet, a decrease in HDL-cholesterol. Moreover, raised levels of triglycerides were recorded in men with lung cancer and women with certain types of tumors.

An elevated blood triglyceride level is known to be caused by hyperinsulinemia. In this context, it is noteworthy that female cancer patients aged 50 or more were often found to have given birth to large babies (weighing 4.0 kg and more) 17 to 31 years before the first clinical manifestations of malignancy (Table 17-4) (Berstein 1973). Weight of the fetus is determined to a considerable degree by insulin level, which tends to rise when tolerance to carbohydrates is reduced (see Chapter 21). Hence, metabolic disturbances may occur well in advance of the first appearance of cancer.

The concomitance of moderate hypercholesterolemia and hypertriglyceridemia in cancer patients corresponds to Type IIb of hyperlipoproteinemia characterized by hyperinsulinemia (Tzagournis et al 1972). It is known that an enhanced blood insulin level leads to an intensification of the somatomedin activity of blood (Daughaday et al 1976). Accordingly, an enhanced somatomedin activity of blood was found in patients exhibiting Type IIb of hyperlipoproteinemia (Table 17-5).

Thus metabolic changes occurring in cancer, atherosclerosis, obesity, and maturity-onset diabetes mellitus are very similar, their common feature being the predominant utilization of free fatty acids as an energy supply. This metabolic shift is caused by the same mechanisms that operate in the process of normal aging, a fact consistent with the data indicating that obesity is associated with a higher tumor incidence, whereas restricted food intake inhibits carcinogenesis. Several patients with endometrial carcinoma, breast cancer, and some other sites of malignant disease reveal distinct metabolic signs that may be identified as manifestations of intensified aging. Particularly significant in this respect are the data demonstrating decline in glucose tolerance (Dilman 1974b).

However, it should be noted that the foregoing changes do not occur

Table 17-3
Lipid Indices in Cancer Patients

Group	Sex	No.	Mean Age (years)	Deviation from ideal weight (%)	Choles-terol (mg%)	Trigly-cerides mg%	Lipo-proteins (Svedberg units)	FFA (μEq/liter)	HDL-choles terol (mg%)
Control (20–29 years)	M	45		−8 ± 2.5	184 ± 6	109 ± 4	0.382 ± 0.017	–	–
	F	45		+1 ± 0.2	192 ± 4	88 ± 6	0.388 ± 0.014	594 ± 62	–
Control (> 45 years)	M	35	51 ± 1	+5 ± 2	241 ± 5	139 ± 9	0.538 ± 0.024	588 ± 23	53 ± 3
	F	32	52 ± 1	+17 ± 2	257 ± 8	118 ± 7	0.498 ± 0.020	693 ± 26	56 ± 2
Cancer of rectum	M	18	56 ± 2	+5 ± 4	253 ± 8	152 ± 12	0.566 ± 0.029	571 ± 63	48 ± 4
	F	24	55 ± 2	+13 ± 2	243 ± 6	149 ± 11*	0.580 ± 0.021*	695 ± 50	56 ± 3
Cancer of ventriculum	M	22	52 ± 2	+2 ± 3	227 ± 9	238 ± 8	0.542 ± 0.029	580 ± 52	49 ± 4
	F	21	52 ± 2	+8 ± 4	255 ± 15*	152 ± 15*	0.581 ± 0.030*	676 ± 86	51 ± 3
Primary breast cancer	F	48	53 ± 1	+22 ± 3	251 ± 7	156 ± 10*	0.586 ± 0.015*	579 ± 22*	51 ± 1*
Breast cancer (remission)	F	73	56 ± 4	+24 ± 3	261 ± 6	161 ± 6*	0.574 ± 0.020	708 ± 28	57 ± 3
Endometrial carcinoma	F	31	59 ± 1	+40 ± 3	263 ± 5	193 ± 9*	0.645 ± 0.022	–	48 ± 3*
Lung cancer	M	110	56 ± 1	−2 ± 2	219 ± 3	160 ± 4*	0.548 ± 0.017	471 ± 21*	45 ± 2*

*Difference from control group is statistically significant ($p < 0.05$).

Table 17-4
Frequency of Births (%) of Large Babies (> 4kg) in Two Age-Distinct Cancer Groups

	Age at Diagnosis of Cancer (years)	
	20 to 49	*50 +*
Endometrial carcinoma	10.5 ± 6.9	42.6 ± 5.7
Breast carcinoma	23.0 ± 3.6	35.5 ± 4.1
Cancer of colón	31.8 ± 9.9	45.8 ± 5.9
Cancer of stomach	20.0 ± 10.3	43.5 ± 10.2
Melanoma	38.2 ± 12.5	46.7 ± 8.5
Control group	20.1 ± 2.4	14.2 ± 2.9

Source: Berstein 1973.

in all patients with breast or endometrial carcinoma. Hormonal and metabolic shifts characteristic of diseases of compensation are more frequent in middle-aged patients, usually after menopause. Therefore, I have suggested that two major pathogenic types of cancer should be distinguished: early-onset and late-onset cancer. Assays should be performed in each case to establish hormonal and metabolic conditions under which tumors develop. This is important because early-onset cancer may occur in middle-aged and old patients, and late-onset cancer in juveniles. Tests used for biologic age determinations may establish these conditions (see Chapter 10). Regarding endometrial carcinoma and breast cancer, the proposed distinction allows a more adequate specification of tumor promoting conditions to be made than the existing distinctions between the premenopausal and postmenopausal types (Hems 1970) or the ovarian and adrenal types (De Waard et al 1969), since the latter are established on the basis of an assessment of steroid production alone. Moreover, the notion of late-onset or hypothalamus-dependent cancer includes not only breast and endometrial carcinoma but many other types whose development is facilitated by age-associated changes of metabolic pattern.

Changes in the Adaptive System in Cancer Patients

As discussed in Chapter 3, the hypothalamic threshold of sensitivity to feedback suppression in the adaptive homeostat gradually rises in the course of hormonal aging. This is manifested by a decrease in the inhibitory effect of dexamethasone with the advance of age. Similar changes in breast cancer patients have been reported by a number of authors. It also has been shown that the dexamethasone-induced suppression of 11-hydroxycorticosteroid levels in the blood is insufficient in cancer patients

Table 17-5
Level of Blood Somatomedin Activity in Patients with Breast and Endometrial Cancer

Group	Type of Hyperlipidemia	Mean Age (years)	Overweight (%)	Somatomedin Activity (units)	Blood Cholesterol (mg%)	Blood Triglyceride (mg%)
Breast cancer	–	49.3 ± 4.9	+ 28.1 ± 9.2	0.68 ± 0.2	197.2 ± 12.6	129.4 ± 5.5
	IIa	47.4 ± 2.7	+ 11.4 ± 6.0	0.43 ± 0.1	257.7 ± 9.1	123.2 ± 14.6
	IIb	55.6 ± 2.8	+ 19.5 ± 3.9	2.92 ± 0.8*	266.0 ± 11.9	190.0 ± 9.3
Endometrial carcinoma	–	51.7 ± 4.2	+ 33.7 ± 10.8	0.41 ± 0.1	216.1 ± 4.9	110.1 ± 8.7
	IIa	51.8 ± 3.5	+ 46.8 ± 10.4	0.81 ± 0.3	269.0 ± 11.9	107.0 ± 10.4
	IIb	58.2 ± 1.6	+ 44.4 ± 5.8	2.1 ± 0.6*	269.0 ± 9.8	202.8 ± 16.2

*$p < 0.02$.

who relapse rapidly, or who do not show any improvement after primary treatment (Saez 1974). On the basis of results that show that resistance to dexamethasone suppression increases as the tumor progresses (Bishop and Ross 1970), it was concluded that the elevation of the hypothalamic threshold is influenced by progression of the tumor process (Saez 1974). Although tumors do exert such an effect, there is every reason to believe that primary hypothalamic changes also influence the elevation of the sensitivity threshold to feedback suppression in the adaptive homeostat in cancer patients. This is supported by the following data showing a greater resistance to dexamethasone inhibition in breast and endometrial cancer patients of the reproductive age compared with menopausal patients (Table 17-6).

Table 17-6
Effect of Dexamethasone* Suppression on Steroid Hormone Excretion in Breast Cancer Patients

	Reproductive Patients (mean age 41 ± 1.0 years) (n = 28)	Menopausal Patients (mean age 59.5 ± 1.4 years) (n = 17)
17-Ketosteroids (mg/24 h)		
Before	6.9 ± 0.8	4.5 ± 0.8
After	4.2 ± 0.3	2.5 ± 0.3
Inhibition (%)	−23.6 ± 5.0	−16.8 ± 5.0
17-Hydroxysteroids (mg/24 h)		
Before	5.9 ± 0.5	4.6 ± 0.7
After	3.3 ± 0.4	4.7 ± 0.7
Inhibition (%)	−35.0 ± 4.8	−2.2 ± 8.8
Phenolsteroids (μg/24 h)		
Before	60.9 ± 5.4	50.0 ± 6.4
After	72.0 ± 8.4	55.8 ± 4.7
Enhancement (%)	+13.8 ± 11.8	+24.6 ± 12

*Dexamethasone (0.015 mg) was administered four times a day for two days.

Hence it may be concluded that changes in the hypothalamic threshold in the adaptive system in this group of cancer patients are identical to those observed in the course of normal aging (see Chapter 3). The degree of relevant changes in cancer is much greater, however, and therefore may be interpreted as an indication of intensified aging. Data presented in Table 17-6 are interesting from still another point of view. They show that total phenolsteroid excretion is somewhat increased rather than decreased in the dexamethasone test. Mention should be made of the data showing a much higher than normal rise in 17-hydroxycorticosteroid excretion in response to the blocking of cortisol synthesis by administration of metyrapone in breast cancer patients (Saez 1974). Such a reaction is consistent with the increased reactivity of the hypothalamus following the use of stimulating drugs, when the hypothalamus is resistant to inhibition (Dilman 1968, 1971).

Another conclusion that can be drawn on the basis of the data in Table 17-6 is that in menopausal patients dexamethasone-induced suppression is greater for 17-ketosteroid excretion than for 17-hydroxycorticosteroids. It can be suggested that the production of hormones of these two types is independent of each other, and that this dissociation offers an explanation for the much faster decline with age of 17-ketosteroid excretion compared to 17-hydroxycorticosteroids (see Chapter 3). This would shift the balance toward hydroxysteroids. Moreover, the predisposition to breast cancer, the duration of the so-called free interval, and the effectiveness of hormone therapy were found to be correlated with the ratio of 17-hydroxycorticosteroid excretion to 17-ketosteroids, or more precisely, to the excretion of androsterone and etiocholanolone (Bulbrook et al 1971, Bulbrook 1972). If this ratio, or the so-called index of discrimination of Bulbrook, is less than unity, which is the case in the predominant production of hydroxysteroids, the likelihood of breast cancer, and accelerated cancer at that, is increased. The significance of the index of discrimination also was shown for endometrial carcinoma (De Waard et al 1969) and cancer of the lung (Rao 1972). In the latter case the decreased excretion of androsterone was recorded in 90% of patients. Decreased excretion of 17-ketosteroids in conjunction with a gain of body weight also is a manifestation of the predisposition to breast cancer (De Waard 1973) and possibly some other types of cancer.

As age increases, the tendency toward negative 17-ketosteroid/17-hydroxycorticosteroid ratio is increased (see Chapter 3). This shift manifests the age-associated decrease in anabolic 17-ketosteroid output. Hence, on the basis of this ratio it may be concluded that each individual more than 55 years of age is cancer-prone. Also, the higher the blood cortisol level, the more cell-mediated immunity reactions are inhibited; therefore, the shorter the survival period of breast cancer patients (MacKay et al 1971). These data are consistent with concepts of the protective role of the connective tissue (Kavetsky 1962) and immunologic systems (Good 1972) in carcinogenesis.

It should be noted that the central type of homeostatic failure in the adaptive homeostat triggers a series of metabolic disturbances. Among other things it stimulates gluconeogenesis, reduces glucose uptake by muscle tissue, and tips the metabolic balance toward the predominant utilization of free fatty acids as a source of energy. This in turn intensifies similar changes in the energy homeostat (see Chapter 6).

Changes in the Reproductive Homeostat in Cancer Patients

Data on the condition of the reproductive system in carcinogenesis discussed here were obtained largely from studies of breast and endometrial carcinoma, although there is some information concerning cancer of the lung, prostate, and cervix uteri (Marmorston et al 1966, Dilman 1974a). A number of investigations show a tendency toward increased gonadotropin excretion in breast cancer patients (Dilman 1960, 1968; Coleman and Lederis 1965). This phenomenon is most frequently observed in menopausal patients (Table 17-7).

Table 17-7
Excretion of Total Gonadotropins, Follicle-Stimulating Hormone, and Luteinizing Hormone in Menopausal Patients with Breast Cancer

Group	Total Gonadotropins (muu/24 hrs)*	FSH (mg/1 h equivalent)†	LH (IU of human chorionic gonadotropin)
Control (menopause)	194.8 ± 13.0	15.7 ± 1.3	21.6 ± 3.1
Breast cancer (menopause)	273 ± 9.8	14.2 ± 0.8	36.6 ± 6.4
Significance *(p)*	< 0.001	< 0.2	< 0.95

*muu – mouse uterine units.
†FSH was determined by the Steelman and Pohley (1953) method, and FSH value was estimated as the difference between the weights of the ovaries in experimental and control groups of animals per one hour equivalent of 24 hours of urine output.

Increased secretion of gonadotropins may be caused by a decrease in ovarian hormone output, ie, it may occur by the mechanism of a peripheral type of homeostatic failure (see Chapter 2). However, a high level of gonadotropin excretion also is observed in patients with normal menstrual cycles (Dilman 1960). On the basis of these data the conclusion can be drawn that a primary increase in hypothalamic-pituitary activity occurs with breast cancer, since the menstrual cycle may be maintained at an excessive level of gonadotropin production only if there is a compensatory elevation of ovarian function (see Chapter 4). Accordingly, patients with breast and endometrial cancer often reveal a hyperplasia of the ovarian thecal tissue and an increased output of nonclassical phenolsteroids (Figure 17-3). This provides an explanation for a later than normal onset of menopause in these patients (see Chapter 4).

Hypothalamic resistance to inhibition in breast cancer patients also may be demonstrated on the basis of data showing that the therapeutic administration of daily doses of 10 to 20 mg of stilbestrol fails to fully inhibit total gonadotropin excretion (O'Conner and Skinner 1964). This dose is several times greater than the estrogen level required to inhibit gonadotropin secretion in healthy women (see Chapter 4).

The status of the reproductive homeostat in patients with endometrial carcinoma is still more complicated. Indirect evidence points to a primary increase in hypothalamic activity in such patients. They often reveal hyperplasia of the ovarian thecal tissue and the endometrium with late-onset menopause; however, the level of classic estrogen excretion is not enhanced (Charles et al 1965, Berstein 1967). This discrepancy may be accounted for by the data obtained in our laboratory on the elevation of total phenolsteroid excretion in endometrial carcinoma patients during menopause (Berstein 1967). Such a possibility also seems to be indicated indirectly by the findings of Charles et al (1965). They show that ovariectomy in menopausal women with endometrial carcinoma is followed by a compensatory intensificiation of adrenal function despite the absence of a decrease in classic estrogen excretion. These data may be interpreted as an indication of the role of nonclassic phenolsteroids in the pathogenesis of endometrial carcinoma (Dilman 1961, Dilman et al 1968; see Chapter 4). At the same time a direct determination of the level of excretion of total gonadotropins and FSH showed the decrease in the excretion of these hormones (Table 17-8).

Ovarian hyperfunction unaccompanied by any hyperproduction of gonadotropins can be interpreted in light of the changes in the spectrum of secreted isohormones of gonadotropins. In our laboratory we found differences in the concentrations of sialic acids, hexosamines, and total

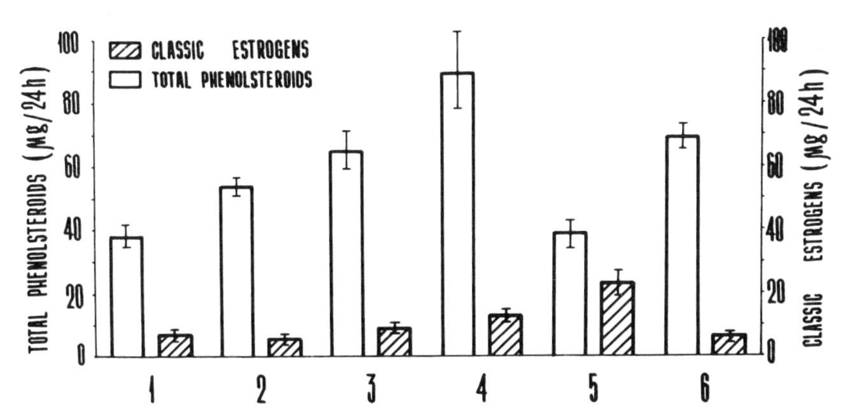

Figure 17-3 Excretion of classic estrogens and total phenolsteroids in normal menopausal women and in menopausal female patients with different types of cancer. Groups: 1: Menopausal women (control); 2: Endometrial carcinoma; 3: Cancer of breast; 4: Cancer of corpus uteri; 5: Patients with cancer of corpus uteri (reproductive age) before x-ray castration; 6: Same patients after x-ray castration.

Table 17-8
Excretion of Total Gonadotropins, FSH, LH, Total Phenolsteroids, and Estrogens in Menopausal Patients with Endometrial Carcinoma

	Control (Menopause)	Endometrial Carcinoma (Menopause)	Significance *(p)*
Total gonadotropins (muu/24 hr)*	194.8 ± 13.0	114.1 ± 9.5	< 0.001
FSH (mg/1 hr equivalent)	15.7 ± 3.3	12.7 ± 0.8	> 0.05
LH (IU/HCG) (biologically active)	21.8 ± 3.4	25.6 ± 2.8	> 0.1
Classic estrogens (μg/24 hr)	7.0 ± 0.7	6.4 ± 0.4	> 0.05
Total phenolsteroids (μg/24 hr)	38.5 ± 2.7	52.8 ± 2.4	< 0.001

*muu: mouse uterine unit.
FSH was determined by the Steelman and Pohley (1953) method, and FSH value was estimated as the difference between the weights of the ovaries in experimental and control groups of animals per 1-hr equivalent of 24 hr of urine output.

hexoses in the gonadotropic residues from the urine of patients with endometrial cancer (Ostroumova 1970). The induction of changes in the spectrum of secreted FSH by pituitary hyperfunction has been reported recently by several investigators (Peckham et al 1973, Diebel et al 1973). Changes in the properties of gonadotropins in patients with cancer of the lung, and mammary and prostate glands also have been observed (Marmorston et al 1966). Recently, Benjamin and Deutsch (1976) documented the increase in endogenous estrogen and the decrease in FSH blood levels in patients with endometrial carcinoma, using more specific and sensitive techniques. These authors concluded that "these higher levels may be etiologically related to the development of endometrial neoplasia and may explain our previously demonstrated excessive growth hormone secretion in these cases. Furthermore, the excessive growth hormone response, as well as the marked FSH suppression and moderate prolactin elevation, strongly supports the theory of hypothalamic dysfunction in this disease, as previously suggested by Dilman and associates (1968)."

In light of present-day concepts that the elevation of prolactin level may be determined by the decline in dopamine concentration in the hypothalamus (see Chapter 7), of interest are our findings indicating that surgical stress causes a dramatic rise in blood prolactin in endometrial carcinoma patients. We presume that the deficit of catecholamine in the hypothalamus is typical of such patients. Thus, the effect of operative stress may result from the addition of the stress changes to the underlying impairment of dopamine function.

Changes in the Thyroid Homeostat in Cancer Patients

The cancer-prone condition also is characterized by a decline in thyroid function (Stoll 1965, Mittra and Hayward 1974). Our results show that, in their youth, the potential cases of fibroadenomatosis and breast cancer are characterized by an elevated threshold of hypothalamic-pituitary complex sensitivity to feedback inhibition by T_3 (Table 17-9). These findings may be interpreted as an indication of intensified aging, because elevation of the hypothalamic threshold starts in healthy women at a relatively late age. However, it should be repeated that the factors underlying the differences in the data on age-associated changes in the sensitivity threshold of the thyrostat in rat and man are not yet clear (see Chapter 7).

Table 17-9
Triiodothyronine Suppression Test in Healthy Women and in Patients with Benign Mastopathia or Breast Cancer

				Blood Thyrotropin Levels (μU/ml)		
Group	Mean Age (years)	Over-weight (%)	Serum T_4 μg%	*Before T_3 Test*	*After T_3 Test*	Inhibition (%)
Healthy women	32.0±2.6	+1.3	9.75±1.8	7.5±1.2	5.2±0.9	−31.0
	55.0±3.3	+9	7.30±0.7	11.3±1.0	9.2±1.2	−18.5
Benign mastopathia	34.6±2.2	+2.1	6.70±0.6	6.9±0.8	5.6±0.7	−18.7
	51.0±2.0	+7.2	5.00±1.0	12.3±1.2	11.2±2.0	− 9.0
Breast cancer	37.8±3.6	+5.5	6.30±0.7	7.0±1.2	5.1±1.0	−27.0
	54.5±2.1	+9.8	7.80±1.2	12.3±1.3	11.0±1.4	−10.0

Changes in Immune Homeostat of Cancer Patients

The problem of changes observed in the immunity of cancer patients is discussed in numerous other publications. Still, it is important to stress that metabolic immunodepression often occurs in endometrial and breast cancer patients, and phenformin treatment of breast cancer patients improves their cell-mediated immunity indices (see Chapter 15). The phenomenon of metabolic immunodepression is probably also present with other tumor sites, eg, cancer of the rectum, since disturbances in metabolic pattern are apparent in many such patients.

Considering the data available on the effects of metabolic immunodepression on the appearance of autoantibodies (see Chapter 16), the high rate of antithyroid antibody with many sites of cancer may be regarded as another proof of metabolic immunodepression in those cancer patients who exhibit a corresponding metabolic pattern. Table

17-10, presenting the results of our examinations of more than 300 cancer patients and 120 healthy subjects, shows a considerable increase in the frequency of identifying antibodies to thyroglobulin in female patients with cancer of the breast, sigmoid colon, and stomach, and a tendency to such increase in endometrial carcinoma and some other tumor sites.

Table 17-10
Incidence of Autoantibodies to Thyroglobulin in Cancer Patients and Control Subjects

Group	Age (years)	No. Cases	Percentage of Incidence of Antibodies to Thyroglobulin: *In a Titer of 1/10 and More*	*In a Titer of 1/80 and More*
Healthy females (F)	20–49	38	34.2±7.7	5.3±3.5
	>50	21	52.3±10.9	9.5±6.4
Healthy men (M)	20–49	49	8.2±3.9	2.0±2.0
	>50	21	42.9±10.8	9.5±6.4
Breast cancer	20–49	34	67.7±7.8*	38.2±8.3*
	>50	41	63.5±7.6	34.2±7.4*
Cancer of the lung (M)	20–49	11	45.5±14.9*	—
		40	57.5±7.3	6.5±3.6
Cancer of the lung (F)	>50	5	60.0±22.0	—
Ovarian cancer	>50	28	53.6±9.4	25.0±8.2
Fibroma of the uterus	>50	22	40.8±10.4	13.6±7.3
Endometrial carcinoma	>50	12	58.3±14.2	25.0±12.5
Cancer of the stomach (M)	>50	15	40.0±12.6	6.7±6.5
Cancer of the stomach (F)	>50	14	50.0±13.4	35.7±12.8*
Cancer of the sigmoid colon (M+F)	>50	10	80.0±12.6	50.0±15.7*
Bone tumors (M+F)	>50	13	53.7±13.9	23.0±11.7

*Difference as compared with controls is significant ($p < 0.05$)

At present there is no explanation for the elevated titer of normal antibodies involved in many types of cancer. If we consider that tumor patients often exhibit metabolic shifts, which may be interpreted as typical of an intensified aging, it may be supposed that the syndrome of metabolic immunodepression promotes autoimmune disturbances inherent in cancer as it does in diabetes mellitus and obesity (see Chapter 16). It is possible that autoimmune disturbances, particularly the increased titer of antithyroid antibodies, may aid tumor progression by suppressing the activity of the thyroid gland. Such a situation resembles a relationship between the autoimmune lesions of the thyroid gland and atherosclerosis.

Data show that in cancer patients the main homeostatic systems often reveal changes that may result from an elevation of the hypothalamic sensitivity threshold. These shifts are similar to changes inherent in diseases of compensation and include inadequate inhibition of growth hormone secretion by glucose, decreased sensitivity of the muscle tissue to insulin, intensified lipolysis, diminished tolerance to carbohydrates, compensatory increase in insulin output, obesity, decreased thyroid function, increased blood levels of cholesterol and triglycerides and decreased HDL-cholesterol, absolute and relative increases in cortisol level, decreased output of 17-ketosteroids, lowered cell-mediated immunity with enhanced expression of autoimmunity, and increased production of gonadotropins and nonclassic phenolsteroids (Dilman 1974a).

The above shifts indicate intensified aging in many cases. However, at present it is impossible to specify precisely in what manner they contribute to carcinogenesis because the mechanism of malignant transformation is not yet clear. It would be desirable to study factors promoting the development of malignant tumors.

There are many arguments supporting the essential role of two such factors. First, whatever factor may be actually responsible for the malignant transformation of cells, it is certain that an increase in the pool of proliferating cells contributes to the rise in cancer incidence. Second, the decline in cellular immunity vigor aids carcinogenesis. Let us discuss the data available on the role of these conditions in tumorigenesis. The effect of the first factor, the increase in the proliferating cell pool, is clearly manifested in so-called hormonal carcinogenesis.

There is a large body of experimental evidence showing that disturbed hormonal self-regulation is associated with an increase in tumor incidence. For example, an unbalanced hormonal homeostasis results in a sharp increase in tumor incidence (Lipschutz 1957). Following the transplantation of one ovary into the spleen of an ovariectomized rat, tumors arise in the transplanted ovarian tissue. The mechanism in this phenomenon has been described adequately. Hormones produced by the transplanted ovary pass directly to the liver via the portal system where estrogens are inactivated. As a consequence the inhibitory effect of estrogens on the hypothalamic-hypophyseal system is reduced, thus increasing gonadotropin secretion. This in turn causes a hyperplasia of the ovarian tissue at the initial stage and, if the experiment is of sufficiently long duration, a tumor arises in the thecal and granulosa tissues. Conversely, the administration of an antigonadotropic serum or estrogens arrests development of these tumors. This effect has been obtained by means of immunization with analogs of gonadotropic hormones (Dilman and Blok 1962, Dilman 1968). In addition to the above case of transplanation of the ovary into the spleen, this phenomenon also is supported by the results of a comprehensive study on the development of thyroid tumors by the blocking of thyroid function in some strains of rats (Napalkov 1965).

In such cases a decreased inhibitory effect of the peripheral hormone leads to homeostatic failure and subsequent intensification of the cell division of the thyroid epithelium. Moreover, while excessive thyrotropic hormone induces thyroid carcinoma, and the excess of estrogens induces endometrial carcinoma (Knab 1977), thyroid hormones and progestins produce an antitumor effect in patients with papillary carcinoma of the thyroid gland and the endometrium, respectively.

Many investigators believe, however, that these experimental and clinical data are relevant in hormonal carcinogenesis only, but such a conclusion would be erroneous. It should be noted that hormonal shifts that promote tumor development cannot induce the malignant transformation of cells directly because hormones alone do not alter the unique composition of DNA (Lipsett 1969). It is thought that hormones exert a cocarcinogenic effect through an increase in the pool of proliferating cells. This means that hormones cannot cause the malignant transformation directly, yet certain hormones are responsible for tumors; the relationships established in the studies of hormonal carcinogenesis point merely to the factors that generally promote carcinogensis, such as an increased pool of proliferating cells. Although hormones that intensify cell division have been studied for the so-called hormone-dependent tissues only, cell division processes in any tissue are undoubtedly controlled by certain factors.

One such factor is cholesterol. Cholesterol is a unique and major lipid component of the plasma membrane of mammalian cells. All the cell cultures studied so far synthesize cholesterol when they are grown in a sterol-free medium. The depletion of membrane cholesterol in cells will result in cessation of growth, and ultimately cell death (Chen et al 1978). On the contrary, the studies with lymphocytes stimulated to blastogenesis by phytohemagglutinin show that the cycle of cholesterol synthesis precedes that of DNA synthesis and cell division (Chen et al 1975). It should be pointed out that all cells except neurons in the adult brain can synthesize cholesterol (Bortz 1973). Perhaps this is the reason why neurons in the adult brain never divide or become malignant.

Chapter 15 cited data showing that somatic cells either synthesize cholesterol themselves (in the kidney, intestine, and skin) or are supplied with it from low density lipoproteins carried by the circulating blood. Taking into consideration that the mechanism of self-regulation is intended to maintain the cell concentration of cholesterol at a constant level, it would appear that the elevation of the cholesterol level in the internal environment should not influence cellular metabolism and behavior, ie, it should not stimulate cell division and cancer development. However, this supposition is at variance with the experimental data avialable on induction of tumors of the intestine. As is known, the intestinal mucosa is an important site of cholesterol synthesis and contributes to serum cholesterol concentrations (Dietschy and Wilson 1970).

Moreover, Nigro et al (1977) showed that accumulation of cholesterol in rat intestines increases the yield of intestinal tumors induced by dimethylhydrazine. Therefore, the elevation of cholesterol concentration in the internal environment, despite its high basal level in the intestinal mucosa, promotes carcinogenesis. In this context, it is noteworthy that patients with familial polyposis and those with colon cancer show an increase in cholesterol excretion (Reddy et al 1977).

Considering that cholesterol concentration in tissues, eg, lymphocytes, rises with increasing age (see Chapter 15), the age-associated elevation of blood cholesterol may be regarded as a cancer-promoting factor.

Dilman and Bobrov (1976) found an elevated blood cholesterol level in many patients with carcinoma of the uterus, stomach, large intestine, and breast. A report by Barclay and Skipski (1975) showed that high-density lipoproteins (HDL) are deficient in cancer patients. These data gain particular importance in the light of the so-called HDL theory of atherosclerosis. According to this hypothesis, the body cholesterol pool size shows a strong negative correlation with HDL concentration. Theoretically, this could reflect a function of HDL in the removal of cholesterol from tissue (Boudjers and Bjørkern 1975). As the decline in HDL-cholesterol level aids atherosclerosis (see Chapter 12), it may promote carcinogenesis, despite the absence of pronounced hypercholesterolemia (Barclay and Skipski 1975). In this respect, of particular interest are the data obtained in our laboratory (see Table 17-3). Data show that a cholesterol deficient diet produces a retarding effect on tumor growth (Szepsenwol 1966) and provide additional proof in support of the hypothesis that cholesterolemia contributes to carcinogenesis. However, there are two different aspects to the problem under study: the significance of disturbances in the internal environment, particularly of hypercholesterolemia in the formation of tumor-prone conditions; and uncontrolled synthesis of cholesterol in transformed cells. Normal cells typically exhibit a suppression of cholesterol biosynthesis after exposure to external cholesterol. In contrast, neoplastic cells almost universally lack this response and may synthesize cholesterol at rates so rapid as to lead to cellular cholesterol enrichment (Heiniger et al 1976). It was observed in particular that hepatotropic carcinogens disturb the mechanism of self-regulation of cholesterol synthesis. After exposure to such carcinogens, exogenous cholesterol fails to inhibit the synthesis of cholesterol in the liver and its output increases severalfold (Sobine 1976). Cells transformed as a result of exposure to viruses were found to exhibit a sharp increase in cholesterol synthesis (Howard and Kritchevsky 1969). This points to the role of hypercholesterolemia for carcinogenesis as a whole, ie, a factor that is not only required for cell proliferation but, under certain conditions, promotes tumor cell division. Some transplantable tumors, eg, Ehrlich's carcinoma, almost completely rely on LDL as a source of cholesterol (Brennerman et al 1974). If similar pathologic mechanisms operate in some human tumors, the growth of the latter may be inhibited by reducing the blood level of LDL-cholesterol (probably increasing that of high density lipoproteins).

Finally, it is necessary to consider still another aspect of this problem which did not receive attention in the brilliant review of Chen and colleagues (1978). Gonzalez and Dempsey (1977) showed that sterol synthesis in cultured cells of human genital carcinoma is influenced by serum lipoprotein concentration in the medium. This evidence is at variance with the results of in vivo experiments, in which the lack of regulation of cholesterol synthesis was described as characteristic of malignancy (Siperstein et al 1966). This discrepancy between the behavior of tumor cells in culture and in vivo suggests that disturbances in the mechanism of self-regulation of cholesterol synthesis may be related to overall regulatory changes, similar to those involved in age-dependent modifications of enzyme induction (Adelman 1978). These findings support the premise that a high cholesterol concentration in somatic cells is necessary for the acceleration of their division. On the other hand, excessive accumulation of cholesterol in the plasma membrane of lymphocytes inhibits blast transformation (Waddell et al 1976, Alderson and Green 1975) and, therefore, cell division.

I suppose that in this respect somatic cells should be subdivided into two groups, lymphoid and nonlympoid cells. The division of cells in nonlymphoid tissue is activated by cholesterol accumulation in cells, while cell division in lymphoid tissue (or more precisely that of T lymphocytes) is suppressed by excessive accumulation of cholesterol in the plasma membrane. As a result of the analysis of this problem, I suggested that the opposite effects of the saturation of the cell membranes of lymphoid and nonlymphoid cells with cholesterol may occur in tumor cells (Dilman 1978a). Indeed, some observations show that the concentration of cholesterol per cell surface area in transformed cells is higher than in normal cells. This assumption holds only for nonlymphoid tissue: human diploid cell strain WI-38, and the line derived from it by SV40 transformation (Howard and Kritchevsky 1969); human breast cancer tissue (Hilf et al 1970); and transplanted Morris rat hepatoma (Synder et al 1969). The Ehrlich ascites tumor is able to derive most of its cholesterol from very low density lipoproteins that are abundant in the ascites fluid (Brennerman et al 1974). In conclusion, it may be said that hypercholesterolemia or, more precisely, an elevated level of LDL, is probably one of the factors promoting carcinogenesis.

Let us consider some other such factors. Experimental data show that insulin or insulin-like substances, eg, somatomedin, are indispensable for cell division in cultured tissue (Temin 1969, Morell and Froesch 1973). The findings of our laboratory show that the somatomedin-like activity of plasma increases in the course of normal aging and is more pronounced in individuals with obesity, atherosclerosis, or diabetes mellitus. It may be inferred then that excessive insulin and insulin-like activity are factors of higher risk of cancer because they promote an increase in the pool of proliferating cells (see Table 17-5). Insulin deprivation inhibits the growth of 7,12-dimethylbenzanthracene-induced mammary carcinoma (Heuson and Legros 1972).

The other side of the relationship between the blood levels of insulin and cancer, which relates to accelerated development, is of interest (see Chapter 21). Hyperinsulinemia also aids fat accumulation, thus creating favorable conditions for enhanced synthesis of cholesterol. Obesity is often accompanied by an increase in the blood level of FFA. At the same time, unsaturated fatty acids stimulate the growth of tumor cells directly (Holley et al 1974, Spector 1975). Thus, it may be suggested that such metabolic factors as hypercholesterolemia, low HDL-cholesterol level, elevated somatomedin activity, hyperinsulinemia, and enhanced utilization of FFA promote the division of nonlymphoid cells. Hence, since all these indices increase with advancing age, the said metabolic pattern contributes to the augmentation of the pool of proliferating somatic cells, thus increasing the likelihood of their malignant transformation. Particular mention should be made of the fact that the same metabolic shifts cause the development of metabolic immunodepression (see Chapter 15).

Therefore, both these factors, which increase the risk of tumor development, namely, the increased pool of proliferating cells and decreased cellular immunity, may be related to the same metabolic shifts. The opposite-directed influences of these metabolic factors on somatic nonlymphoid cells and T-dependent lymphocytes and macrophages are conducive to the formation of the syndrome of metabolic cancer susceptibility (Dilman 1978a). Hence, cancer susceptibility denotes a syndrome caused by specific metabolic shifts, rather than a general proneness to carcinogenesis. In more general terms, it may be maintained that the cancer susceptibility syndrome develops whenever a shift toward the predominant utilization of FFA as a source of energy occurs.

On the basis of the concept of such a syndrome, I suggested that phenformin should be studied with regard to its ability to suppress tumorigenesis (Dilman 1967, 1971). Several experiments in this field have been performed in our laboratory. First, it was shown that phenformin treatment reduces the incidence of DMBA-induced tumors of the mammary gland in rats (Dilman 1974a, 1974b; Dilman et al 1978). Second, it was found that phenformin treatment lowers the incidence of mammary gland tumors in the C3HA strain of mice (Table 17-11). It should be mentioned that the treatment resulted in a longer life span of experimental animals and a lower incidence of leukemia. Third, the antitumor effect of cyclophosphamide on transplantable squamous cell cervical carcinoma, on hepatoma-22a, and on Lewis lung tumor was found to be enhanced considerably when phenformin and cyclophosphamide were administered in combination (Table 17-12). Fourth, phenformin treatment potentiated the antitumor effect of hydrazine sulfate on Walker's carcinoma-256 (Table 17-12). Fifth, phenformin treatment alone inhibits the growth of Ehrlich's carcinoma.

Table 17-11
Effect of Phenformin and Dilantin Treatment on Life Span and Tumor Incidence in Female C3H Mice

	Control (n = 30)	Phenformin (n = 25)	Dilantin (n = 23)
Mean life span (days)	450±19	555±32*	558±28*
No. tumor-bearing mice	24 (80%)	5(20%)*	8 (34.8%)*
Adenocarcinoma of mammary gland			
No. mice	19 (63%)	4 (16%)*	7 (30.4%)*
Total tumors	30	4	7
Mammary tumors per mouse	1.58	1.00	1.00
Leukemia (no. mice)	4 (13.3%)	1 (4%)	2 (8.7%)
Other tumors	5	1	0

*Difference is statistically significant, $p < 0.05$.

Lack of space prohibits a detailed description of the data that indicate that the effects of pineal polypeptide extract (epithalamin) have much in common with those of phenformin. It also was found to exert an antitumor effect on mouse transplantable tumors (mammary cancer, squamous cell cervical carcinoma, hepatoma-22a, and lympholeukemia L10-1), to reduce the incidence of DMBA-induced mammary adenocarcinoma in rats, and to extend the life span of rats by 25% (Dilman and Anisimov 1975, Anisimov et al 1973b).

Naturally, the question arises as to what extent the available data may be interpreted as proof supporting the above concept of a cancer susceptibility syndrome. As mentioned, it is supposed that this syndrome is characterized by two components: an increased pool of proliferating somatic cells, and metabolic immunodepression. Metabolic immunodepression can be annulled by treatment with phenformin (see Chapter 15), and probably epithalamin (Dilman 1977). As to the increased pool of proliferating cells, the antitumor effect of phenformin via action on this component still has to be established. Proceeding from the concept of the cancer susceptibility syndrome, it should be supposed that the metabolic pattern concomitant with normal aging should promote cell division. This supposition is further supported by the evidence showing that hyperlipidemic blood serum contains a certain element that helps trigger DNA synthesis and cell division in aortic tissue culture (Florentin et al 1969; Chen et al 1977a, 1977b; Bierman and Albers 1975). The concomitance of hypocholesterolemia and some types of anemia may also be [illegible] Action of Cyclophosphamide or Hydrazine Sulfate

Species	Line	Tumor Strain	Drug	No. Animals	Average Weight of Tumor (mg)	Inhibition of Tumor Growth (%)	p*
Mice	BALB/c	SCC	Control†	16	951 ± 101	–	
			Phenformin	17	775 ± 118	19.4	> 0.05
			Cyclophosphamide	17	599 ± 78	37.7	< 0.01
			Phenformin + Cyclophosphamide	18	353 ± 81	63.6	< 0.01‡
	BALB/c	Sarcoma 180	Control†	10	2355 ± 186	–	
			Phenformin	9	1886 ± 290	19.9	> 0.05
			Cyclophosphamide	10	823 ± 163	65.1	< 0.01
			Phenformin + Cyclophosphamide	10	589 ± 135	75.0	< 0.01
	C3HA	Hepatoma-22a	Control†	12	990 ± 86	–	
			Phenformin	10	698 ± 112	29.5	> 0.05
			Cyclophosphamide	11	438 ± 59	55.8	< 0.01
			Phenformin + Cyclophosphamide	12	189 ± 51	80.9	< 0.01‡
	C57BL/6	Lewis lung tumor	Control†	16	424 ± 136	–	
			Phenformin	14	225 ± 79	46.9	> 0.05
			Cyclophosphamide	16	91 ± 62	78.5	< 0.05
			Phenformin + Cyclophosphamide	15	32 ± 27	92.5	< 0.01
Rats	Noninbred	Walker carcinoma-256	Control†	11	17,536 ± 1354	–	
			Phenformin	11	14,073 ± 999	19.7	> 0.05
			Hydrazine Sulfate	10	8310 ± 1182	52.6	< 0.05
			Phenformin + Hydrazine Sulfate	10	5150 ± 664	70.6	< 0.01‡

*Difference from control data.

†Control animals were treated orally with tap water and i.p. with normal saline.

‡Difference from the data for animals treated with cyclophosphamide or hydrazine sulfate only is statistically significant, $p < 0.05$.

considered as an indication of the key role of cholesterol in cell division (Westerman 1975). In diabetic rats, ie, in states characterized by an intensified utilization of FFA, an increase in the proliferative pool of mucosal cells in the small intestine was observed (Miller et al 1977a).

Meanwhile, it is generally believed at present that aging entails a decline in the proliferative pool of cells (Baserga 1977).[1] If this is true, it is desirable to know why aging inhibits cell division, although the number of the cell division-stimulating factors of the internal environment increases.

It may be suggested that the formation of the cancer susceptibility syndrome increases the risk of cancer because of the following factors and mechanisms, which at different stages may operate separately or in combination with each other:

1. Metabolic immunodepression. It is possible that the potentiation of the antitumor effect of hydrazine sulfate by phenformin treatment is caused by the ability of hydrazine sulfate (Gold 1970) and phenformin (Dietze et al 1978) to inhibit gluconeogenesis and thus to alleviate metabolic immunodepression.
2. Increased pool of proliferating cells as compared with the level typical of each tissue. Here, an analogy with the increased yield of intestinal tumors as a function of the enhanced cholesterol concentration in this tissue (Nigro et al 1977) seems to be justified.[2]
3. Development of conditions favoring tumor cell division. For example, FFA is utilized by tumor cells as a source of energy (Holley et al 1974) and inhibits lymphocyte activity at the same time (Turnell et al 1973). The inhibition of Ehrlich's ascites tumor by phenformin treatment is probably caused by the availability of the cholesterol contained in plasma VLDL for utilization by Erhlich tumor cells (Brennerman et al 1974).
4. Development of conditions promoting tumor nodule growth. For example, the metabolic pattern of cancer susceptibility contributes to platelet aggregation (see Chapter 12), thus promoting metastatic spread.

---

[1] When the influence of age on cell division is investigated in in vitro experiments, the same medium is used regardless of the age of the cultured cells; this is at variance with the age-dependent shift of the internal environment.

[2] The initiation of carcinogenesis and appearance of a tumor are spaced by a latent period; accordingly, the metabolic patterns of these states may be different. Taking into account the negative correlation between the shift in metabolic pattern and the decrease in DNA repair, one cannot neglect the influence of this mechanism pertinent to age-associated cancer susceptibility.

Hence, the pathways corresponding to (1), (3), and (4) occur at the stage of promotion, while those of (2) occur at the stage of inhibition of carcinogenesis. Taking into account the above, a "metabolic" explanation for the age-associated rise in cancer incidence may be given.

Metabolic Model of Age-Related Carcinogenesis

Mutations and related phenomena, for instance the integration of a viral genome or derepression of a cancer genome, taking place in the cells, make a major contribution to carcinogenesis (Knudson 1977). Metabolic shifts inherent in aging stimulate the division of somatic, nonlymphoid cells, thus presenting a higher risk of malignant transformation. At the same time, aging creates a metabolic pattern that causes metabolic immunodepression. Therefore, in the mechanism of carcinogenesis we must take into account both the phenomenon of genuine carcinogenesis caused by mutations and related phenomena, and the conditions promoting tumor development.

Under normal conditions, ie, when metabolic immunodepression does not occur, new antigens resulting from mutations or the newly developed properties of transformed cells stimulate lymphocyte division and, eventually, macrophage activity (Alexander 1976). As a result, malignant transformed cells are generally eliminated. The equilibrium gradually becomes upset on completion of body growth because the elevational mechanism leads to development of homeostatic failure. Finally, constancy of the internal environment becomes more and more disturbed. Since lymphocyte division processes depend on the condition of the internal environment, a metabolic immunodepression sets in, and transformed cells may escape from immunologic surveillance.

Thus, the same metabolic factors in different ways influence T lymphocytes on the one hand, and nonlymphoid somatic cells and tumor cells on the other. In particular, the division of T lymphocytes is controlled by antigens or mitogens that act on the plasma cell membrane. Thus the accumulation of cholesterol in the plasma cell membrane of T lymphocytes decreases (or abolishes) the lymphocyte proliferation in response to mitogen or antigen stimulation, thus causing metabolic immunodepression. On the contrary, the same metabolic factors (in particular, the increased blood insulin level and, correspondingly, the activation of the membrane glucose transport) act as an onset of the signal for cell division, which then increases the probability of the malignant transformation of somatic cells. It can be suggested that the decrease in cyclic AMP concentration and cholesterol synthesis intensification are induced by the increased glucose uptake in the cell and are the essential components of the cascade signal for cell division.

Finally, I believe the behavior of a transformed cell is determined by the so-called effect of insulinization of the cell. This phenomenon is brought about by the transforming protein (Karess et al 1979, Baumann and Hand 1979, Collett et al 1979) whose transformation mechanism may be determined by two factors: 1) the increase of cell membrane sensitivity to insulin and insulin-like serum factors, followed by the increase of glucose transport to the cell; and 2) phosphorylation of the main glycolytic enzymes, which increases their activity. Combination of these events provides both the division signal appearance and the increased internal concentrations of nutrients in the cell, thus being the crucial condition for cell growth, according to the version suggested by Holley (1972). The increased glycolysis produced by this transforming protein is believed to be responsible for the other properties of a transformed cell (Ash et al 1976, Lau et al 1979, McClain et al 1978). From this point of view a transforming protein may be defined as "an internal insulinizing factor." Many external environmental factors may aid carcinogenesis by stimulating different components of this mechanism, including an intensified cell division of normal and transformed cells caused by the increased blood level of insulin and insulin-like factors.

Many external environmental factors may promote carcinogenesis by influencing different components of the elevational mechanism. For example, excessive food intake and resultant overweight raise the levels of insulin, free fatty acids, and cholesterol in the blood. It was shown experimentally that a fat-rich diet may intensify carcinogenesis (Wynder 1976). Tobacco smoking (nicotine) and coffee drinking enhance lipolysis. Ionizing irradiation increases the number of mutations and raises FFA and cholesterol levels (Moroz and Kendich 1975). Many hormones promote an increase in the pool of proliferating cells, thus raising the risk of mutations. Since the metabolic pattern of cancer susceptibility has much in common with that of normal aging, pregnancy, and stress, it becomes clear that this pattern is identical to those of all basic diseases of compensation. For example, depressive illness is characterized by the resistance of the hypothalamic-pituitary complex to inhibition by glucocorticoids (see Chapter 14) and, as a consequence, metabolic shifts, typical of the cancer susceptibility syndrome, develop (Brown et al 1975). Moreover, some data show that depressive illness contributes to carcinogenesis and intensifies tumor development (Stoll 1976). The concepts of metabolic cancrophilia and compensation diseases can provide explanations of a relatively higher cancer incidence in patients with essential hypertension as compared with subjects with normal arterial pressure (see Chapter 13), as well as the correlations between blood glucose levels and cancer proneness (Cheraskin et al 1968). In other words, any compensation disease is concomitant with higher incidence of cancer.

Finally, it can hardly be denied that the metabolic pattern

characteristic of cancer susceptibility can act as a trigger mechanism causing malignant transformation or derepression of a preexisting cancer genome. In particular, Hradec (1975) presented evidence on the role of cholesteryl 14-methylhexadecanoate in gene expression. Normal aging also involves a specific mechanism thought to be responsible for the rise in tumor incidence in the so-called hormone-dependent tissues. In such cases, the increased secretion of proliferative hormones, as a result of the development of the central type of feedback failure in the main homeostatic systems of the organism, increases the pool of proliferating cells. For example, gonadotropin secretion in healthy women increases nearly sixfold in the period from 25 to 45 years of age. If this finding is compared with the similar data on animals following the transplantation of an ovary into the spleen, it becomes apparent that a cancer-promoting background is gradually formed in the course of normal aging.

Secondary Syndrome of Metabolic Cancer Susceptibility

As far as the influence of tumors is concerned, on reaching a certain size, they in turn cause secondary hormonal-metabolic shifts that correspond to the syndrome of cancer susceptibility to a considerable degree, if not completely (Dilman 1974a). My associates have observed that tumor transplantation results in an elevation of the hypothalamic threshold in the reproductive system of the rat (Anisimov and Yermoschenkov 1975). These findings are consistent with the decrease in the inhibitory effect of dexamethasone on the hypothalamic-pituitary-adrenal system as tumor growth progresses (Bishop and Ross 1970, Saez 1974). An elucidation of the mechanism by which tumors influence the hypothalamus is of particular interest. It has been observed that carbohydrate tolerance is decreased in rats with transplanted tumors (Figure 17-4), with blood insulin level rather high. This state fits the pattern of age-associated metabolic shifts and should stimulate gluconeogenesis. Following inoculation of experimental animals with tumors, the cholesterol level in lymphoid cells increases progressively (Kigoshi and Akiyama 1975), which may contribute to further metabolic immunodepression.

At present, it is possible to test the hypothesis on the cause of all the manifestations of the secondary syndrome of cancer susceptibility, from the elevation of the hypothalamic threshold of sensitivity to feedback suppression to lymphocyte enrichment with cholesterol.

To a certain extent, changes related to "accidental" or genetic defects, which finally bring about the formation of the metabolic pattern typical of this syndrome, may be referred to as the secondary syndrome of cancer susceptibility. In particular, it is known that cancer incidence is relatively high while the blastogenic response of lymphocytes to PHA declines in patients with Down's syndrome. Of some interest in this connection are our findings demonstrating cholesterol level in Down's syndrome to be 1.75 $\mu g/1 \times 10^6$ cells, as compared with 1.1 ± 1 $\mu g/1 \times 10^6$ cells in healthy controls ($p < 0.01$) (Schwarz et al 1978). It is not yet clear whether it is possible to eliminate metabolic immunodepression and the cancer susceptibility syndrome in these patients by improving the lipid profile of blood.

Some types of familial hyperlipoproteinemia (types IIb and IV) (Frederickson et al 1967) with concomitant hyperinsulinemia may be responsible for the secondary syndrome of cancer susceptibility. There is also much in common between this syndrome and disturbances caused by many carcinogenic substances in vivo. Apart from causing damage to cells, ie, producing a mutagenic effect, such carcinogens, as DMBA, dimethylhydrazine, nitrosamines, and aflatoxin diminish glucose utilization, thus tilting the balance toward the predominant utilization of FFA. This eventually produces a syndrome that may be described as carcinogenic aging.

In light of the latter concept, more pathways of the action of carcinogenic chemicals on the organism may be identified (see Chapter 20). But until this problem is tackled, it is advisable to cite the data revealing

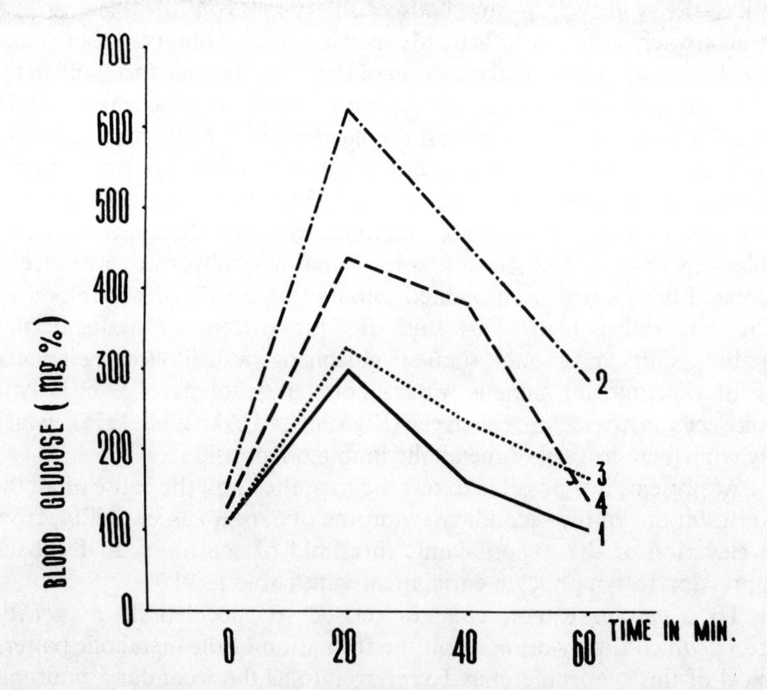

Figure 17-4 Effect of tumor transplantation on glucose tolerance in rats, measured after administration of glucose (3 g/kg body weight). 1: Control; 2: Walker carcinoma 256; 3: Pliss lymphosarcoma; 4: Sarcoma 45.

that, in genetically susceptible C3H/H1J female mice carrying the Bittner mammary tumor virus from birth, tumor incidence was dramatically reduced from about 80% in mice housed under sustained stress to less than 10% in mice housed in specially designed protective antistress conditions (Riley et al 1976). It is also significant that mammary gland tumors were not detectable on day 500 in C3H mice on a diet with a 40% reduction in calorie content, while in controls on a free diet, tumor incidence rate was as high as 70% in the same period (Fernandes et al 1976). Perhaps, had both experiments been carried on for a longer period, the effect of carcinogenesis inhibition by diet control would have declined. For instance, our findings demonstrate that treatment with phenformin and epithalamin can considerably lower the incidence of tumors induced by chemical substances (Dilman et al 1978) or virus (see Table 17-11). However, if these drugs are administered during the whole lifetime of animals, tumors will probably arise at later stages, frequently outside the mean life span limits characteristic of control animals. Thus, if we can neutralize the effects of the genetic heterogeneity of the human population which manifest themselves by familial hyperlipoproteinemia or other random defects, and the syndrome of cancer susceptibility becomes manageable by drugs, the age-associated increase in cancer incidence will be so slow that the probable date of cancer onset in many cases may shift outside the mean life expectancy limits of modern man.

18 Physiologic Aging as a Normal Disease

It is certain that people do not die of old age as such, but rather of the disease incident to it. Even if this disease cannot be diagnosed, aged people still die of diseases because aging is a disease or a confluence of diseases of homeostasis.

Suppose there is an ideal external environment that precludes exposure of the organism to any unfavorable factors. Still, certain age-associated changes will inevitably occur in this organism even in such a strictly conditioned environment. For instance, it is certain that reproductive function will be switched off at a predetermined age. Therefore, a normal disease related to specific disturbances in reproductive homeostat, the climacteric, will inevitably occur, regardless of external environmental factors (see Chapter 4). Relevant age-associated changes take place in the other main homeostatic systems, too: the adaptive, energy, caloric, and thyroid homeostats (see Chapters 3, 5, 6, and 7). Any persistent disturbance in the stability of the internal environment is a disease. Therefore, normal aging should be referred to as a confluence of diseases of homeostasis, or diseases of compensation.

If aging is a disease or a confluence of diseases, what are their symptoms and manifestations? As shown in Chapters 3–7 all main homeostatic systems are characterized by the same pattern in this regard. All the disturbances occurring in the different homeostats accumulate to form a perpetual cycle of interdependent metabolic shifts. In the energy homeostat regulatory disturbances lead to a compensatory age-connected rise in insulin secretion. This hyperinsulinemia becomes a key factor in the age-associated gain of body weight and rise in the blood levels of VLDL, triglycerides, LDL, and cholesterol (see Chapter 6). Increased resistance to the action of glucose and insulin in the hypothalamic system controlling food intake and fat stores is followed by overfeeding and adiposity (see Chapter 5).

The adaptive system experiences a rise of resistance to feedback suppression in the hypothalamic-ACTH-glucocorticoid system which leads to a relative excess of glucocortiocoids (see Chapter 3). The output of androgen-like steroids drops off. Consequently the metabolic process shifts toward an intensified catabolism. Gluconeogenesis is accelerated; the insulin-antagonistic action of growth hormone is potentiated; tolerance to carbohydrates declines; and immunologic defense mechanisms are inhibited, particularly those of cell-mediated immunity (see Chapter 15).

In the reproductive system, elevation of the hypothalamic threshold in the tonic region of the sex center produces intensification of gonadotropin secretion (see Chapter 4). The compensatory increase in sex hormone output contributes to the maintenance of cyclic reproductive function as the hypothalamic threshold gradually rises. In the course of this compensatory process, however, there occurs an excess of both central hormones (gonadotropins) and peripheral (estrogen-like) hormones). This has an untoward effect on the target tissues of the reproductive system. Later, the age-associated switching-off of reproductive function results in decreased secretion of classic estrogens.

As age advances, the blood level of triiodothyronine declines, which causes several metabolic disturbances, eg, hypercholesterolemia. However, the drop in triiodothyronine level does not cause a compensatory intensification of thyroid activity because the sensitivity of the hypothalamic-pituitary system that controls this activity rises with advancing age (see Chapter 7).

To summarize, the metabolic pattern of aging is characterized by the following complex of disturbances: decreased sensitivity to insulin; hyperinsulinemia; decline in tolerance to carbohydrates; obesity; increased lipolysis and utilization of fatty acids; high blood levels of VLDL, triglycerides, LDL, and cholesterol; relative excess of cortisol secretion; decreased output of androgen-like hormones (17-ketosteroids); decreased cellular immunity; increased secretion of total gonadotropins and total phenolsteroids; lowered output of classic estrogens; elevation of blood pressure; decreased function of the thyroid; and a high titer of auto-antibodies such as thyroglobulin antibodies.

The formation of such hormonal and metabolic patterns in the course of normal aging lies at the basis of age-specific pathology that develops in humans. Following are eight diseases known to be the cause of death in about 85% of middle-aged and older persons: atherosclerosis, cancer, essential hypertension, maturity-onset diabetes mellitus, obesity, lowered resistance to infection (dysadaptosis), psychic depression, and autoimmune disorders. The frequency of these pathologic states rises with advancing age, and their hormonal and metabolic conditions are identical to those of normal aging (see Chapters 11–17). These diseases often manifest signs of the metabolic shifts characteristic of intensified aging, but generally it requires only normal age-associated changes to trigger their development. Some of these diseases are masked, thus producing a false impression that the decline in life vigor is determined by aging. Latent development is particularly characteristic of atherosclerosis; still, the lipid levels in the arterial wall show an increase in each individual as age advances.

We can account for all this by citing the age-associated deviation of homeostasis which in turn is connected with the shift of the hypothalamic threshold of sensitivity to homeostatic signals. At this point we should summarize the main data and consider the mechanisms which are likely to underlie the elevation of the hypothalamic threshold of sensitivity to feedback control.

Biogenic Amines and Other Neurotransmitters

The level of biogenic amines is one of the most important factors of hypothalamic sensitivity to feedback control. Therefore, one should agree with those authors who identify disturbances in the balance between the adrenergic and serotonergic systems as the cause of homeostatic disorders, rather than the simultaneous decrease in the activity of these systems.

However, the specific roles of the adrenergic and serotonergic mechanisms in the functioning of main homeostatic systems seem to differ. For instance, the adrenergic mechanisms are of major importance for the implementation of age-associated changes in the reproductive homeostat (see Chapter 4). Conversely, treatment with tryptophan and L-dopa improves the sensitivity of the adaptive homeostat to feedback suppression (see Chapter 3).

As age advances, the level of biogenic amines in the brain and, particularly, in the hypothalamus declines (Finch 1973, Robinson 1975, Robinson et al 1977). It was found in our laboratory that the age-associated decline in catecholamine levels is determined by the diminished concentration in noradrenaline, while that of dopamine remains unchanged (see Chapter 4). This is matched by a decrease in the levels of serotonin and 5-hydroxy-indolacetic acid, though, judging by the data of Robinson (1975), the concentration of serotonin in the hypothalamus becomes relatively higher with respect to that of catecholamines. It should be taken into consideration that the effect of biogenic amines and other neurotransmitters on the secretion of pituitary hormones (Smythe 1977), and on the threshold of sensitivity of the hypothalamic-pituitary complex to homeostatic stimuli, manifest different aspects of their action.

Reduction in Hormone Receptor Concentration

Many tissues are characterized by a decrease in the concentration of hormone receptors and in the binding ability of cell membranes with increasing age (Larson et al 1972; Freeman et al 1973; Roth et al 1978a, 1978b). The decline in the concentration of some hormone receptors inevitably occurs in the course of aging. Therefore, there is no reason to believe that brain cells, specifically those of the hypothalamus, are exceptions. Lower concentration of hormone receptors may be expected to result in the decline in the sensitivity or even resistance of relevant structures to regulatory stimuli. However, it should be emphasized that this phenomenon is not an irreversible defect under all conditions, and sometimes is caused by functional disturbances, eg, shifts in the level of biogenic amines. The following data should be considered in this connection.

Neonatal treatment with testosterone is known to cause continuous estrus in rats. It was shown that the treatment results in a reduction in the concentration of estrogen-binding receptors in the hypothalamus (Flerko and Mess 1968). The resumption of the estrous cycle in the androgenized rats was attained by noradrenaline administration (Flerko 1974). Age-associated decrease in the catecholamine level in the brain may affect adversely the hypothalamic ability to bind estrogens (Peng and Peng 1973) and, therefore, may contribute to the elevation of hypothalamic threshold.

Changes in Monoamine Oxidase Activity

Changes taking place in monoamine oxidase activity are likely to be directly responsible for relevant changes in biogenic amine levels with increasing age. It was shown that the levels of activity of these enzymes in the brain rise with aging both in animals and in humans (Robinson et al 1972, Robinson 1975). Such changes in different areas of the brain, primarily the hypothalamus, are accompanied by a decrease in catecholamine levels and, to a lesser degree, in the serotonin level. However, it is not clear yet what is actually responsible for the decline in monoamine oxidase activity.

Changes in Tissue Sensitivity to Hormones and Other Factors of Feedback Control

Aging is accompanied by the decline in the sensitivity of many tissues to hormones. To specify, the time required to induce the synthesis of some hepatic enzymes increases in direct proportion with age. Previously, it seemed that these data supported the concept of aging processes on cellular and tissue levels. Now, it has been shown that such shifts are brought about by regulatory factors (Adelman 1976, 1978). For example, under specific experimental conditions, no age dependence is demonstrable for the increase in glucokinase activity following treatment with insulin (Adelman 1970). Indeed, as far as the effect of hormone concentration is concerned, the hypothalamus is a peripheral tissue. Meanwhile, the decline in hypothalamic sensitivity to homeostatic inhibition may be determined to a considerable degree by changes in hormonal environment.

Decreased Secretion of Pineal Hormones

Melatonin and related compounds have received study thus far. On the whole, melatonin has an inhibitory effect on some systems of the hypothalamic-pituitary complex (Wurtman 1970, Axelrod 1974). However, a growing amount of data show that the pineal gland also secretes polypeptides (or even protein hormones) (Milcu et al 1963, Morozov and Khavinson 1971, Benson et al 1972, Chazov et al 1972, Ostroumova and Dilman 1972, Chazov and Isachenkov 1974). It was suggested that some pineal polypeptides act as modulators that change hypothalamic sensitivity to regulatory endogenous stimuli (Dilman 1970a). From this point of view, it was easier to explain the broad spectrum of the effects exerted by the pineal gland. The hypothesis on the ability of polypeptides to raise hypothalamic sensitivity to regulation was later confirmed for the adaptive (Ostroumova and Dilman 1972) and reproductive homeostats (Anisimov et al 1973a). The level of melatonin output seems to decrease with aging (Pelham et al 1973). It is likely that, as age advances, the production of pineal polypeptides is decreased. This is suggested by indirect evidence pointing to a low level of antigonadotropic factor excretion observed in some types of cancer (Ostroumova 1972; Table 18-1).

Table 18-1
Frequency of Antigonadotropic Factor Detection in Healthy Women and Patients with Breast Cancer or Endometrial Carcinoma

Group	Frequency of Detection (%)	*p*
Menopausal controls	80.0	
Breast cancer	33.5	< 0.02
Endometrial carcinoma	11.8	< 0.001

Source: Ostroumova 1972.

Some data suggest the pineal origin of the antigonadotropic factors. This is supported by a lower weight of the pineal gland in cancer victims (Tapp and Blumfield 1970). It should be noted that pineal extract raises sensitivity to estrogens in old rats, ie, in cases of elevated hypothalamic threshold, and fails to exert a similar effect in younger animals (Anisimov et al 1973a). The same treatment also brings about the resumption of cyclic ovarian function in old rats with constant estrus (see Figure 4-1). There is a recent report indicating that aqueous extracts of rat pineal glands are more potent than melatonin in blocking compensatory ovarian hypertrophy (Orts et al 1974). The age-associated elevation of the hypothalamic threshold of sensitivity and longer reaction to stress in old age may be at least partially accounted for by the decline in the functional activity of the pineal gland (see Chapter 3). However, there remains much to be explained in the mechanism of pineal polypeptide effect. Changes in the regulation of the rate of energy processes may provide one possible mechanism.

Shifts in Energy Processes

One of the fundamental concepts of the elevational model of development and aging is that the supply of energy required during growth and accelerated aging is ensured by prevalent utilization of free fatty acids (see Chapters 1 and 8). Use of this concept seems to be justified when the mechanism of hypothalamic threshold elevation is studied. Generally speaking, aging is characterized by disturbances in the rhythm of control systems and, therefore, probably by an intensification of energy processes taking place in the hypothalamus itself. For instance, it was shown that hypothalamic tissue takes up more oxygen in an old rat than in a young one (Panksepp and Reilly 1975); the same occurs in humans (Kushima et al 1961). However, pineal polypeptides raise hypothalamic sensitivity and inhibit respiration in an isolated culture of mitochondria (Kondrashova et al 1977).

The relationship between hypothalamic sensitivity to feedback control and energy processes is further exemplified by the results obtained by Kennedy and Mitra (1963) in experiments on rats and the statistical data of Frisch (1973), showing that the age at which reproductive function is switched on, is determined, to a considerable extent, by reaching a certain "critical" body weight. If the switching-on of reproductive function is dependent upon the increase in hypothalamic resistance to inhibition by sex hormones (Donovan and Van der Werff ten Bosch 1959), it points to a relationship between the hypothalamic threshold of sensitivity and body fat accumulation, the latter being an indication of a certain stage of metabolic processes. It should be particularly emphasized that estrus was found to commence in the rats on a high-fat diet at an earlier age than in those kept on an isocalorically equivalent low-fat diet (Frisch et al 1975).

However, it may be emphasized that administration of not only L-dopa but also pineal polypeptide extract, phenformin, Dilantin, and succinic acid, raises the sensitivity of the hypothalmic-pituitary complex to stilbestrol action (see Figure 4-3). And the same effect can be produced by injecting L-dopa and pineal extract into the third ventricle of the brain, which suggests that these drugs do exert their effect on the hypothalamic level. Our present knowledge is not sufficient for an adequate description of the mechanism of the effects of all these preparations. Still, there is evidence that each of them exerts its effect via metabolic processes. To illustrate, succinic acid was found to stimulate metabolic processes in Krebs cycle (Kondrashova et al 1977). Dilantin, which raises hypothalamic sensitivity to inhibition by estrogens (Figure 4-3), seems to exert its effect through the catecholamine mechanism, taking into account the Dilantin-induced stimulation of hypothalamic binding of dopamine (Hadfield 1972). Also, the Dilantin-induced intracellular accumulation of potassium ions (Escueta and Appel 1971) should be taken into consideration because this phenomenon may reduce the activity of the regulatory system as the result of a shift to synthetic anabolic processes (Laborit 1965).

The effect of phenformin is difficult to explain because it is customarily assumed that glucose transfer to nerve cells is not controlled by insulin. However, phenformin-induced normalization of a number of metabolic parameters, eg, the decrease in blood levels of 11-hydroxycorticosteroids, cholesterol, and β-lipoproteins, as well as diminished gonadotropin excretion (see Chapter 24), points to a much wider-than-expected therapeutic range of this drug. It is possible that there is still another as yet unknown mechanism of lowering the hypothalamic threshold and therefore normalizing the metabolism. This mechanism may be similar to the one by which prepubertal weight gain leads to age-associated switching-on of the reproductive function. In this connection it may be mentioned that, even in cases of secondary (central) amenorrhea, spontaneous resumption of the menstrual cycle is followed by a short-term increase in body weight (Frisch and McArthur 1974). Moreover, phenformin may affect metabolism of the neuroglia where, according to Laborit (1965), metabolic processes required for neuronal function take place.

This analysis of possible mechanisms for the changes in hypothalamic feedback systems by some pharmacologic agents suggests the functional origin of the age-associated deviation of the hypothalamic set point of sensitivity.

It should be stressed that the above data bear only on the role of biogenic amines in the mechanism of homeostatic deviation during aging. However, these results should be evaluated with great caution with respect to the role of a particular neurotransmitter, because the species-specific peculiarities and interactions of the neurotransmitter system cannot be assessed in most cases (see Chapter 3). Some data available on the role of biogenic amines in the mechanism of changes in the sensitivity threshold of these homeostats are discussed in other chapters.

The hypothalamus-induced changes in the levels of peripheral hormones and metabolites seem in turn to affect the hypothalamus by causing changes in biogenic amine concentration. The following data illustrate this point. Sex hormones affect the uptake of biogenic amines in the brain (Wirz-Justice et al 1974) as well as catecholamine metabolism in the hypothalamus (Cardinali et al 1975). Moreover, there are indications that in the hypothalamus estradiol and estrone are converted to catechol estrogens, and the latter are competitive inhibitors of O-methylation of catecholamines by catechol-O-methyl transferase. This finding establishes a biochemical link in the central nervous system between estradiol and neurotransmitters (Fishman and Norton 1975).

It has been suggested that the level of sensitivity of hypothalamic centers to glucose may be reduced by glucocorticoids (Franchimont et al 1970), and the latter may influence serotonin metabolism in the brain (Neckers and Sze 1975). It is also necessary to mention the data showing that L-dopa stimulates the secretion of serotonin (Ng et al 1970), while 5-hydroxytryptophan stimulates secretion of noradrenaline in the brain (Okada et al 1972). The brain seems to contain a decarboxylase that takes part in the synthesis of both serotonin and catecholamines (Dairman et al 1975). Finally, the insulin-induced rise in the blood free tryptophan level influences an extremely wide range of parameters, including the brain level of serotonin.

Thus there is a rather impressive body of evidence of functional changes to support the supposition that the hypothalamic threshold is elevated in the course of normal development and aging. This conclusion is also consistent with the observation that the number of neurons in the hypothalamus is not decreased unless the brain is damaged by arteriosclerosis (Finch 1973). These functional changes may be caused by at least the following factors:

1. An age-associated decrease in catecholamine and serotonin levels in the hypothalamus, as well as a change in the balance between them due to a less pronounced decrease in serotonin (Dilman 1978).
2. An increase in the level of MAO activity in the midbrain (Robinson et al 1977).
3. A decrease in the quantity and binding ability of the hypothalamic receptors of hormones. This process may depend partially on the reduction in biogenic amine concentration.
4. A decrease in the secretion of pineal polypeptide hormones capable of decreasing hypothalamic sensitivity to homeostatic stimuli, as well as a decrease in serotonin and melatonin levels.
5. A decreased utilization of glucose in the direct pentose oxidative pathway, which determines the effectiveness of the so-called potassium pump. The raised threshold of hypothalamic sensitivity following Dilantin administration may be caused partially by the rise in intracellular potassium concentration under the influence of this drug.
6. A rise in the rate of metabolic processes. It is possible that the increase in body mass (observed both in periods of growth and in age-associated fat accumulation) results in an initial elevation of the hypothalamic threshold, which is conducive to a further increase in the fat content of the body.

If in some degree this approaches an adequate description of the mechanism of deviation, it still does not reveal the causes of the regular age-dependent development of all the factors responsible for hypothalamic sensitivity regulation. One therefore turns to the genetic program of age-associated changes, since this would be consonant with the fundamental biologic significance of hypothalamic threshold elevation. But, before we can consider the problems pertinent to such a genetic program, we must take up one other matter.

On completion of growth the elevation of the hypothalamic set point leads to deviations from the constancy of the internal environment of the organism, and thus to the formation of diseases of compensation. What happens to the steadily changing hypothalamic sensitivity threshold, however, when the genetic growth period, ie, the development of sexual maturity, is complete? It seems logical to assume that on termination of the growth period the set point of hypothalamic sensitivity would stabilize at a permanent level. But the data obtained in our study on age-associated changes in the adaptive system show that this does not happen (see Chapter 3). Why is the hypothalamic sensitivity threshold not stabilized?

First, stabilization of the hypothalamic threshold would require an additional mechanism to come into play on completion of the reproductive period. But natural selection does not seem to have promoted the formation of such a mechanism. Instead, elevation of the hypothalamic threshold, which continues after the onset of the reproductive period, assures the age-associated switching-off of reproductive function by the same mechanism used earlier to switch it on (see Chapter 4). (Here the biological role of elevation of the hypothalamic threshold becomes apparent.) Finally, natural selection is probably not able to remove harmful late-acting genes from the population (Medawar 1952). This is because evolution selects features only during the reproductive phase of life.

Any of these three reasons would account for the lack of stabilization in the hypothalamus on completion of the organism's growth. However, it appears likely that all may be responsible for this phenomenon. At the same time it is evident that this process results inevitably in a deterioration of those optimal physiologic conditions established in the period immediately after the completion of growth. Consequently the stability of the internal environment is upset, and this eventually leads to age-specific pathology since any persistent state at variance with the normal parameters of the internal environment is a disease. Therefore, aging is at the same time a normal physiologic process and a disease, or rather a confluence of homeostatic diseases. There is no distinction, in other words, between so-called normal aging and diseases associated with aging; rather we consider normal aging itself to be a form of disease. Thus the compensatory intensification of the activity of some endocrine glands, physiologically indispensable when the hypothalamic threshold is rising, creates at the same time a mechanism for the formation of diseases inherent in aging. Such diseases originally were designated as diseases of compensation (Dilman 1968, 1971, 1974a). Initially I implied by this term only a compensatory increase in peripheral endocrine activity. However, the same principal applies to the intensification of hormonal activity in the pituitary which immediately follows elevation of the hypothalamic threshold. The increased output of pituitary hormones may inhibit the secretion of hypothalamic hormones directly through the short loop of hormonal feedback (see Chapter 2).

The type of age-specific pathology is determined chiefly by two factors: specific age-associated changes in the organism's main homeostatic systems, and certain features of these systems that are peculiar to the specific organism. Accordingly, different species of animals have different features in their age-specific pathology, but on the whole the metabolic patterns of such pathology are similar. Like humans, for instance, rats feature an age-associated gain of body weight, decreased tolerance to carbohydrates, hyperinsulinemia, raised blood levels of cholesterol and triglycerides, and hypercorticism (Wexler 1976, Lewis and Wexler 1974). Similar changes occur in the Pacific salmon (see Chapter 1).

All the foregoing suggests the conclusion that aging is characterized by a confluence of diseases of compensation. However, it is well known that such changes may develop at any age, independent of age-associated processes, often as a result of external factors. Stress, diet, toxic factors, even the general quality of life, can all be primary causes for diseases of compensation like obesity, atherosclerosis, late-onset diabetes, reduced resistance to infection, and cancer. Consequently these diseases often are referred to as "diseases of civilization." Since there is an obvious discrepancy between the interpretation of age-specific pathology as a consequence of internal factors on the one hand, and external factors on the other, it is necessary to compare the mechanisms of action of both these factors. Such a comparison will be the subject of Part III of this book, in which the most influential external factors, stress, chemical carcinogens, and overfeeding, will be discussed.

PART III
External Environment and Diseases of Aging

Civilization does not cause the so-called diseases of civilization, it rather introduces uncertainty into the predetermined mechanism of formation of diseases of aging.

---

19 The Relationship between Diseases of Compensation and Diseases of Adaptation

Adaptation to stressor factors is not feasible unless certain homeostatic disturbances in the internal environment of the organism have occurred. In turn, a homeostatic disturbance cannot persist throughout the period required for defense, unless hypothalamic threshold of sensitivity to feedback control is elevated. Thus, acceleration of aging and diseases of aging are the price we pay for defense against stressors.

It is natural that the hormonal mechanism of adaptation to various stressors should be assured by a relevant intensification of energy processes. Moreover, little attention has been paid to the contribution made by the energy supply in the stress reaction to the mechanism of formation of diseases of adaptation.

During stress, out of the two available energy-producing substrates, glucose and FFAs, the latter are used predominantly. As a result, stress switches on a mechanism that ensures the uptake of FFA rather than glucose by target tissues. One of the features of this mechanism is the elevation of hypothalamic activity, followed by a rise in the levels of secretion of such lipolytic and contrainsulin hormones as adrenaline, growth hormone, ACTH, and prolactin (Noel et al 1972). Simultaneously, the hyperadrenalinemia-induced inhibition of insulin secretion (Kansal et al 1977) intensifies the lipolytic action of these hormones.

An intensified lipolysis leads directly to a decrease in the uptake of glucose by muscle tissue within the glucose fatty acid cycle (Randle 1965). This effect is contributed to by excessive cortisol, which eventually results in the predominant utilization of FFA for energy supply. It should be pointed out that the mechanism responsible for the enhanced utilization of FFA for energy supply promotes gluconeogenesis. This is also effected by an excessive cortisol level and the direct action of FFA, which act to switch on the metabolic pathway in the direction toward gluconeogenesis (Weber et al 1966). Simultaneously, high levels of cortisol, and probably free fatty acids, cause the lysis of lymphocytes (Turnell et al 1973). This causes a soaring in the level of glycogenic amino acids, precursors of glucose synthesis. Finally, such an interaction leads to the formation of a metabolic pattern that produces the syndrome of metabolic immunodepression (see Chapter 15).

It should be emphasized that during stress reaction the level of blood cholesterol is increased (Rothfeld et al 1974), although triglyceride synthesis is inhibited by stress (Robertson and Smith 1975). Moreover, a shift toward the predominant utilization of FFA as a source of energy must necessarily result in disturbances inherent in normal aging, ie, in compensation diseases, if the stress situation continues for a long period of time.

The mechanism of reaction to stress is actuated by the intensification of activity of the hypothalamic-pituitary-adrenal complex. Subsequently, it was found that stress causes the activation of other hypothalamic-pituitary complexes as well. However, it was overlooked that the elevation of hypothalamic-pituitary activity could not persist long enough, ie, for a period when defense against the stressor is needed, unless the resistance of the hypothalamic-pituitary complex to inhibitory stimuli were raised (Dilman 1971, 1972). Indeed, stress reaction involves such disturbances as increased blood levels of cortisol, free fatty acids, and glucose. Because of the negative feedback mechanism, a rise in blood concentrations of these substances would inhibit the hypothalamic-pituitary complex and thus decrease the said parameters, unless hypothalamic threshold to inhibition in stress were simultaneously elevated. In other words, elevation of the hypothalamic threshold makes possible the mechanism of defense against stressors.

Fortunately, stress does involve a rise in the hypothalamic threshold to inhibition following the intensification of hypothalamic activity. This concept may be illustrated by the findings of Zimmerman and Critchlow (1969), who showed that where only 10 μg/100 g body weight of dexamethasone is required to suppress adrenal function in rats under normal conditions, a dose ten times that much is necessary to obtain the same effect in rats 15 minutes after the onset of stress induced by a three-minute application of ether. Similar data have been obtained in our laboratory (Ostroumova 1978). It may be supposed that a similar situation exists in the other homeostatic systems, ie, those involving growth hormone and glucose regulation.

An exposure to chronic stress caused, for instance, by an increase in the size of an animal population, is also characterized by relevant rises in ACTH and corticosteroid output (Christian 1968). Such shifts raise animal death rates from infections, tumors, and glomerulonephritis, and suppress the reproductive system, thus maintaining an optimal size of the population (Solomon et al 1974; Christian 1968, 1976).

Naturally, there is a problem as to the nature of processes underlying the mechanism of the stressor-induced elevation of the hypothalamic set point. It is important to note that there is considerable neuropharmacologic evidence for a brain noradrenergic system that exerts tonic inhibition of ACTH secretion (Gruen 1978). Stress intensifies catecholamine metabolism in the brain, leading to a decrease in their concentration in the hypothalamus (Scapagnini et al 1973). This relieves the tonic inhibition of ACTH secretion, raising its level in blood. The decrease in catecholamine level is, at the same time, one of the cardinal factors of hypothalamic threshold elevation (see Chapter 18). This may be accounted for by the results of Scapagnini et al (1973), which indicate that the sensitivity to dexamethasone suppression during stress reaction was restored by iproniazid administration.

The insusceptibility of growth hormone secretion to inhibition in stress is determined largely by the adrenergic mechanisms of its regulation, which are not controlled by energy metabolites (Vigneri et al 1973).

Serotonin metabolism undergoes considerable changes, too. Short-term stress lowers serotonin concentration in the hypothalamus (Vermes et al 1973) by enhancing the rate of its metabolism. The increased effect of serotonin is immediately responsible for the rise in ACTH, growth hormone, and prolactin secretion. Yet, stress of longer duration (60 to 180 minutes under experimental conditions) results in a rise in the hypothalamic content of serotonin (Telegdy and Vermes 1975). The turnover of serotonin is similarly increased (Morgan et al 1975, Scapagnini et al 1973). The decline of serotonin level in the hypothalamus may also be supposed to be among the factors causing the elevation of the hypothalamic set point to feedback suppression during stress. This assumption can be supported by the data showing that both L-dopa and L-tryptophan improve the sensitivity of the limbic-hypothalamic-pituitary-adrenal complex to dexamethasone suppression (see Table 3-8). The assumption of similarity between hypothalamic alterations occurring in chronic stress and those observed in mental depression seems to be of interest from still another point of view. One of the obscure problems directly related to the general adaptation syndrome is why the organism fails to maintain the same level of resistance to stress throughout the life span. Hans Selye (1952) put forward the concept of "some adaptive energy required to perform adaptive work and manifested by the resistance of the organism to chronic stress." The amount of adaptation energy was believed to be finite and subject to exhaustion under the influence of stress (Selye and Tuchweber 1976).

In this context, the following proposal can be made. If the realization of a chronic stress reaction is not feasible unless the hypothalamic set point is steadily elevated, the factors determining the elevating mechanism should play an important role in the decline of adaptive capacity in the course of aging. With advancing age, a constant decrease takes place in the concentration of biogenic amines in the hypothalamus (Robinson 1975), which is one of the key factors determining the age-related elevation of the hypothalamic set point to feedback control in the adaptive homeostat (see Chapter 3). As a result, the state of the adaptive homeostat, with advancing age or when unaffected by stress, is similar to that in chronic stress. Time is a natural stressor.

In addition, the pool of biogenic amines becomes increasingly exhausted because of the influence of environmental stressors. Together, the influences of intrinsic (aging) and extrinsic (stress) factors form in the course of aging a pattern that in many respects corresponds to that of mental depression (Sachar 1975; see Chapter 14).

In this connection, it is noteworthy that sedatives, specifically diazepam and phenazepam, exert a normalizing influence on the diurnal rhythm of cortisol secretion as well as on the threshold of sensitivity to dexamethasone suppression (Table 19-1).

Table 19-1
Influence of Phenazepam (Benzodiazepine Derivative) on Diurnal Rhythm of Blood 11-Hydroxycorticosteroids and on Dexamethasone Suppression Test in Patients with Depressive Illness*

	Before Phenazepam Treatment (n = 27)	After Phenazepam Treatment (n = 27)	% Change
Blood 11-hydroxycorticosteroid level			
9 AM	20.8 ± 1.4	14.9 ± 1.3	28
11 PM	11.7 ± 1.2	7.6 ± 1.3	35
After dexamethasone test	14.4 ± 1.1	6.7 ± 0.9	53
Inhibition (%)†	−24 ± 8	−55 ± 5	129

*For short-term dexamethasone test procedure see Table 3-4. Phenazepam was administered in doses of 2 to 3 mg/day for seven to nine days.
†Inhibition of secretion of 11-hydroxycorticosteroids.

Another method that theoretically affects favorably the stores of "adaptive energy" is the prevention of an excessive stressor reaction. As has been shown by Hess and Riegle (1972), chronic ACTH injections result in decreased responsiveness to ether vapor stress in young male and female rats, while the responsiveness of the older rats is not reduced. Based on their experiments, these investigators concluded that "the decreased responsiveness of the young rats to stress suggested that the hypothalamic-pituitary corticotropin control mechanism of the young rats was responding differently to the elevated blood corticoid levels following prolonged adrenocortical activation then that of the old rats." Thus, the great amount of "adaptive energy" peculiar to the young animals corresponds, as was expected (see Chapter 3), to the higher sensitivity in the hypothalamic control mechanism to feedback suppression.

Pineal polypeptide extract (epithalamin) raises the hypothalamic sensitivity to feedback suppression (Ostroumova and Dilman 1972, Anisimov et al 1973a). This may restore equilibrium in many homeostatic systems immediately. Our findings show that pineal polypeptide extract lowers blood corticosterone in rats subjected to ether-induced stress (see Table 3-9). It is probable that under natural conditions in post-stress periods, pineal gland function is activated; this is probably the most potent factor limiting metabolic shifts induced by stress. In this connection, it is of interest that pineal polypeptide extract causes such effects as increased carbohydrate tolerance and decreased blood triglyceride levels; it also improves cellular immunity and acts as a tumor-preventing factor (see Chapter 17). The intensity of stress reaction can also be decreased with the aid of ACTH anahormone (see Chapter 24).

This fully applies to the stress-dependent acceleration of specific age pathology. The development of diseases of compensation is determined by two interconnected factors: elevation of the hypothalamic threshold, and enhanced utilization of FFA. Therefore, all external environmental factors that raise the hypothalamic threshold, the whole spectrum of stress factors, for instance, may promote diseases of compensation. In other words, diseases of adaptation are similar to those inherent in normal aging; the difference lies only in the sequence of disturbances. In normal aging elevation occurs in the hypothalamic set point which leads to intensified hypothalamic activity. In disorders brought on by external factors such as stress, however, it is just the reverse. Initially, the stress factors promote an increase in hypothalamic activity, and this increase then leads to an elevation of the hypothalamic threshold. Then, reaction to stress may be considered a particular case of the elevational mechanism of aging. Such an approach adequately accounts for the intensification of aging processes in stress (Selye and Tuchweber 1976).

It is certain that the mechanism of diseases of compensation have features distinct from those of adaptational diseases. To balance mechanisms stimulating metabolic shifts under conditions of stress, mechanisms intended to restrict these shifts are probably also switched on. Such a promoting factor is provided, for example, by the suppression of insulin secretion. This intensifies lipolysis by reducing the antilipolytic effect of the hormone. Recently a new interpretation of the stress-induced rise in growth hormone secretion also has been put forward that points to a connection between this phenomenon and the mechanism of reparative processes in the lymphoid tissues (Chatterton et al 1973). In this interpretation lymphocyte function is released from glucocorticoid-induced inhibition by the anabolic effect of growth hormone. Growth hormone also is found to stimulate thymic function (Fabris et al 1972). And stress is known to suppress gonadotropin secretion, thus curbing reproductive ability, a biologic requirement under stress conditions. In a study on population stress (Christian 1968) gonadotropin secretion was shown to be inhibited to a considerable degree. This differs from the mechanism in diseases of compensation, which features an enhanced activity of the reproductive system pathogenic for target tissue (see Chapter 4).

The data presented in Table 19-2 show that the changes involved in normal aging and stress coincide with respect to the first ten parameters, and point to many features that diseases of compensation and those of adaptation have in common. For example, both aging and stress are characterized by metabolic changes that may induce atherosclerosis (see Chapter 12).

However, mechanisms of aging and those of stress may not play equal parts in the formation of human age-specific pathology. We can determine that the mechanisms of aging, and therefore diseases of compensation, are more important than diseases of adaptation in the formation of this pathology by considering the following factors:

First, the development of diseases of compensation is related to normal physiologic aging, not to accidental events such as those causing stress. Diseases of compensation develop at a certain rate even under theoretically ideal conditions free of stress. There are some other limitations to the pathologic influences of stress. For example, thyroid function and growth hormone secretion are increased after stress. Therefore, unlike the processes of aging, stress involves certain pathology-limiting reactions.

Second, the spectrum of hormonal and metabolic disturbances intrinsic to normal aging and the formation of diseases of compensation is broader than in stress, as shown in Table 19-2 (see Noradrenaline through Pineal gland activity).

Third, the intensity of the stress reaction or, to be more precise, the time required for it to subside, is increased in the course of aging because of changes in hypothalamic sensitivity (Riegle 1973, Blichert-Toft 1978). Thus the regular mechanism of aging modifies the nature of the stress reaction. And since stress reactions and aging both employ the same mechanism that activates the neuroendocrine mechanism of the developmental program, it can be said that stress actually is a means of intensifying mechanisms of aging.

Table 19-2
Comparison of Hormonal and Metabolic Shifts Inherent in Aging, Diseases of Compensation, and Stress

Parameter	Normal Aging and Diseases of Compensation	Stress
Glucocorticoids	Relative and absolute increase	Increased
Growth hormone	Relative and absolute increase	Increased
Sensitivity to insulin	Decreased	Decreased
Blood free fatty acids	Increased	Increased
Glucose uptake by muscle tissue	Decreased	Decreased
Gluconeogenesis	Intensified	Intensified
Cholesterol	Increased	Increased
Triglycerides	Increased	Decreased
Prolactin	Decreased (in women)	Increased
Thrombogenesis	Intensified	Intensified
Noradrenaline	Normal	Increased
Insulin	Increased	Decreased
Gonadotropins	Increased	Decreased
Phenolsteroids	Increased	Decreased, with increased output of adrenal hormones
Thyroid function	Decreased	Decreased, followed by increase
Immunologic defense	Lowered	Decreased, followed by normalization
Pineal gland activity	Decreased*	Decreased, followed by increase

*There is no direct evidence for an age-associated decline in pineal gland function. However, considering that the hypothalamic threshold to inhibition is elevated with aging, and pineal polypeptide hormones are capable of reducing the hypothalamic threshold of sensitivity, at least a relative decrease in pineal gland function may be presumed to exist.

20 Carcinogenic Aging

That exposure to chemical environment promotes aging seems to be a decisive argument showing that chemical agents do act as carcinogens.

At present, many oncologists believe that the environmental factors and, particularly, chemical carcinogens are responsible for 70% to 80% of cancer incidence in humans (Doll and Peto 1976). From this point of view, the age-associated rise in cancer incidence is attributed to the increase in exposure to carcinogenic environment with aging (Peto et al 1975). Indeed, the probability that a human will develop cancer during the next five years is only 1 in 700 if he is 25 years old, whereas it is 1 in 14 if he is 65 (Peto et al 1975).

There are numerous carcinogens of different chemical classes and the number is growing. Therefore, it is not likely that malignant transformation of the cell, which lends it new specific properties, may occur by numerous different mechanisms, peculiar to different carcinogens. The very diversity of carcinogens is hardly compatible with the final common pathway mediating cancerogenesis. This statement can be proven by the fact that most of the tumors induced by carcinogens contain individually distinct tumor-specific rejection-type antigens. Considering these data, it is possible that the carcinogenic effect of chemical agents promotes the natural selection of transformed cells which have become malignant because of some other factor, eg, mutation. However, there is no general agreement on the nature of a selecting mechanism induced by exposure to a genuine carcinogen. I would like to put forward some arguments in support of a point of view that carcinogenic aging is this mechanism.

Some years ago, an editorial in *Lancet* (1976) discussed three hypotheses which might account for the association between advancing age and carcinogenesis, namely, a hypothalamic hypothesis (Dilman 1971), an immunologic hypothesis (Burnet 1970a), and a theory of accumulation of carcinogen-induced cell shifts (Kahn 1966). However, these three mechanisms should not be discussed independently. Suffice it to recall that chemical carcinogens are known to be immunosuppressive themselves (Kroes et al 1975). In addition, obesity contributes to cancer incidence in men, just as a high calorie diet does to tumor yield in experimental chemical carcinogenesis (Tannenbaum 1959). Thus the induction of cancer is determined by the dosage of chemical carcinogen, time of exposure, and by the metabolic pattern, characteristic of, for example, obesity and, therefore, aging, because the metabolic patterns involved in these two states are much alike.

Recently, Pitot (1977) summarized the data available on the effects of the organism itself on chemical carcinogenesis development. The review compares the process of aging and that of neoplasia. The author cites data demonstrating how hormonal status modifies carcinogenesis. But there is still another aspect of the relationship between chemical carcinogenesis and aging missed in this review. Not only is the effect of chemical carcinogens modified by hormonal status, but chemical carcinogenic agents modify hormonal status, too. Such a situation suggests searching for a common tie between the carcinogenic effect of chemical agents on the cell and that on metabolism and on the immune system. Recent studies by our group have shown that exposure to numerous chemical carcinogens causes the development of the syndrome of premature aging in experimental animals and, what is still more important, carcinogenic aging. Let us consider some data demonstrating the similar nature of changes taking place during normal aging and during chemical carcinogenesis.

Normal aging is accompanied by a decline in the hypothalamic levels of biogenic amines, particularly that of dopamine (Robinson 1975). Table 20-1 shows that 1,2-dimethylhydrazine treatment brings about a decrease in the hypothalamic level of biogenic amines in experimental animals.

At the same time, our experimental findings demonstrate that a decrease in catecholamine level in the hypothalamus is responsible for an elevation of the hypothalamic threshold of sensitivity to inhibition by estrogens (see Chapter 4). Figure 4-6 shows that exposure to chemical

Table 20-1
Effect of a Single Dose of 1,2-Dimethylhydrazine on Biogenic Amine Level in Rat Hypothalamus*

Time after DMH treatment (hours)	Noradrenaline (μg/g tissue)	Dopamine (μg/g tissue)	Serotonin (μg/g tissue)	5-Hydroxy-indolacetic acid (μg/g tissue)
0	1.67 ± 0.08	0.75 ± 0.20	0.99 ± 0.12	0.79 ± 0.11
0.5	1.05 ± 0.08†	0.60 ± 0.12	0.84 ± 0.07	0.95 ± 0.20
12	1.32 ± 0.08	0.60 ± 0.33	0.66 ± 0.08	0.83 ± 0.08
24	1.11 ± 0.06†	0.24 ± 0.02†	0.70 ± 0.09	0.45 ± 0.17

*1,2-Dimethylhydrazine (DMH) was injected subcutaneously (21 ng/kg of body weight).
†$p < 0.05$.

carcinogens also produces this hypothalamic response (Anisimov and Dilman 1974). Although elevation of the hypothalamic threshold was studied in the system of the reproductive homeostat only, it is likely that the same phenomenon occurs in the other main homeostatic systems because treatment with 1,2-dimethylhydrazine and dimethylbenzanthracene causes metabolic shifts similar to those of normal aging (Anisimov et al 1975). An exposure of rats to 1,2-dimethylhydrazine was followed by a decrease in glucose tolerance with a concomitant increase in reactive insulinemia (Dilman 1978b). As mentioned in Chapter 18, such a shift occurs in normal aging, prediabetes, and maturity-onset diabetes mellitus, and is generally concomitant with hypertriglyceridemia and hypercholesterolemia. Besides, there is also a considerable amount of evidence that prolactin levels are elevated during the administration of carcinogenic agents (Dao and Sinha 1975), which may be attributed to the decrease in dopamine concentration in the hypothalamus.

As mentioned above, chemical carcinogens are immunosuppressive. Yet, the mechanism of immunosuppression caused by carcinogens remains to be elucidated. At least for some carcinogens, this mechanism is related to metabolic immunosuppression (see Chapter 15), because administration of phenformin eliminates an immunosuppression induced by 1,2-dimethylhydrazine (Table 20-2).

Thus, chemical carcinogens lower the hypothalamic concentration of biogenic amines, raise the threshold of sensitivity of the hypothalamic-pituitary complex to regulatory stimuli, decrease tolerance to carbohydrates, increase blood concentrations of insulin, free fatty acids, triglycerides, and cholesterol, and cause the formation of metabolic immunosuppression. The above data are sufficient for the formulation of the concept of "carcinogenic aging." The introduction of this notion is

Table 20-2
Abolition by Phenformin Administration of Metabolic Immunodepression Caused by 1,2-Dimethylhydrazine (DMH) in Rats*

	Treatment		
Test	*Control*	*DMH*	*Phenformin + DMH*
Blastogenic response of lymphocytes			
Spontaneous (imp/min)	1315 ± 391	294 ± 155	1059 ± 423
PHA-induced (imp/min)	27,350 ± 7949	1080 ± 652	34,757 ± 13,103
Lipopolysaccharide-induced (imp/min)	2142 ± 740	388 ± 221	2587 ± 852
Titer of antibodies to sheep erythrocytes (complement fixation)	156 ± 62	58 ± 14	147 ± 62
Percentage of macrophage ingestion of *Staphylococcus albus*	28.2	16.0	30.7

*DMH was administered in dosage of 21 mg/kg per body weight once a week for four weeks; phenformin was administrated 2 mg/day for four weeks.

not a purely phenomenologic generalization, to a considerable degree similar to that of the generally accepted concept of "radiation aging." The significance of carcinogenic aging is determined by many factors; some of them are listed below.

First, metabolic shifts induced by chemical carcinogen treatment, and particularly hyperinsulinemia, contribute to the augmentation of the pool of proliferating cells. Since nondividing cells do not undergo malignant transformation, exposure to chemical carcinogens results in the development of a metabolic pattern suitable for cell proliferation in the formation of prerequisites for cell transformation, and causes cell impairment. Metabolic shifts induced by chemical carcinogens also predetermine the development of metabolic immunodepression, an important factor in the formation of a cancer susceptibility syndrome.

Second, the concept of carcinogenic aging draws attention to the fact that, apart from inducing cancer, carcinogen treatment should intensify the development of the diseases concomitant with aging. For example, chemical carcinogens induce atherosclerosis, and it is suggested that atherosclerotic plaques should, perhaps, be thought of as multiple benign leiomyomas (Albert et al 1977). However, it is possible that the carcinogen-induced proliferation of smooth muscle cells is also caused by relevant metabolic shifts, which are caused by the effect of the same carcinogenic agent. In this connection, it seems desirable to explore the possibility of testing the effects of carcinogens on the body, eg, their atherosclerotic effect. Such an approach has certain advantages over studies of mutagenic and carcinogenic effects because in the latter cases, the effect is determined by unknown events that can only be measured in terms of probability. Meanwhile, carcinogen-induced metabolic shifts occur regularly and are probably dose-dependent. This may prove useful for evaluating the "threshold hypothesis" of the action of chemical carcinogenic compounds.

Third, considering the mechanism of carcinogenic aging, it may be supposed that chemical carcinogens may accelerate development. To solve this problem, it is necessary, in particular, to establish whether an accelerated puberty of rodents can be induced by administering low doses of carcinogens. In this context, it may be of interest that DDT treatment results in obesity development in rats (Tomatis et al 1972).

Fourth, the possibility of induction of carcinogenic aging by an exposure to chemical carcinogens opens up new vistas for the modification of carcinogenesis. For instance, phenformin was found to lower the incidence of tumors induced by DMBA (Dilman et al 1978) and the yield of neoplasms induced by 1,2-dimethylhydrazine (Anisimov et al 1978). It was shown recently that postnatal treatment with buformin halved tumor incidence in rats subjected to transplacental administration of methylnitrosourea (Napalkov and Alexandrov 1978).

Hence, the suggested concept of carcinogenic aging provides more available means for cancer prevention, because relevant prophylactic measures may be taken not only with a view to controlling the carcinogenic environment but to effecting individual prophylaxis (individual anticancerogenesis) as well, which should rely on improvement of metabolism as a means of decelerating the process of aging. It should be mentioned in this connection that, for instance, tobacco smoking stimulates adrenaline secretion, thus promoting an intensified utilization of free fatty acids for energy supply, a characteristic feature of aging and age-specific pathology. Also, menopause sets in at an earlier stage in smokers than in nonsmokers (Daniele 1978). It was shown that the incidence of lung cancer induced by tobacco smoking is much higher among smokers with hypercholesterolemia (Stamler et al 1968). On the other hand, daily cigarette smokers had higher serum cholesterol levels than nonsmokers (Hjermann et al 1976).

Peto et al (1975), attempting to distinguish experimentally between environmental and aging mechanisms for the increased incidence of neoplasms with age, utilized skin tumor induction by benzpyrene in mice as a model system in which to study this process. Their studies showed that cancer incidence increased as a power of the duration of exposure to the carcinogen. However, when distinguishing between the roles of environmental and aging factors in carcinogenesis, it is necessary to bear in mind that chemical carcinogens can intensify the aging process. Moreover, the choice of the model that assures tumor induction in 100% of animals seems to be hardly justified for an evaluation of relationships between environmental and aging mechanisms.

Therefore, whenever thorough statistical and epidemiologic studies show that the cancer incidence is directly proportional to the time of exposure to chemical carcinogens, it is important to remember that, apart from the duration of exposure, in patients exposure time flies faster because of the intensification of normal aging processes.

21 Pregnancy and the Acceleration of Development in Light of the Concept of Diseases of Compensation

Acceleration of development is acceleration of aging and the diseases of aging at the same time.

The term acceleration denotes a number of processes, of which the spurt of linear growth and an earlier sexual development receive most attention. The chief factor promoting this acceleration is thought to be the influence of external environment, since growth is so sensitive to malnutrition and other detrimental environmental factors. It has been noted that children grow faster, reach a greater final size, and show a downward secular trend in the age of menarche as environmental and social conditions of a country improve. For instance, some countries showed a downward trend in the age of menarche of as much as three to four months per decade in the period from 1840 to 1960 (Tanner 1973). Although the causes of this secular trend are not fully understood, it seems likely that better nutrition, particularly in infancy, is chiefly responsible. Another explanation links this acceleration with prolonged exposure to artificial light. According to this hypothesis increased illumination inhibits the pineal gland, resulting in a decreased antigonadotropic and antigrowth action of the pineal hormones, and subsequent acceleration of the organism's development (Jafarey et al 1970, Wurtman 1975).

In contrast to these theories, however, it is our belief that acceleration of development is an endogenous process that has much in common with diseases of compensation. Note that food intake, or its correlate, metabolic rate, may act as the normal signal initiating puberty (Kennedy and Mitra 1963). If this is so, then it can be supposed that growth acceleration is brought on by the intensification of aging, primarily through metabolic shifts.

In the maternal organism we can propose two additional aspects of an acceleration mechanism: first, that acceleration commences during pregnancy, and second, that this acceleration is intensified further by the normal age-associated metabolic shifts of pregnancy. Let us consider these two suggestions.

The immune reactions of normal pregnancy are very complex. Burstein and Blumenthal (1969) suggested that "immune responses in pregnancy, like many other biologic phenomena, operate on a homeostatic principle, with the protective and injurious components in balance until term." Burnet (1969) emphasized a feature common to pregnancy and cancer from an immunologic point of view: in both cases foreign antigens (the fertilized ovum and malignant cells, respectively) are supposed to be rejected because of immunologic mechanisms. Hence, there should be some factors which suppress transplantation immunity during pregnancy and carcinogenesis. What I suggest is that these factors constitute an element of a more general mechanism that provides metabolic conditions for a rapid increase in cell mass during pregnancy.

In order to clarify the relationship between the intensification of metabolic processes indispensable for cell mass growth and immunodepression, it is necessary to ascertain whether both phenomena may be induced by the same mechanism. A number of hormonal factors which are at work during pregnancy do produce an immunodepression effect, partially in very early pregnancy. As was shown by Strelkauskas and colleagues (1978), in all cases an inversion of T and B cell levels was observed, ie, T cell levels were decreased and B cell levels were increased. Such a pattern is characteristic of the pattern of metabolic immunodepression. A most characteristic feature of such a pattern is the shift toward the predominant utilization of FFA for energy supply (see Chapter 15). Let us discuss the way in which this metabolic shift is realized.

During pregnancy the output of chorionic somatomammotropin, which has the properties of growth hormone, reduces the level of glucose utilization in the pregnant organism. In general, normal pregnancy induces a state of insulin resistance and consequently some impairment of glucose utilization despite enhanced pancreatic insulin responsiveness. Generally the tissue sensitivity to insulin is reduced by as much as 80% in normal pregnancy (Sutherland et al 1975). This is followed by compensatory hyperinsulinemia that leads to body fat accumulation (Pedersen and Mølsted-Pedersen 1971), the latter resulting in intensified lipolysis in the second half of pregnancy (Knopp et al 1973). The FFA does not pass through the placental barrier (Felig 1977). Therefore, with the high level of FFA utilization in the maternal organism, a secondary decrease in the muscle utilization of glucose occurs (Randle 1965), and FFA become the chief source of energy supply. This shift leads to intensified synthesis of cholesterol in the maternal organism. Cholesterol is transported to the fetoplacental unit where it is utilized for cell formation and steroid hormone synthesis. This mechanism of hypercholesterolemia is supported by our data demonstrating that administration of phenformin to pregnant rats reduces blood cholesterol level (Table 21-1; Berstein and Alexandrov 1976). I believe that simultaneously, in the maternal organism, hypercholesterolemia or, more precisely, the increased blood level of LDL in conjunction with the elevated blood level of FFA, cortisol etc, causes suppression of T cell function, and bring about metabolic immunodepression.

Table 21-1
Influence of Phenformin Administration on Metabolic Parameters in Pregnant Rats

	Nonpregnant Rats (n = 10)	Pregnant Rats (n = 12)	Pregnant Rats treated with Phenformin† (n = 17)
Blood cholesterol (mg%)	49.5 ± 1.7	63.90 ± 3.3*	46.3 ± 1.9*
Blood phospholipids (mg%)	101.6 ± 5.0	150.1 ± 6*	120.4 ± 8*
Free fatty acids (μEq/liter)	270 ± 33	605 ± 56*	251 ± 19*
11-Oxycorticosteroids (μg%)	12.1 ± 0.5	17.1 ± 0.8	17.9 ± 1.0

*$p < 0.02$.
†Phenformin (15 mg/day) was administered per os, beginning from the eighth day of gestation to the end of the term.

Thus, pregnancy is incompatible with the maintenance of constancy of internal environment of the organisms, inasmuch as the development of the organism is incompatible with homeostatic stability. The indispensable metabolic disorders occurring during pregnancy are nothing but a programmed disease. In this respect I feel it necessary to mention the data showing that women who have produced large families have an increased risk of diabetes mellitus, directly related to the number of pregnancies: women who bear seven children are six times more likely to develop diabetes than those who have had none (Pyke 1956). Thus, a decrease in glucose tolerance, ie, "diabetes of pregnancy," is a condition necessary for the normal course of pregnancy.

However, the intensity of diabetes of pregnancy is determined not only by the level of production of placental hormones, but also by the state of the maternal organism. It can be expected a priori that the older the pregnant woman, the more pronounced the shift toward the intensification of metabolism may be or, the stronger the pressure of external environment, the more pronounced the "programmed disease of pregnancy." It is the intensification of the normal disease of pregnancy that is actually a disease, ie, it is an excess over the indispensable level of disorders that are necessary to provide for fetal growth. In accordance with physiologic correlations, this excess can cause an intensification of growth of the fetus (Baird 1969), ie, it is able to cause an acceleration of development. The mechanism of accelerated development will be discussed in the light of this assumption (Dilman 1975).

It is known that the number of adipose cells and the fat content of these cells are increased as a consequence of hyperinsulinemia (Sjöström 1972, Brook et al 1972), and the fetus grows heavier as the insulin level grows higher (Mølsted-Pedersen 1972). Therefore a large fetus is generally a "fat" fetus, and its biologic age may be much greater than its chronologic age (Klimek 1974). These relationships are supported by numerous observations showing that prediabetic women often give birth to heavier babies (Jackson 1960), a coincidence so common that a large baby now is considered to be a symptom of prediabetes; in fact, normal infants weighing 4 kg or more do show a higher insulin level at birth than do infants of a lower weight (Pedersen and Mølsted-Pedersen 1971). Data obtained in our laboratory serve as additional arguments in favor of these relationships. Three to four months after alloxan administration to rats (240 mg/kg body weight), those animals that developed hyperglycemia were selected for further observation (Berstein et al 1977). From the eighth day of gestation the animals were divided into two subgroups: controls and those treated with phenformin (10 mg/day) until the end of gestation. It is evident from Table 21-2 that administration of phenformin caused a statistically significant decrease in blood levels of insulin, FFA, and cholesterol, as well as a decrease in the weight of the fetus at birth.

The birth of a large baby represents another stage in the mechanism of acceleration. It has been reported that the more adipose cells and the greater the weight of the infant, the more rapid is the gain in body weight. Excessive weight gain during the first six months of life also is associated with an increased incidence of obesity in later childhood (Brook et al 1972). Moreover, Frisch (1973) has observed that the age at which the sexual cycle is switched on is determined by body weight. This critical body weight is about 48 kg for girls in the United States. The earlier onset of puberty within the last several decades may be explained by the fact that the critical weight is attained at an earlier age. For instance, 125 years ago girls in the United States reached 48 kg body weight

Table 21-2
Influence of Phenformin Administration on Fat-Carbohydrate Metabolism and Fetal Weight in Pregnant Rats Pretreated with Alloxan

Gain of body weight (g)	− (n = 13)	104 ± 6
	+ (n = 12)	80 ± 9
Weight of fetus (g)	− (n = 105)	5.29 ± 0.05
	+ (n = 98)	4.92 ± 0.06*
Blood sugar (mg%)	− (n = 12)	179 ± 15
	+ (n = 12)	154 ± 19
Cholesterol (mg%)	− (n = 12)	106 ± 13
	+ (n = 12)	72 ± 7*
Phospholipids (mg%)	− (n = 12)	153 ± 20
	+ (n = 11)	113 ± 12
FFA (μEq/liter)	− (n = 12)	528 ± 34
	+ (n = 12)	394 ± 23*
Insulin (μU/ml)	− (n = 9)	93 ± 20
	+ (n = 7)	49 ± 10*

−: control rats.
+: rats treated with phenformin with oral daily dose of 10 mg/day from the eighth day of gestation.
*Significant difference between + and −; $p < 0.05$.

by the age of 16, but today they reach it by the age of 12.5 (Frisch and McArthur 1974).

According to Frisch and Revelle (1970), reaching critical body weight causes a change in the metabolic rate, which reduces the hypothalamic sensitivity to estrogens, thus altering ovarian-hypothalamic feedback. Therefore, postadolescent diabetic patients tend to have an earlier inception of the menarche than controls consisting of their nondiabetic sisters-in-law with no family history of diabetes (Post and Arbor 1962). On the other hand, a decreased carbohydrate tolerance was observed in pregnant patients with early menarche (Loffer 1975).

The process of acceleration does not cease once sexual maturity is reached at this earlier stage. It is well known that blood insulin rises in direct proportion to body weight (Bagdade et al 1968, Woods and Porte 1978). Compensatory hyperinsulinemia, accelerated by relative obesity then becomes a key factor in the mechanism of further weight gain and the resulting earlier onset of age-associated pathologic processes. As reported by Wertelecki and Mantel (1973), children with leukemia had significantly greater birth weight than expected. A positive correlation between frequency of leukemia and growth rate in children (Vorontsov et al 1973), as well as findings in our laboratory of high growth hormone and insulin levels in children with some kind of tumor, may be significant in this regard (see Table 17-2). Besides, it has been shown that, at the time of onset of diabetes mellitus in childhood, diabetic boys may be taller than average for their age (Dragar 1974).

The increased mean blood cholesterol level in populations of healthy subjects, reported recently in several countries, also seems to be determined by factors of acceleration in accordance with the model discussed in Chapter 8. This holds true particularly for men, since there is no phase of stabilization in their metabolic development, and it accounts for the comparatively intensified development of age-specific pathology and higher death rates observed in middle-aged men. Thus, acceleration of the organism's development is at the same time acceleration of the age-related pathology.

The pattern of acceleration is different in women. It has been reported recently that an earlier switching-on of the reproductive cycle contributes to the increase of breast cancer incidence in young women. According to McMahon et al (1973), this pathogenic effect is more pronounced in women who bear children late. Though the switching-on of reproductive function has a stabilizing effect, conditions promoting a steady accumulation of fat still persist, and during pregnancy they may give rise to a metabolic pattern that leads to the birth of a large baby and the start of a secondary acceleration. Such a development results in the build-up of accelerational momentum and an earlier onset of metabolic changes leading to age-specific pathology.

In the female organism the estrogen level also is raised in obesity (De Waard 1973), inhibiting the development of age-associated atherosclerosis, which explains the gap in death rates from atherosclerosis between men and women. This mechanism also explains the later onset of menopause reported in recent decades, since the estrogens maintain the feedback mechanism in the reproductive homeostat for a longer time, thus extending the reproductive period (see Chapter 4).

Hence acceleration is characterized in the female organism by an earlier onset of menarche and a later onset of menopause (Hofman and Soergel 1972). However, excessive estrogens also increase cancer incidence in the reproductive system, particularly breast and endometrial carcinoma; accordingly, there is an increase in the reports of cancer accompanying this later onset of menopause (McMahon et al 1973). Thus, a prolonged reproductive period caused by later-onset menopause, accelerates development, increases the frequency of age-specific pathology, and therefore should be included with premature puberty, earlier-onset adolescent growth spurt, and greater linear growth as a phenomenon associated with acceleration. Consequently, acceleration is a dual phenomenon: it increases both the probability of an accelerated development of age-specific diseases in the accelerates and the probability of developing these diseases in adults. For example, women who give birth to large babies are likely to become obese and to develop diabetes in later life (Fitzgerald et al 1961). In this context it is interesting to note that women with clinical manifestations of malignancy (at age 50 years or older) had frequently given birth to large babies 17 to 31 years before their disease (see Chapter 17). It has also been reported that patients with Hodgkin's disease are taller than the subjects in a control group (Hancock et al 1976). There are also data indicating that survival rates were the lowest for those women with breast cancer who had very early menarche (Juret et al 1976).

The possibility of an accumulated potential for acceleration is of particular interest (Figure 21-1). At birth an obese infant possesses a potential for reproducing acceleration in the following generation. This does not mean a hereditary transfer, of course. Instead, it implies the development of a metabolic pattern that promotes acceleration in the following generation. Hence premature menarche, a primary accelerate, often is followed by the delivery of a large baby, which then is recognized

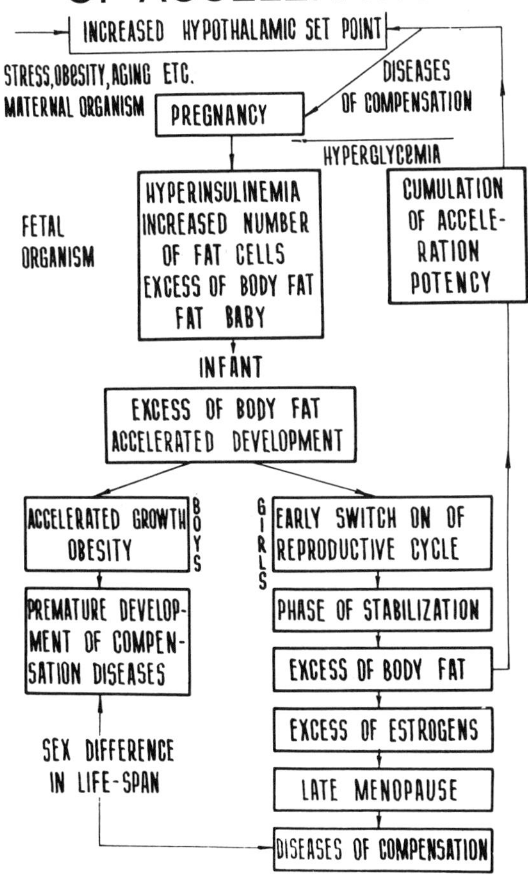

Figure 21-1 Scheme of elevational mechanism of acceleration of development and of age-specific pathology.

as a secondary accelerate. Some external factors also contribute to this process of acceleration. For example, DDT treatment of rats causes as fast a gain of body weight in the first generation as in the animals initially treated (Tomatis et al 1972). In Chapter 20 it was shown that DDT as well as some other carcinogens can raise the hypothalamic threshold. This property may be responsible for the accelerational effect of external environmental factors, including exposure to intense illumination, which inhibits pineal activity and thus causes the hypothalamic threshold to elevate, and overfeeding results from impairment of the appetite control system.

The model of the elevating mechanism of acceleration makes it possible to interpret as elements of a single mechanism the influences of various acceleration-promoting factors. It also suggests that we can expect an increased frequency of such phenomena as acceleration of development and premature age-specific pathology in the future. For example, the social factors and extended reproductive period, which are leading to a higher frequency of late pregnancies, may bring about a situation in which cases of pregnancy with advanced metabolic disorders become more frequent.

It should be particularly noted that the thicker the skin folds, the greater the weight of the infant at birth. The measurements of the skinfold thickness in the suprailiac site in pregnant women showed that in women aged up to 21 years the gain was 3.8 ± 0.8 mm, while in those more than 25 years old it was 8.5 ± 0.7 mm. Taking into account the fact that the increase of skinfold thickness during pregnancy is highly correlated with calculated estimates of body fat (Taggart et al 1967), it may be concluded that as early as 25 to 31 years of age there develop certain metabolic disturbances which, combined with the shifts characteristic of the normal disease of the pregnant organism, lead to more intensive fat accumulation. Such a trend would suggest a further accumulation of accelerational momentum in the generations to follow, which in turn would produce an acceleration of age-specific pathology.

The common features of pathogenic mechanisms inherent in pregnancy, acceleration of development and age-specific pathology, are illustrated by a comparison of the hormonal and metabolic patterns of pregnancy, normal aging, stress, and cancer (see Table 1-3). The formation mechanism of the hormonal and metabolic conditions common to all these processes is described in earlier chapters.

22 Diseases of Compensation: Specific and Nonspecific Features of their Pathogenic Mechanism

Normal diseases and natural death of higher organisms, man included, should be considered regulatory ones.

In preceding chapters we discussed the key role played by deviation of the hypothalamic threshold in implementing the neuroendocrine program of development, aging, and age-specific pathology. Accordingly, it can be shown that the same complex of mechanisms is responsible for producing such outwardly different processes as growth and development, pregnancy, acceleration, normal aging, the climacteric age-associated obesity, dysadaptosis, prediabetes and late-onset diabetes mellitus, atherosclerosis, metabolic immunodepression, autoimmune disturbances, cancrophilia, essential hypertension, and age-connected depression. These mechanisms also include the hormonal and metabolic patterns responsible for adaptation in acute and chronic stress.

All the physiologic and pathologic processes mentioned here are characterized by two indispensable features: shift of the hypothalamic set point of sensitivity, and a compensatory intensification of the peripheral endocrine gland function and rise in the levels of such energy-producing substrates as glucose and free fatty acids. Based on the concept of the elevating mechanism, all these processes are included in the group of diseases of compensation and are listed in four metabolic stages of postnatal ontogenesis: pre-prediabetes, stabilization, prediabetes, and involution (see Chapter 8). Since diseases of compensation all have an identical mechanism, their peculiar features have the following in common:

A pathogenic connection with the neuroendocrine mechanism of organism development Diseases of compensation are associated with this mechanism, and this is precisely what distinguishes them from other diseases encountered in the aged. Therefore, diseases of compensation and normal aging feature closely related and similar hormonal and metabolic shifts. The spectrum of age-specific pathology is determined by the functional structure of the main homeostatic systems or, more precisely, by programmed determined dysregulation in the energy, adaptive, and reproductive homeostats.

A pathogenic dependence on the degree of compensatory response For example, the higher the compensatory hyperinsulinemia is, the more marked and extensive are obesity, atherosclerosis, and possibly cancer, and the more intense is the acceleration of development.

The inevitable development of diseases of compensation under the influence of internal environmental factors during ontogenesis If diseases of compensation do not occur at a certain period of ontogenesis, it points to a failure of the normal mechanism of development and aging.

The interaction of diseases of compensation This is determined by the concurrent age-associated shift of the hypothalamic threshold of sensitivity to homeostatic stimuli in all major homeostatic systems, as well as by the interaction of many compensatory reactions. For instance, a premature age-associated gain in body weight is accompanied by an acceleration of the formation of other diseases of compensation. This relation provides a rational basis for the development of so-called risk factors of diseases. Hyperinsulinemia, prediabetes, and latent late-onset diabetes mellitus are risk factors in atherosclerosis and cancer, for example, and they may trigger a chain of interdependent disturbances. Metabolic disorders taking place in pregnancy also promote an acceleration of development which promotes the formation of age-specific pathology and eventually shortens life.

A shift to free fatty acid utilization as a source of energy, and the utilization of glucose for lipogenesis. This is observed particularly in pregnancy, acceleration of development, latent diabetes, prediabetes, atherosclerosis, and cancer.

Changes in the spectrum of secreted hormones These are likely to be caused by overstimulation of the endocrine glands (Dilman 1961, 1968; Diebel et al 1973; Pelham et al 1973). Such disturbances cause independent, uncompensated shifts to occur in the neuroendocrine system. However, the significance of this phenomenon probably extends further.

It is quite possible that the age-associated increase in the frequency of autoimmune diseases is caused not only by the accumulation of errors in the course of protein synthesis, but also by certain changes that appear in the spectrum of secreted proteins when some organs are overstimulated. Such a proposal seems likely in regard to lipoproteins, for example (see Chapter 12). This approach could explain the age-associated rise in cancer incidence that is associated with the decline in immunologic defense mechanisms, as well as explain this simultaneous increase in frequency of autoimmune processes, as a consequence of the hyperactivity of the immunologic system (see Chapters 15 and 16). Therefore, it is possible that the pathogenesis of certain autoimmune diseases, those of the thyroid, for example, is related to the mechanism of diseases of compensation.

The cyclic development of diseases of compensation The formation of disturbances such as pre-prediabetes starts at an early phase of ontogenesis. It then regresses in the phase of stabilization of females, returns at the period of prediabetes, and regresses again in involution. During involution, regression is accompanied by a loss of body weight, decrease in cholesterol level, and probably some other changes in hypothalamic activity. Hence, the peak frequency of diseases of compensation occurs in prediabetes, a fact which must be considered in the development of relevant therapy.

A relative nonspecificity If elevation of the hypothalamic threshold arises from pathologic rather than age-associated processes, diseases of compensation may occur at any age. For instance, young patients with endometrial carcinoma reveal disturbances that are inherent in diseases of compensation: obesity, arterial hypertension, diabetes mellitus, and sterility (Dockerty et al 1951). Similar changes have been observed by us in rats in the course of aging, following long-term continuous exposure to light and carcinogen administration (see Chapter 20).

Considerable dependence on external environmental factors This feature does not contradict the idea that diseases of compensation are caused by internal factors. External environmental factors such as stress, which raises the hypothalamic threshold, or excessive food intake, which intensifies the compensatory response, are conducive to the premature and more active development of diseases of compensation; and by contrast, those external stimuli which reduce hypothalamic activity or compensatory responses decelerate age-associated changes and the development of diseases of compensation.

Clinical similarity to syndromes involving non-hypothalamic disturbances of homeostatic systems For instance, symptomatic atherosclerosis is similar to atherosclerosis as a disease of compensation as far as the final stage of development is concerned, because hyperlipoproteinemia occurs in both instances.

Initial disturbance in regulation Diseases of compensation are caused by initial disturbances in regulation, and therefore may be controlled effectively at this stage by both spontaneous and therapeutic influences. For example, climacteric bleedings may be followed by periods of recurrent ovarian function. Generally speaking, the natural death of higher organisms, including humans, should be considered to be a regulatory one.

Response to the same therapeutic influence despite differences in clinical manifestations This pecularity seems to be conditioned by common mechanisms underlying shifts of the hypothalamic threshold and compensatory reactions. For example, metabolic parameters of obesity and other metabolic disturbances inherent in both atherosclerosis and cancer may be returned to normal by means of the same antidiabetic preparation, phenformin (see Chapter 24).

PART IV
An Approach to Integrated Medicine in Light of the Law of Deviation of Homeostasis

From separate discoveries—to the once lost and ever fleeting integrity of human perception of Nature.

23 Current Theories in Gerontology and the Law of Deviation of Homeostasis

To explain the identity of the metabolic patterns observed in pregnancy, stress, normal aging, and specific diseases of aging is the problem that any theory of aging is expected to provide an answer to.

The author naturally cannot assume the responsibility of assessing the merits and limitations of the basic theories of aging. Therefore, the present chapter attempts to show that the hypothalamic theory of aging expounded by me since 1955 may be instrumental in explaining some factual evidence pertinent to other hypotheses and theories of aging. The many hypotheses advanced fall into two principal categories, according to whether extrinsic or intrinsic causes of aging are postulated. At present, there are sufficient data to disregard the hypotheses postulating extrinsic causes, including the stress theory of aging, because extrinsic factors can either accelerate or decelerate aging but cannot cause it.

As to the intrinsic theories of aging, they fall into two categories: 1) random, and 2) control theories (Lints 1971). At present, the following are the most popular theories of the random type: a somatic mutation theory (Szilard 1959, Curtis 1966, Burch 1978), an error catastrophe theory (Orgel 1963), an immunologic theory (Burnet 1969, Walford 1969), a free radical theory (Harman et al 1976), a cross-linkage theory (Verzár 1957, Bjorksten 1968), and others (for review see Everitt 1976).

Many arguments may be adduced for each of these concepts. However, all of them have limitations. It should be pointed out that, for instance, according to mutation or error theory, aging is regarded as a stochastic process. However, aging is characterized by a striking constancy of manifestations. The regular development of such metabolic shifts as age-associated fat accumulation, hyperinsulinemia, and hypercholesterolemia, or such hormonal shifts as the climacteric, makes it clear that aging is governed by certain regular rather than probability factors that promote a specific pattern of aging and age pathology.

As to the control theories, two groups of concepts may be distinguished: cell control theories of aging, according to which control mechanisms operate on the cellular level, and those which deal with extracellular regulatory mechanisms. The best-known version of the cell control theory of aging at present is based chiefly on the concept of the so-called limit of Hayflick, which sets certain limits to the number of possible cell divisions in each species of animals (Hayflick 1965, 1975). The death of cells in the course of aging and, therefore, many manifestations of aging, are attributed to the attainment of the genetic limit of cell division processes.

On the other hand, changes occurring in the regulatory systems, particularly the hypothalamus, cannot be related to the limit of Hayflick, because neurons do not divide in the adult organism, and even the quantity of neurons in many areas of the brain, unaffected by pathologic, ie, atherosclerotic, processes, remains nearly the same with advancing age (Finch 1973, Franks et al 1974, Brody and Vijayashankar 1977). Another version of the cell control theory is the immunologic theory of aging. Burnet (1969) suggested the role of clonal exhaustion, in which thymus cells with a genetically programmed clock mechanism for self-destruction die after undergoing a fixed number of divisions.

The immunologic theory provides some explanation of the development of such processes as cancer (Burnet 1976) and age-associated autoimmune phenomena (Blumenthal 1967, Walford 1974, Kent 1977), but it fails to account for the formation of such functional processes as the climacteric or mental depression.

There are also different variants of extracellular regulatory theories (Cannon 1942, Shock 1952, Verzár 1957). Comfort (1964) stresses the possibility of aging as a continuous deviation from homeostasis that increases by itself. However, there were virtually no hypotheses attempting to explain the inevitable and uniform character of disorders of homeostasis inherent in aging.

In 1958 (Dilman 1958) hypothalamic function was evaluated on the basis of indirect evidence; however, some of the conclusions are worth considering. First, the concept of a hypothalamic mechanism of aging was advanced. Second, it was claimed that the advancement of age involves an elevation of activity of some hypothalamic centers, whereas, previously, the mechanism of aging had been invariably associated with a decline in the activity of some system. Third, the paper drew attention to those features which the hypothalamic mechanism of aging and formation of age-specific disease share in common. The latter point calls for an explanation even now. Conventionally, normal physiologic aging is strictly differentiated from age-associated pathology. Such a distinction, however, is not apparent in some cases. For example, the climacteric is a typical manifestation of normal aging, and a pathologic process (considering the homeostatic disturbances involved) at the same time. Baranov and Dilman (1949) claimed that climacteric neurosis is caused by primary disturbances in hypothalamic function rather than by an estrogen deficit, as was generally believed at the time (Isaacs and Havard 1978). The lack of a strict distinction between age-associated and pathologic phenomena has proved to be a common feature of all those pathologic processes, the development of which depends on an elevation of hypothalamic activity to a considerable degree. Therefore, some later publications (Dilman 1958, 1968, unpublished data) discussed a special group of age pathology diseases characterized by elevation of hypothalamic activity.

Reviewing the earlier research, it should be stressed that this system of concepts was formed gradually. This played a certain role both in the choice of terminology used at different stages of the development of the concept and in the selection of experimental and clinical data. It should be pointed out that previously the age-related elevation of hypothalamic activity was considered to be the main factor of the regulatory mechanism of aging. This still holds for the reproductive homeostat, because the rise in the output of gonadotropins, particularly FSH, occurs prior to the switching-on of reproductive function and continues throughout the whole reproductive period (Dilman 1961; see Chapter 4). Later, the concept of elevation of hypothalamic activity was transformed into that of elevation of hypothalamic threshold of sensitivity to negative feedback control (Dilman 1971).[1] The mechanism of the stressor reaction may be used to illustrate the distinction between the elevation of hypothalamic activity and that of hypothalamic sensitivity threshold (see Chapter 19). Hence, the term "elevation of hypothalamic activity" was replaced by "elevation of the hypothalamic threshold of sensitivity to regulatory homeostatic stimuli" (Dilman 1978b).

[1]The term "set point of hypothalamic sensitivity" instead of "hypothalamic threshold" may be encountered in the recent literature (Smelik and Papoikonamon 1973).

Later, Stoll (1972) suggested that the decrease in the hypothalamic level of dopamine raises the hypothalamic threshold, and he administered L-dopa to increase the sensitivity to the action of estrogens in breast cancer patients. This hypothesis is supported by findings from our laboratory (Dilman and Anisimov 1975; see Chapters 3, 4, and 14). Normal aging was found to involve a decline in the level of biogenic amines (Robinson et al 1972, Robinson 1975), particularly dopamine turnover (Finch 1973), in the hypothalamus. It was an important landmark in the investigations of the role of biogenic amines in the regulation of the rate of aging and development of age-related diseases. The reports on the resumption of ovarian cyclicity in old rats with constant estrus as a result of treatment with L-dopa (Quadri et al 1973), as well as the data showing that L-dopa administration extended the life span of mice (Cotzias et al 1974, 1977), have proved to be of considerable importance for the development of our concept.[1]

Recently, Finch (1976) advanced an idea that the decline in the activity of the dopaminergic system of the brain, specifically the hypothalamus, is a key factor in the consequent development of a cascade of regulatory disturbances. The latter include changes in the target tissues, particularly endocrine glands, which in turn contribute to the development of regulatory disturbances in the brain, thus forming a vicious circle.

However, since direct measurements of the biogenic amine levels in the human hypothalamus are impractical, the required data may be obtained by means of hypothalamus inhibition tests. To illustrate, the decreased level of hypothalamic biogenic amines found in patients with depressive illness corresponds to the elevation of the hypothalamic threshold of sensitivity to dexamethasone suppression (see Chapter 14). Subsequently, an analysis of the problem as a whole showed considerable evidence that suggests that in the course of postnatal ontogenesis the set point of hypothalamic sensitivity to feedback stimuli undergoes two different types of changes. In the adaptive homeostat, as evaluated by the dexamethasone suppression test, and the reproductive homeostat (both operating by negative and positive estrogen feedback [Lu et al 1977]), the hypothalamic threshold of sensitivity is elevated with aging (see Chapters 3 and 4). At the same time the age-connected shift in the thyrostat develops in the opposite direction: the threshold of sensitivity of the hypothalamic-pituitary-thyroid complex to inhibition (as evaluated by the T_3 and T_4 suppression test in hemithyroidectomized rats) shows a decrease with advancing age (see Chapter 7).

The age-connected changes in the energy homeostat are character-

---

[1]The prolonged life span in tryptophan-deficient animals (Segall and Timiras 1976) is inconclusive in this respect because tryptophan deficiency has an effect on the developmental program rather than aging proper.

ized by a dual pattern: the hypothalamic threshold of sensitivity to suppressive action of glucose on growth homrone (GH) secretion is elevated with aging, while the hypothalamic threshold of sensitivity to free fatty acids (FFA) diminishes (see Chapter 6). Therefore, the co-occurrence of high blood levels of FFA and GH is observed in childhood, while on completion of maturation, ie, at ages 20 to 25 years, the suppression of GH secretion by FFA is obvious. This peculiarity of age-related hypothalamic changes is responsible for the age-associated switching-on of reproductive function and the high levels of GH, FFA, and thyroid hormones at the developmental stages of ontogenesis, ie, it plays a specific part in the realization of the program of organism development.

Finally, according to Aschheim (1976), cycling rats often respond to estrogen treatment by pseudopregnancy as age advances. This is a manifestation of the age-associated decline in the hypothalamic threshold of sensitivity in a system that contributes to the regulation of prolactin secretion.

The above findings allow the formulation of a more universal concept of the regularities that form the basis for the elevational model of development, aging, and diseases of aging. In a new context, hypothalamic alterations occurring in the course of ontogenesis provide a mechanism by which the implementation of the Law of Deviation of Homeostasis is ensured (see Chapter 1).

Therefore, it does not really matter that the threshold of sensitivity to regulation signals may be elevated (which happens to be the case very often), or that, in some systems, the threshold of sensitivity to homeostatic signals may be lowered. What actually matters is that in both cases a programmed deviation of homeostasis takes place.

Moreover, I do not believe it essential that regulatory changes occur mainly in the hypothalamus. Of fundamental importance is the fact that, in order to obey the Law of Deviation of Homeostasis, a relevant homeostatic system undergoes changes in the direction required. If the functional structure of a system is such that its regulation undergoes changes both in the hypothalamus and in other areas of CNS, then, naturally, changes required for implementation of the Law of Deviation of Homeostasis can also be brought about by mechanisms other than those in the hypothalamus. Therefore, at present it seems justified to use the term "elevational model of mechanism of development, aging, and age-related pathology." This term points to the fact that all these states have one characteristic feature in common, namely, the increase in the vigor of the main homeostatic system, whereas previously the mechanism of aging and age-related pathology was invariably associated with the decline in the activity of a particular system. In addition, this term points to the shift in metabolic processes toward an intensification of utilization of FFA as fuel (see Chapters 5 and 6).

It is evident from the above that the concept based on the Law of Deviation of Homeostasis encompasses many other recent regulation-type hypotheses of aging. However, the approach based on this concept is not at variance with others evolved on completely different principles. Let us consider some examples.

A persistent elevation of the blood level of follicle-stimulating hormone (FSH) almost invariably results in the develpment of ovarian tumors in rats (see Chapter 17). If carcinogenesis is really caused by somatic mutations, this example is proof of a direct correlation between the size of the pool of proliferating cells and the probability of mutation. However, since the increased FSH secretion in aging women is related to the primary elevation of the hypothalamic threshold of sensitivity to inhibition by estrogens (see Chapter 4), this example simultaneously points to a relationship between the Law of Deviation of Homeostasis and the risk of mutation development. If somatic mutations (or other related events) do play a certain role in the mechanism of aging, the same example also suggests a relationship between age-connected regulatory shifts in the hypothalamus and changes in genes and cells.

Similar reasoning seems to be applicable in the interpretation of the hypothesis that regards the inevitable decrease in the efficiency of the DNA repair system as a key factor in aging and carcinogenesis (Vilenchik 1977, Hart et al 1979). The inhibitory effect of phenformin treatment (as much as a calorie-restricted diet) on both chemical- and virus-induced carcinogenesis (see Chapter 17) is indicative of a correlation between metabolic pattern and DNA repair system efficiency. Equally, the metabolic pattern has an appreciable influence on the development of autoimmune disorders (see Chapter 16) which are assigned such a great importance in aging processes by the immunologic theory (Walford 1969).

Recently, it has been demonstrated that hypophysectomy interferes with collagen cross-linkage (Everitt 1976). Hence, this process so frequently regarded as a tissue-dependent one is actually governed, to a considerable degree, by metabolic and, therefore, regulatory factors.

It cannot be ruled out that the same holds true for such cell-dependent phenomena as the limit of Hayflick. It is not yet clear which factors determine the time intervals between two successive cell divisions. Therefore, it is possible that the intermitotic interval may be shortened by processes controlled by the elevating mechanism. There is a possible analogy here to the effects of GH and other hormones capable of a proliferative stimulation, which increases the likelihood of carcinogenesis as well as the cell division-stimulating influences of hypercholesterolemia and hyperinsulinemia (see Chapter 17). Hence, it seems justified to suggest that the in vivo rate of progress toward the Hayflick limit is controlled by regulatory mechanisms. If this suggestion proves true, the biologic significance of the elevating mechanism probably will be enhanced. Finally, the free radical mechanism of aging (Harman et al 1976, Emmanuel and Obukhova 1978) is undoubtedly subject to the influence of metabolic processes. In particular, it is subject to the effects of an enhanced utilization of FFA as fuel. Therefore, some fundamental biologic phenomena, somatic mutations included, may contribute to the pattern of aging and natural death. For instance, *Neurospora crassa* is known to be essentially immortal. However, its recessive mutant, characterized by elevated levels of lipid autooxidation and associated free radical reactions (Munkres and Minssen 1976) has lost this property.

Thus, many of the phenomena described in vitro as signs of aging on cellular or tissue levels have proved to be related to regulatory shifts in the system. In particular, age-connected changes in the induction of the hepatic enzyme glucokinase (Adelman 1970) and thyroxine aminotransferase (Finch et al 1969) "appear to result from alterations in extrahepatic hormones rather than from an intrinsic failure of liver hormone target cells to respond" (Finch 1976). It is probable that a similar situation occurs in connection with the age-associated decline in hormone receptor concentration. For instance, Roth and colleagues (1978a) claim that the altered ability to respond to hormones is an important manifestation of aging. Earlier, Finch (1976) suggested that the regulation of steroid receptor level by hormone status could lead to changes in the threshold for stimulation, which, in the hypothalamus, could result in altered feedback sensitivity. Such a possibility seems to be still more likely with regard to hyperinsulinemia as a factor that reduces insulin receptor concentration on the plasma membrane of target cells.

Thus, many phenomena previously described as primary may actually be secondary ones, the in vivo sequence of events permitting a description in terms of the elevational model in many cases. Let us consider this point, using the example of the emotional stress reaction, which in many respects corresponds to the mechanism of aging. Exposure to stress increases the activity of the hypothalamic-pituitary system, and the latter phenomenon is known to occur in the adaptive and, partly, energy homeostats, with advancing age (see Chapters 3 and 6). An increased turnover of neurotransmitters, particularly biogenic amines, indispensable for the implementation of the stressor reaction, reduces their concentration in the brain (hypothalamus), which in turn leads to the elevation of the hypothalamic threshold of sensitivity to homeostatic stimuli (see Chapters 4 and 19). Thus, the decline in biogenic amines (which fits the concepts of Finch [1973, 1976], Cotzias and collegaues [1974, 1977] and Samorajski [1977]) appears to be a biochemical equivalent of the physiologic mechanism of hypothalamic threshold elevation. This change is followed by such shifts as the decrease in carbohydrate tolerance and enhanced utilization of FFA, the latter corresponding to changes taking place in the energy homeostat in the course of aging. The numerous consequences of these shifts are discussed in Chapter 25. In particular, it may be supposed that these shifts, via elevation of concentrations of LDL-cholesterol, insulin, and somatomedin, result in the increase in the proliferative pool of cells, as was shown for the arterial wall (see Chapter 12) and intestinal epithalium (Miller et al 1977a). This in turn increases the likelihood of mutations (a link to the mutational theory of aging) and accumulation of errors at the post-translational level (theory of error catastrophe). Moreover, enhanced lipolysis causes metabolic immunodepression (see Chapter 15), auto-immune disturbances probably being intensified by the suppression of T suppressors (see Chapter 16) (a link to different versions of the immunologic theory of aging); enhanced lipolysis also promotes atherosclerosis, particularly in brain vessels (a link to the theory of death of brain neurons); raises the level of free radicals (free radical theory); and stimulates the cross-linkage of macromolecules, particularly in connective tissue (cross-linkage theory).[1] In the final analysis, metabolic disorders induced by hypothalamic shifts of regulation cause certain changes in cells.

Hence, if the disturbances in hypothalamic regulation are considered from a physiologic point of view, the key factor in their cause appears to be the elevation of the threshold of hypothalamic sensitivity to feedback control in the three superhomeostats: energy, adaptive, and reproductive. From the neurophysiologic standpoint, the key role is played rather by the decline in the hypothalamic levels of biogenic amines that render the hypothalamus less sensitive to homeostatic stimuli. A biochemist, however, would rather see the main cause of aging and age disease formation as the shift toward a predominant utilization of FFA for energy supply, and would say that humans burn down in the flames of fats.

A pathologist would probably point to another remarkable feature of aging and age diseases, ie, reactive hyperinsulinemia, which occurs in response to the decrease in carbohydrate tolerance. This was one of the reasons why I designated age-specific pathology as diseases of compensation, and referred to normal aging as a disease (see Chapter 10).

A therapist might note that all diseases of compensation are characterized by very similar hormonal-metabolic patterns. As a result, for example, obesity increases the risk of premature development of other diseases of compensation: the climacteric, atherosclerosis, maturity-onset diabetes mellitus, metabolic immunodepression, cancer, and essential hypertension.

A philosopher might discern the dialectic unity of the mechanism of

---

[1] It is possible that the accelerated aging of human collagen in patients with diabetes mellitus (Hamlin et al 1975) is a partial manifestation of this relationship.

development, and aging and diseases of compensation, because the key role is invariably played by an accumulation of the shifts that are responsible for the implementation of the organism's developmental program.

A biologist might be interested to see that the regulatory type of natural death may be interpreted as a consequence of the evolutional development of complex homeostatic systems that ensure a better adaptation of higher organisms to the pressure of internal and external environmental factors.

A scholar of comparative physiology would notice that the transformation of the program of development into that of aging and natural death may take place at a site other than the hypothalamus in the species in which homeostatic regulation is not confined to the hypothalamus.

A gerontologist, who seeks an integrated approach to the problem of aging, might appreciate the sequence of interrelated changes shown for the whole animal organism. In particular, proceeding from the Law of Deviation of Homeostasis it is possible to distinguish features common to such seemingly different phenomena as pregnancy, stress, normal aging, and cancer (see Table 1-3). These phenomena, accordingly, characterize one of the integral components of the elevational model: developmental, environmental, intrinsic, and pathophysiologic.

Using current terminology, it may be said that the elevational model mirrors the developmental,[1] dysregulatory,[2] CNS-cybernetic,[3] and reversible[4] mechanisms of implementation of the Law of Deviation of Homeostasis. And it is precisely in these contexts that the advantages of this model become apparent: it points to some yet unknown regularities in the mechanisms of normal ontogenesis and age-specific pathology, although some details of the model structure are still missing.

---

[1]According to Lints (1978), "the developmental hypothesis of aging argues that aging and death are the ultimate, programmed, stages of development and differentiation."

[2]Some scholars advance the dysregulatory hypothalamic theory as a separate concept (Everitt 1976), although it is quite obvious that elevation (or any changes) of the hypothalamic threshold of sensitivity to regulatory stimuli results in the dysregulation of the relevant controlling mechanisms in the hypothalamus.

[3]Meier-Ruge (1975) refers to such theories, put forward after my concept was formulated, as the cybernetic CNS pacemaker theory of aging.

[4]Recently, Denckla (1977) suggested that "death appears to be a regulated function" and advanced a hypothesis of specific pituitary mechanisms of natural death.

24 Therapy for Aging and Diseases of Compensation in Light of the Elevating Mechanism of their Development

Aging is a disease or, more precisely, the confluence of the diseases of homeostasis. Therefore, the traditional point of view that therapy for aging is useless should be reconsidered.

It follows from the concept of a stable norm that the state of normality inevitably is lost in the course of normal aging. This is caused largely by the age-associated elevation of the hypothalamic threshold, with some influence from various external factors, primarily those which raise the hypothalamic threshold or intensify compensatory mechanisms. These external factors include stress, overfeeding, decreased physical activity, the influence of many carcinogens, exposure to intense solar or artificial light, and ionizing irradiation. It is practially impossible to prevent exposure to many of these factors. But since the homeostatic systems have evolved as a natural response to the damaging influence of such factors, these systems also may be able to respond to stimuli which are designed specifically to delay the aging process. This chapter, therefore, deals with some possibilities regarding therapy for aging.

It is necessary to stress that there is a current tendency to draw a demarcation line between the mechanism of aging and that of diseases associated with aging. However, the concepts of the author suggested some time ago (Dilman 1971) as well as those in this book, and the results of the studies made by Blumenthal (1974), may lead to a conclusion that measures which might retard physiological aging might also retard the development of age-associated pathology.

Proceeding from the concept of the elevating mechanisms of aging and development of diseases of compensation, homeostatic regulation, and therefore metabolic processes, may be returned to normal either by normalizing the threshold of hypothalamic sensitivity to feedback control or by reducing the degree of compensatory response. Thus, possible therapeutic measures should proceed in the following directions:

1. Restore the hypothalamic threshold of sensitivity to homeostatic signals.
2. Reduce hypothalamic-pituitary activity.
3. Inhibit the compensatory increase of peripheral endocrine gland function and associated metabolic shifts.
4. Counteract hormonal effects on target tissues.
5. Use substitution therapy wherever the output of some hormone is insufficient.

Let us examine some of these potential therapies.

Therapy Aimed at Normalizing the Hypothalamic Threshold to Feedback Control

Little is being done in this area at present because pharmacologists have yet to develop new drugs which can raise hypothalamic sensitivity to feedback control. Yet, if the concept of diseases of compensation has validity, such drugs should be feasible, and research on developing them should begin.

Of the available drugs, pineal polypeptide extract (epithalamin), phenformin, diphenylhydantoin, levodopa, and to a lesser degree, succinic acid and tryptophan, can decrease the hypothalamic threshold of sensitivity to feedback control (see Chapter 18). Let us consider some experimental and clinical data pertaining to these drugs.

Pineal hormones It is well known that pinealectomy is followed by an increase in hypothalamic-pituitary activity. In animals this manifests itself in premature puberty, enlargement of the adrenals and thyroid, and intensified growth. Similar effects are produced by long-term exposure to continuous lighting, which inhibits pineal gland activity (Wurtman 1970).

The most popular theory regarding the functional role of the pineal gland is that its hormonal effect is determined by melatonin. Many effects of melatonin are similar to those of the pineal gland. For example, melatonin inhibits the secretion of growth hormone (Smythe and Lazarus 1974), insulin, and gonadotropins. It also suppresses the action of somatomedin (Smythe et al 1974) and lowers MSH concentration in the pituitary (Kastin and Schally 1967). Melatonin-like substances have been found in the plasma of human males (Pelham et al 1973).

Additional evidence points to the synthesis by the pineal gland of a hormone (or hormones) of polypeptide nature. These hormones not only produce the main effects of the pineal gland but are more active than melatonin. A polypeptide has been extracted from the pineal gland, which inhibits synthesis of growth and luteinizing hormones, intensifies prolactin synthesis, and increases blood potassium concentration (Chazov and Isachenkov 1974, Cheesman and Forsham 1974). Polypeptide extracts obtained by other researchers (Morozov and Khavinson 1971) and in our laboratory by Ostroumova and Dilman (1972) reveal a pronounced hormonal activity.

But the spectrum of effects produced by the pineal gland cannot be accounted for solely on the basis of its inhibitory action on the hypothalamic-pituitary system. An analysis of effects observed during both stimulation and suppression of pineal gland function suggests that its hormones can raise hypothalamic sensitivity to the action of peripheral hormones (Dilman 1970a). Data presented in Table 24-1 demonstrate such an effect (Ostroumova and Dilman 1972).

Table 24-1
The Effect of Polypeptide Extract of Pineal Gland on Sensitivity of the Hypothalamic-Adrenal System to Inhibition by Prednisolone in Rats

Treatment	Blood Corticosterone Level (μg%)	
	Before Administration	*After Administration*
Prednisolone	22.8 ± 3.8	22.2 ± 2.6
Prednisolone and pineal gland extract	22.0 ± 3.6	11.1 ± 2.8

Prednisolone (0.05 mg/100 g body weight) was administered intraperitoneally at 10 AM. Pineal gland extract (1 mg) was administered intraperitoneally at 9 AM and 10 AM on the same day. Blood samples were taken at 12 noon.

Table 24-1 shows that prednisolone fails to inhibit the hypothalamic-pituitary system, while combined administration of prednisolone and pineal gland extract (which also fails to affect blood corticosterone concentration when used alone) results in a decrease of the hypothalamic threshold to inhibition by prednisolone. Similar data were obtained in experiments involving the use of pineal gland extract to raise hypothalamic sensitivity to estrogens (see Chapter 4; Dilman et al 1973). Following treatment with pineal polypeptide extract, cyclic estral function was resumed in old rats (Anisimov et al 1973a).

These properties of polypeptide extracts of the pineal gland support the suggestion that this gland controls hypothalamic sensitivity to feedback regulation (Dilman 1970a, 1971) and superintends the mechanisms of cyclicity of the hypothalamic-pituitary system (Quay 1972). Therefore, one way to lower the sensitivity threshold of the hypothalamus would be to develop preparations that could use these processes of adaptation. This conclusion is supported by data obtained in our laboratory on the inhibition of corticosterone hypersecretion by epithalamin in stress (see Table 3-9), and by the findings of a hypoglycemic effect of epithalamin (Ostroumova and Vasiljeva 1976).

These data are in agreement with reports of the inhibition of atherosclerosis as a result of pineal polypeptide hormone administration (Tasca et al 1974). Taking into consideration the ability of epithalamin to alleviate metabolic shifts inherent in metabolic immunodepression (see Chapter 15), and to improve carbohydrate tolerance and reduce blood insulin and triglyceride levels, it would appear that the improvement of cellular immunity (Belokrylov et al 1976, Dilman 1977) caused by epithalamin treatment is connected with the alleviation of the syndrome of metabolic immunodepression. This provides a new aspect to the findings from our laboratory on the oncolytic effect of pineal polypeptide extract (Anisimov et al 1973b; Table 24-2). Epithalamin exerted a pronounced antitumor effect on squamous cell cervical carcinoma (76% of tumor weight inhibition) and transplanted breast carcinoma (80% of inhibition), a weak action on hepatoma-22a (35% of inhibition), and had no effect on Harding-Passy melanoma (Dilman et al 1979). Moreover, epithalamin significantly increased the survival time of SHR mice with transplantable lymphoid leukemia L10-1, but showed no effect on the survival time of (C57Bl/6 × DBA/2)F_1 mice with leukemia L-1210.

These data also are consistent with reports that after pinealectomy the growth and metastatic spread of transplantable tumors are intensified (Das Gupta and Terz 1967, Lapin 1975, Rodin 1963). At the same time, administration of melatonin (Buswell 1976, Anisimov et al 1973a) or pineal extracts (Bergman and Engel 1950, Kitay and Altschule 1954, Lapin and Ebels 1976) suppresses tumor development or tumor growth in animals. As shown by Table 24-3, epithalamin decreases the incidence of mammary adenocarcinoma induced with DMBA in rats (81.1%), while DMBA and epithalamin administration is followed by the induction of adenocarcinomas in 9 out of 35 animals (25.7%). As shown by the data in Figure 1-2 epithalamin treatment results in a longer life span for rats, the life span of the animals treated with 0.5 mg/day being longer than the average by 25%. Therefore, pineal gland hormones should be studied to ascertain whether they are capable of exerting an influence on diseases of compensation, including aging, cancer susceptibility, and metabolic immunodepression. In this connection it should be pointed out that nocturnal peaks of growth hormone secretion are not observed in blind subjects with a supposedly active function of the pineal gland, whereas a high level of nocturnal secretion of the same hormone has been recorded

Table 24-2
The Effect of Polypeptide Pineal Extract (PPE), Melatonin, and Sigetin on the Growth of Transplantable Tumors in Mice

Strain of Mice	Tumor Strain	Treat-ment	Daily Dose (mg)	No. Animals	Tumor Inhibition (%)
BALB/c	SCC*	PPE	1	9	26
			2	18	76
C3HA	RSM†	PPE	1	16	40
			2	28	79
C3HA	RSM†	Melatonin	0.05	10	51
		Sigetin	0.2	10	38
C3HA	Hepatoma-22a	PPE	2	34	35
SHR	Harding-Passy melanoma	PPE	2	25	8

Source: Dilman et al 1979a.
*SCC squamous cell cervical carcinoma.
†RSM small alveolar mammary cancer.

Table 24-3
Effect of Polypeptide Pineal Extract (PPE) on the Incidence of DMBA-Induced Mammary Tumors in Rats

	DMBA + Saline (n = 37)	DMBA + PPE (n = 35)
No. rats with tumors	36 (97.3%)	28 (80.0%)
No. tumors	52 (1.44 per rat)	33 (1.18 per rat)
Mean latent period of tumors (days)	102 ± 11	182 ± 5*
Adenocarcinomas		
No. rats	30 (81.1%)	9 (25.7%)*
No. tumors	43 (1.43 per rat)	10 (1.11 per rat)
Mean latent period (days)	95 ± 6	86 ± 9
Fibroadenomas		
No. rats	3 (8.1%)	12 (34.3%)*
No. tumors	3	12
Mean latent period (days)	81 ± 44	216 ± 21*
Other tumors	5†	9‡

*Difference from control is significant, $p < 0.05$.
†Cancer of Zymbal gland (2), leukemia, (1), adenoma of thyroid (1), cancer of cutis (1).
‡Cancer of Zymbal gland (5), leukemia (4).

in cancer patients (see Figure 17-2). Thus, statistics on cancer incidence in blind subjects would be relevant to these considerations.

Recently, Cohen et al (1978) put forward a special hypothesis on the role of the pineal gland in the etiology and treatment of breast cancer. It should be mentioned that a hypocaloric diet improved the metabolic activity of the pineal gland (Walker et al 1978). These authors conclude: "Based upon the capacity of pineal compounds to alter neuroendocrine feedback sensitivity, life prolongation resulting from feed restriction may in part be due to the persistence of a juvenile type pineal gland in the chronically underfed rat." This suggests that a decreased activity of the pineal gland may provide one of the mechanisms responsible for elevating the hypothalamic threshold. If such a decline does occur in the course of aging, however, a simple confirmation of the relationship between hypothalamic sensitivity and the pineal gland activity would be of little use in attempting to establish the precise mechanism of the interaction, and would pose a problem as to the causes of the age-related changes in pineal function.

Phenformin, metformin, buformin The classification of the antidiabetic biguanides phenformin, metformin, and buformin as preparations that raise the threshold of the hypothalamic-pituitary complex sensitivity to feedback control is recognized to a considerable degree. Muntoni (1974) is right in saying that "biguanides exert their metabolic effects through a single basic mechanism, namely inhibition of fatty acid oxidation." The impaired glucose tolerance, insulin resistance with secondary hyperinsulinemia, and enhanced gluconeogenesis at least partly account for the excessive fatty acid oxidation (Randle 1965, Ruderman et al 1969). Muntoni (1974) presented evidence that biguanides "cause metabolic effects which are the exact opposite of the above changes." Dietze et al (1978) support the view that the hypoglycemic effect of biguanides is caused, at least in part, by inhibition of hepatic gluconeogenesis. Muntoni (1974) also suggests the existence of other mechanisms of biguanide action, eg, that cellular metabolism may be capable of influencing the availability of insulin receptors.

It was also shown by Feldman and Durchen (1975) that phenformin produces the inhibition of monoamine oxidase. Therefore, the effect of phenformin treatment of CNS is probably also caused by the influence of this drug on the hormonal-metabolic pattern. Compensatory hyperinsulinemia is the key factor in acceleration of development, obesity, and metabolic disorders observed in maturity-onset diabetes and atherosclerosis, and it seems to be a significant factor also in carcinogenesis (see Chapter 17). Therefore, it is particularly noteworthy that short-term administration of phenformin to prediabetics results in a lower incidence of overt diabetes mellitus (Wilansky and Hahn 1967). For this reason metabolic disturbances can be counteracted by means of phenformin administration in cases of atherosclerosis and cancer even where there are no clinical manifestations of diabetes mellitus (Dilman 1967, 1968). Figure 24-1 provides an example of phenformin-induced normalization of the blood lipoproteins in a woman with atherosclerosis. Tzagournis et al (1968) showed independently that phenformin treatment lowers blood insulin, triglycerides, and cholesterol levels in young male patients with ischemic heart disease (see Table 15-3). It should be stressed that phenformin treatment produces a decrease in cholesterol level in lymphocytes (see Figure 15-1). This suggests that phenformin is capable of both lowering LDL-cholesterol level in blood plasma and inhibiting cholesterol accumulation in tissues. Metformin has been shown to exhibit a similar effect (Agid et al 1975). However, our preliminary results indicate that clofibrate can sometimes reduce cholesterol level in blood and raise it in lymphocytes.

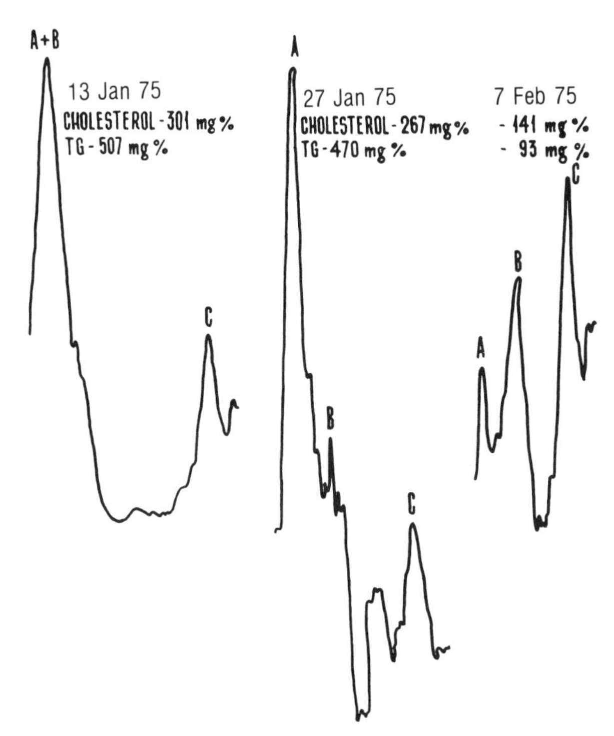

Figure 24-1 Changes in lipoprotein profile of blood serum following phenformin therapy (100 mg/day for 25 days) in patient with ischemic heart disease. A: Pre-β-lipoproteins; B: β-lipoproteins; C: α-lipoproteins. Before treatment (first curve) pre-β- and β-lipoproteins are predominant and do not separate during electrophoresis on polyacrylamide gel. After phenformin therapy (second and third curves) a sharp fall in pre-β- and β-lipoprotein fraction matched by a rise in α-lipoproteins is observed. The dates indicate when the blood was sampled.

Table 24-4 illustrates our findings on phenformin-influenced loss of body weight and drop in insulin, fatty acid, triglyceride, cholesterol, and lipoprotein levels in cancer patients. It also indicates a decrease in blood and urine hydroxysteroids and total gonadotropin excretion, and contains a comparison of results following administration of dilantin and clofibrate.

Note that the effect of clofibrate is not confined solely to a reduction of FFA, triglyceride, and cholesterol levels; it also inhibits gonadotropin excretion. Dilantin has been found to shift the 17-ketosteroid/17-hydroxycorticosteroid ratio toward positive values, which may have a beneficial effect in light of the prognostic significance of the index of discrimination (Bulbrook et al 1971; see Chapter 3). The effects of phenformin and Dilantin treatment on the reproductive homeostat are consistent with our findings on the resumption of estral cycle in old rats following the administration of these drugs (see Chapter 4). Chapters 15 and 20 cite data on the normalizing effect of phenformin on cellular immunity and elimination of 1,2-dimethylhydrazine-induced immunodepression. Treatment with phenformin was followed by a fourfold reduction in the incidence of mammary gland carcinoma in C3H mice, as well as a 25% rise in survival time (see Table 17-11). Moreover, phenformin treatment reduces considerably the incidence rates of mammary gland carcinoma induced with DMBA (Dilman et al 1974, Dilman et al 1978). As mentioned, phenformin also has the effect, in common with hydrazine sulfate, of suppressing gluconeogenesis (Ray et al 1970). These also have an antitumor effect (Gold 1973) which may be the result of a decreased lysis of lymphocytes when gluconeogenesis is suppressed. Phenformin treatment has been shown to increase the antitumor effect of hydrazine sulfate and cyclophosphamide (see Table 17-12). It also should be pointed out that phenformin used in conjunction with anabolic drugs increases blood fibrinolytic activity (Ciswicka-Sznejderman et al 1974), which may be a desirable effect in view of the relation between cancer metastasis and thrombogenesis.

Thus, bearing in mind the two key elements of the elevational mechanism of aging, we can explain now why the antidiabetic drug, phenformin, lowers the blood levels of cholesterol, triglycerides, and lipoproteins in patients with some type of hyperlipidemia (Stout et al 1974; see Table 15-3); delays experimental atherosclerosis (Agid et al 1975, Sirtori et al 1977a); reduces age-associated hyperinsulinemia (Tzagournis et al 1972); raises the sensitivity of the hypothalamic-pituitary complex to inhibition by dexamethasone (see Chapter 3) and estrogens (see Chapter 4); causes the resumption of estral cycle in old rats (see Chapter 3); reduces the fetal weight in animals with chemical diabetes (see Chapter 21); prolongs the life span of mice and rats; improves cellular immunity in atherosclerotic (see Chapter 15) and cancer patients (see Chapter 17)

Table 24-4
Effect of Phenformin, Clofibrate, and Dilantin on Metabolic and Hormonal Parameters in Cancer Patients

	Phenformin (n = 17)		Clofibrate (n = 10)		Dilantin (n = 5)	
	Before *(87.6 ± 3.3 kg)*	*After* *(83.6 ± 3.1 kg)*	*Before* *(77.4 ± 5.8 kg)*	*After* *(77.6 ± 5.5 kg)*	*Before* *(80.0 ± 7.2 kg)*	*After* *(79.8 ± 7.7 kg)*
Blood sugar (2 hr after glucose load)	164 ± 11	132 ± 8	154 ± 14	128 ± 4	134 ± 23	183 ± 3
Cholesterol (mg%)	290 ± 4	217 ± 9	312 ± 16	235 ± 8	242 ± 7*	245 ± 21*
FFA (μEq/liter)	825 ± 71	618 ± 48	928 ± 31	619 ± 81	698 ± 91	866 ± 251
Triglyceride (mg%)	230 ± 15	216 ± 33	364 ± 73	248 ± 31	191 ± 33	215 ± 25
Total lipoproteins (mg%)	719 ± 29	597 ± 37	770 ± 51	647 ± 31	774 ± 58	527 ± 55
Corticosteroids						
11-Hydroxysteroids in blood (μg%)	17.2 ± 0.8	10.2 ± 0.6	10.2 ± 1.1	11.1 ± 0.9	22.0 ± 2.3	16.3 ± 1.7
17-Hydroxysteroids in urine (mg/24 hr)	6.8 ± 0.9	4.2 ± 0.8	5.0 ± 0.7	4.5 ± 1.3	3.3 ± 0.7	1.5 ± 0.4
17-Ketosteroids in urine (mg/24 hr)	5.4 ± 1.4	4.6 ± 0.4	5.0 ± 0.8	4.6 ± 1.3	5.0 ± 1.0	1.8 ± 0.6
Total gonadotropins (mmu/24 hr)†	101 ± 9	50 ± 28	115 ± 26	51 ± 21	...‡	...‡

*In another series of experiments Dilantin was found to decrease blood cholesterol in 15 of 19 cases (from 272 ± 13 to 237 ± 15 mg%).
†mmu: mouse uterine units.
‡The same series showed a decrease in total gonadotropin excretion, from 126 to 44 mmu/24 hr (p = 0.01).

(Dilman et al 1976, Dilman 1978b); cuts down the incidence of DMBA-induced cancer of the mammary gland (Dilman et al 1974, 1978); reduces hypercholesterolemia in pregnancy (Berstein and Alexandrov 1976); raises the activity of some oncolytic agents (Cohen and Strauss 1976, Dilman and Anisimov 1979); diminishes the immunosuppressive effect of such a potent carcinogen as 1,2-dimethylhydrazine (Dilman et al 1977b); suppresses the growth of Ehrlich's carcinoma; effects transplacental carcinogenesis (Napalkov and Alexandrov 1978); cuts down the yield of intestinal tumors induced in rats by 1,2-dimethylhydrazine treatment (Anisimov et al 1978); and lowers the blood somatomedin level in cancer and atherosclerotic patients with Type IIb hyperlipoproteinemia. Thus, phenformin treatment produces a therapeutic effect on age-associated obesity, chemical diabetes mellitus, metabolic immunodepression, and a metabolic pattern typical of many cases of atherosclerosis and cancer. I believe that phenformin is the drug of choice for prevention of premature development of diseases of aging. Moreover, these data suggest the conclusion that drugs capable of "lipostatic action" (Muntoni 1974) are the drugs of choice in attempting to influence the mechanisms of development, aging, and age-associated pathology.

As far as the therapeutic application of phenformin is concerned, it is necessary to consider some limitations. A report of the University Group Diabetic Program shows that treatment with phenformin resulted in a slight increase in the mortality rates from cardiovascular disorders among patients with diabetes mellitus, rather than a decrease.[1] However, treatment with phenformin failed to eliminate hyperglycemia in this study. It may be supposed that this result was caused by extremely high levels of hyperglycemia in most patients. To illustrate, the glycemic square during glucose tolerance test exceeded 575 mg% in most of the patients. Moreover, it may be suggested on the basis of our findings and those of Tzagournis et al (1968, 1972) that phenformin administration may be effective in treating age-related disturbances of metabolism in atherosclerosis and cancer, ie, in diseases characterized by latent chemical diabetes. Moreover, it should be taken into account that the therapeutic effect of a drug may be adequately assessed only on the basis of the metabolic patterns observed on reaching a certain ideal norm. Such an effect is rare when patients with overt diabetes mellitus are treated with phenformin. This drug is more suitable for therapy of age-connected metabolic changes rather than maturity-onset diabetes proper. Therefore, we used phenformin only in patients without overt diabetes mellitus. In addition, the risk of blood lactate increase seems to be negligible.

Using phenformin since 1970 and observing the necessary precautions

[1] *Diabetes* 24(suppl 1). 1975.

with respect to contraindications, we have not had a single case of grave lactate acidosis. Metformin, which possesses the same properties[1] but presents less hazard of lactate acidosis (Luft et al 1978b), seems to offer more advantages. Generally speaking, any other means of treatment which inhibits the accumulation or synthesis of lipids in cells may be used.

Dilantin (diphenylhydantoin) and benzodiazepines As has been reported by Greenblatt and Shader (1974) Dilantin and diazepam have a similar molecular conformation and might interact with the same receptor sites. This hypothesis is consistent with our findings that both Dilantin and phenazepam increase the sensitivity of the hypothalamic-pituitary complex to inhibitory action of estrogens and dexamethasone respectively (see Chapters 3 and 4). Dilantin has a very wide range of effect; in particular, it inhibits gonadotropin secretion (Dilman et al 1971). Dilantin is known to suppress adrenal steroidogenesis as well as insulin and glucogon (Cohen et al 1973). Dilantin also has been used to treat certain forms of cardiac arrhythmia. Its inhibitory influence on atherogenesis in rabbits (Chung 1967) and its beneficial effect on the behavior of aged animals and humans (Gordon et al 1968) also have been reported.

This wide range of action is caused possibly by an associated increase in intracellular concentration of potassium (O'Reilly and MacDonald 1973). This effect also seems to characterize pineal polypeptide hormones (Quay 1972, Chazov and Isachenkov 1974), and provides a basis for administering Dilantin to cancer patients (Dilman et al 1971). One of the advantages offered by treatment with Dilantin, as compared, for example, with aminoglutethimide (an antiepileptic drug) for inhibiting corticosteroid production [Smith et al 1978]) lies in the fact that it does not cause the compensatory elevation of ACTH secretion, probably because of the inhibitory effect of Dilantin on the hypothalamic-pituitary system.[2]

It is noteworthy that statistics show a decrease in tumor incidence in epileptics who receive anticonvulsant therapy (Clemensen et al 1974). The immunosuppressive effect of Dilantin (Kruger and Harris 1972) has not been assessed fully, while our results of evaluation of skin tests with DNCB and tuberculin did not confirm the immunosuppressive effect of Dilantin in breast cancer patients, particularly following long-term administration. The increase of serum high density lipoproteins in Dilantin users (Nikkilä et al 1978) is worth mentioning in light of the report of Glueck et al (1977) demonstrating the frequent co-occurrence of the "syndrome of longevity" and the high level of HDL-cholesterol

---

[1]It was shown in our laboratory that metformin potentiates the antitumor effect of cyclophosphamide in rats with Lewis's tumor.

[2]The assessment of the effects of Dilantin on the adaptive homeostat involves some difficulty because this substance causes changes in cortisol metabolism and disturbs the sensitivity of the hypothalamic-pituitary complex to dexamethasone suppression.

in the blood. Since Dilantin inhibits thyroid function, it seems promising to investigate its effect when combined with the administration of triiodothyronine.

Levodopa and other neurotropic preparations Our findings show that levodopa raises the sensitivity of the reproductive (see Chapter 4) and adaptive (see Chapter 3) homeostats to feedback suppression. Cotzias et al (1974, 1977) produced a prolonged life span in mice treated with levodopa. Some data demonstrate a short favorable response of breast cancer patients during levodopa treatment (Stoll 1972).

It should be emphasized that both drugs for the treatment of parkinsonism (eg, bromocriptine) and some antidepressants and anorexigenic drugs (eg, mazindol) should be studied for their effect on aging and diseases of aging, since they are known to raise biogenic amine levels in the brain.

Since Cushing's syndrome resembles accelerated aging in many respects (Dilman 1961, 1968, 1971, 1974a; Wexler 1971, 1976), it should be noted that cyproheptadine administration produces a beneficial effect in many cases of this disease (Krieger 1978; see Chapter 3). Lamberts et al (1977) put forward the hypothesis of a hypothalamic dopaminergic depletion in Cushing's syndrome.

Blood cholesterol can be lowered by chlorpromazine, a fact indicative of the role the hypothalamic-pituitary activity plays in the pathogenesis of neurogenic hypercholesterolemia. It is possible that this effect is caused by the decreased secretion of growth hormone, and for this reason chlorpromazine also has been administered in the treatment of acromegaly. Chlorpromazine also reduces the death rate of animals from populational stress (Christian 1968, 1976). Neurogenic hypercholesterolemia generally unaccompanied by a rise in triglyceride level may be annulled by administration of other neurotropic drugs (Byers et al 1976).

Therapy Aimed at Decrease in Hypothalamic-Pituitary Activity

Hormones of the peripheral endocrine glands interact with the hypothalamic-pituitary system by negative feedback, and thus can be used to inhibit the activity of this system. The main limitation of this method is the undesirable hormonal action on the target tissues, which restricts the range of application of the peripheral hormones for inhibition.[1] Apart from this well-known problem it should be recalled that

---

[1]This effect also suggests the distinguishing feature between decreasing hypothalamic-pituitary activity as a therapy and the therapy aimed at lowering the hypothalamic threshold to feedback control. As an example of the former, estrogens typically are administered for diseases of compensation that occur during the climacteric. However, the suppression of hypothalamic-pituitary activity is not followed by resumption of the rhythmic functioning of this system.

estrogens, progestins, and glucocorticoids are most frequently used to inhibit hypothalamic-pituitary activity.

Despite their abundance in the organism, estrogens are often administered during the climacteric period, eg, for climacteric bleeding, which is inherent in the central type of homeostatic failure. The same principle lies at the basis of the suggestion that large doses of oxytocin may suppress lactation (Klimek 1968). The effectiveness of estrogen therapy for late-onset breast cancer (though in early-onset breast cancer remission is achieved by ovariectomy) points to the role of elevation of hypothalamic-pituitary activity in the pathogenesis of late-onset cancer (Dilman 1968, 1974a). This also is supported by statistical data showing a sharp fall in the incidence of tumors of the reproductive system following a long-term cyclic treatment with estrogens and progestins (Wilson 1962, Defares 1971). Similarly important is the report of a higher therapeutic effectiveness in the treatment of breast cancer by the use of estrogen when L-dopa is administered (Stoll 1972). The ability to block the growth hormone effect on peripheral tissues is an essential component of the mechanism of estrogen action (Kovaleva et al 1964).

It is possible that the ability of estrogens to reduce age-associated hypercholesterolemia (Oliver and Boyd 1956, Blagosklonnaya 1959) is caused by their antisomatotropic effect. Estrogen treatment results in an improved tolerance to carbohydrates (see Chapter 6; Vishnevsky and Dilman 1972) and a lower blood insulin (Pyorälа and Pyorälа 1971). The effect of estrogen treatment on the metabolic pattern should be distinguished from the action of steroid contraceptive preparations that decrease carbohydrate utilization and raise triglycerides (Spellacy et al 1972). Estrogens also have been shown to affect the development of some types of cancer, atherosclerosis, and late-onset diabetes mellitus. Such a wide range of overlapping effects of the same agent is typical of the therapy for different diseases of compensation, because of the common pathogenic features inherent in their formation.

It should be stressed that many physicians have recently administered estrogens without progestins. The common explanation was that natural rather than synthetic estrogens were given. This practice resulted in an increased incidence of cancer in the reproductive system, particularly that of the endometrium. However, the premise that natural estrogens would present less hazard than synthetic ones was wrong because the risk of carcinogenic hazard in this case is determined by the proliferative effect of estrogens on target tissues. Under the circumstances, there is no essential difference between the effects of natural and synthetic estrogens. It is noteworthy that estrogen therapy in conjunction with progestin administration was followed by a far lower cancer incidence in the reproductive system (Defares 1971).

Progestins, capable of inhibiting growth hormone secretion (Lucke and Glick 1971), raise carbohydrate tolerance in cases of climacteric bleeding and endometrial carcinoma, and therefore may be used in the treatment of certain diseases of compensation.

If derivatives of these hormones are developed, however, the important thing will be to find drugs which retain the inhibitory effect on the hypothalamic-pituitary complex while leaving the peripheral tissues unaffected; although some of these side effects undoubtedly can be eliminated at present, it is not yet clear to what degree their elimination will be feasible without altering the main effect of the hormones. Among the estrogens deprived of their primary effect, a derivative of stilbestrol (sigetin) is of particular interest since it retains some antigonadotropic effect (Dilman 1959). The data presented above in Table 24-2 demonstrate that sigetin inhibits the growth of transplanted tumors of the mammary gland. Some of our findings show that sigetin probably also has an antiestrogen effect. This property deserves particular attention since sigetin and estrogens may compete for the same hormonal receptors.

The possibility of dissociating the properties of polypeptide and protein hormones also must be studied. Earlier I suggested the term anahormone to designate derivatives of protein and polypeptide hormones which have been chemically deprived of their hormonal activity while retaining one of the three main properties of the hormonal protein molecule (affinity for the target tissue, initial antigenicity, or ability to participate in the process of hormonal self-regulation). Thus, three types of anahormones may be developed on the basis of the three main modifications: competitive anahormones, anahormone antigens, and anahormone inhibitors (Dilman 1962, 1966; Dilman et al 1974).

Table 24-5 illustrates the effect of the anahormone inhibitor, acetylated corticotropin, capable of inhibiting stress-induced ACTH secretion.

Table 24-5
Decrease in Blood Corticosterone Levels Following Treatment with Ana-ACTH and Block of Stressor Release of ACTH

Group	No. Rats	Blood Corticosterone (μg%)	Pituitary Level of Corticotropin (mU/pituitary
Control			
Before stress	66	9.0±0.2	36.9±2.0
Ether-induced stress	77	19.0±1.3	23.7±3.4
Ana-ACTH-treated animals			
Before stress	64	7.1±0.2	35.5±3.2
Ether-induced stress	17	14.7±1.3*	39.0±3.7*

*Difference is statistically significant ($p < 0.05$).

Theoretically, the anahormone of ACTH may be used for suppression of adrenal cortical activity in cancer patients, particularly in those cases of breast and prostate carcinoma, which currently are treated with glucocorticoids and show an undesirable immunodepressive effect. Table 24-6 shows that ACTH-anahormone treatment extends the free period following the removal of a primary mammary tumor, and therefore prolongs the survival time of mice of strain C3H/He. Figure 24-2 shows that the administration of acetylated corticotropin decreases the frequency of spontaneous mammary cancer in mice of the C3H/He strain.

Table 24-6
Relationship between Acetylated ACTH Treatment and Postoperative Recurrence of Mammary Cancer and Survival Time of Mice of C3H/He Strain

Group	No. Animals	Average Time from Removal of Primary Tumor to Detectable Recurrence (days)		Postoperative Survival time (days)	
Control	24	41 ± 4.3	$p = 0.03$	86 ± 6.7	$p = 0.02$
Experiment	22	60 ± 8.3		118 ± 9.2	

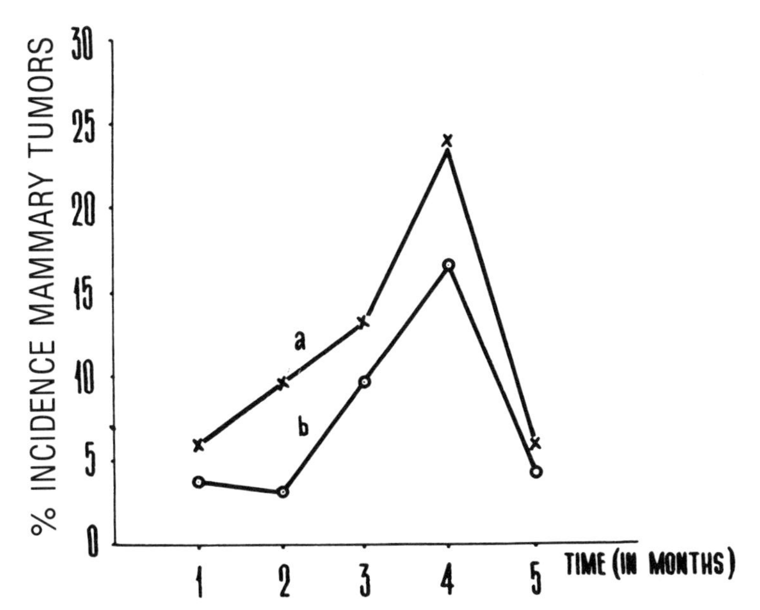

Figure 24-2 Incidence of spontaneous mammary cancer in mice. (Strain C3H/He repeatedly treated with acetylated corticotropin as anahormone). Curve a: Control; Curve b: Experimental animals treated with acetylated corticotropin (anahormone).

Therapy to Inhibit Compensatory Intensification of Endocrine Gland Activity

A relative increase in cortisol output (see Chapter 3), and particularly compensatory hyperinsulinemia (see Chapter 6), constitute the key factors of diseases of aging. Apart from the effect on the hypothalamic-pituitary complex, such drugs as phenformin, Dilantin, and ana-ACTH lower insulin and cortisol levels in blood. Moreover, it has been demonstrated that aminoglutethimide inhibits gonadotropin secretion (Vishnevsky et al 1969). Aminoglutethimide also appears to produce remission in advanced cases of breast cancer (Elubajeva et al 1972, Griffiths et al 1973), and to inhibit corticosteroid production (Fishman et al 1967). However, it causes a compensatory elevation of ACTH secretion and, therefore, combined administration of aminoglutethimide and dexamethasone is usually used in treating breast cancer (Lipton and Santen 1974, Smith et al 1978). Taking this into consideration, we used Dilantin to inhibit adrenal cortical function in cases of cancer.

A carbohydrate-restricted diet or physical exercise may reduce the level of hyperinsulinemia (Björntorp et al 1973), with the blood-cholesterol level showing a particularly dramatic drop (Evans et al 1972, Truswell 1978). It was shown experimentally that diet restriction improves hormonal profile (Pierpaoli 1977). The effect of diet on brain neurotransmitters (Wurtman and Fernstrom 1976) should also be taken into consideration. However, as far as dietary therapy is concerned, there are certain limitations. Polyunsaturated fatty acids used as a component of the complex therapy of atherosclerosis (Kritchevsky 1976) suppress cellular immunity, thus aiding tumor process progression (Meade and Mertin 1978). Therefore, when it is necessary to diminish the compensatory intensification of insulin secretion, therapy should be based on the three following mechanisms which do not overlap completely: diet, increased physical exercise, and medication aimed at normalizing regulatory mechanisms, eg, phenformin or metformin.

Antibodies are an efficient means of hormone neutralization. For instance, an experimental administration of antisomatotropic serum enhanced the effect of chemotherapeutic drugs on transplanted tumors (Anigstein et al 1963, Lazarev and Izotov 1965). A similar effect also has been reported under clinical conditions. Previously we noted a female patient in whom a decrease in hyperglycemia and therapeutic dose of insulin took place following a four-day course of immune serum to growth hormone anahormone (see Chapter 6). Accordingly, active immunization with anahormone-antigens might prove useful. Such an immunization with growth hormone anahormones involves the development of antigens which cross-react with native growth hormone (Dilman et al 1974); this may offer certain advantages over immunization with native growth hormone, even in cases of acromegaly in which antibodies have been induced by native growth hormone (Frantz and Raben 1967).

Among the anahormone-antigens worthy of particular mention are anahormones of luteinizing gonadotropins, placental lactogen, parathyroid hormone, and other so-called anahormone-chimeras, ie, conjugates of heterogenous hormones such as human growth hormone and bovine ACTH (Dilman et al 1974). Development seems particularly promising for anahormones with active hormonal centers or molecular fragments (Sonenberg et al 1969), and for hypothalamic hormones.

It should be noted that an anahormone of chorionic gonadotropin was the first anahormone-antigen produced in our laboratory (Dilman 1962, 1966). Such anahormones are of particular interest now in two respects: first, as a contraceptive preparation (Talwar et al 1976) and, second, because the production of chorionic gonadotropin by many tumors (Acevedo et al 1978) perhaps manifests the role of this hormone as a factor of tumor growth or as a factor that alters the potentially immunogenic antigen expression (Whyte 1978).

Treatment to Counteract Hormonal Influences on Target Tissues

Application of hormonal antagonists, eg, progestins for endometrial carcinoma, or antiestrogens and antiandrogens, is being carried out on a wide scale. Therefore, it is necessary to dwell on some aspects of this problem.

Receptor concentration in tumor tissue is often used as a criterion of choice of the type of hormonal treatment. However, hormone level variation in blood produces a certain effect on receptor concentration both in normal and tumor tissue (Saez et al 1978).

Unlike progesterone, progestins and even contraceptive pills improve the dinitrochlorobenzene sensitization test (Gerretsen et al 1975). We observed the same effect in a patient with endometrial carcinoma treated with 17-hydroxyprogesterone acetate. It is likely that this effect of progestins is caused by their inhibition of the secretion of ACTH and somatotropin, which is used, for instance, in the treatment of menopausal diabetic women (Danowski et al 1975).

Apart from more traditional therapies, there seem to be certain advantages in the administration of nicotinic acid to cancer patients to counteract metabolic disturbances. Large doses of nicotinic acid suppress lipolysis and thus lower blood cholesterol and triglycerides. Of particular interest also are some derivatives of nicotinic acid which are characterized by prolonged action. Anahormones of growth hormone and prolactin inhibit the lipolytic effect of growth hormone (Kovaleva et al 1972). Earlier, acetylated thyrotropin was shown to counteract the effect of active thyrotropin (Sonenberg and Money 1957). Iodinated derivatives of insulin, deprived of hypoglycemic effect, also inhibit lipolysis (Dilman and Vasiljeva 1971).

Substitution Therapy

This therapy may be employed in diseases of compensation to compensate for the deficit of some hormones. For instance, dehydroepiandrosterone is administered for atherosclerosis to counteract the insufficient output of androsterone and etiocholanolone metabolites (Fassati et al 1970). Since androsterone and dehydroepiandrosterone lower blood cholesterol (Oliver 1962, Ben-David et al 1967), it is desirable to test the effectiveness of such drugs, including etiocholanolone, in oncology. The effect of deoxycorticosterone on the immune system also deserves study (Seifter et al 1974).

Thyroid hormone therapy may be important, considering the age-dependent decline in thyroid function (see Chapter 7). For instance, administration of thyroid hormones reduces hypercholesterolemia in patients with premyxedema. Successful therapy for latent hypothyroidism returns the production of androgen-like hormones excreted by the adrenals to normal levels, and may contribute to a reduction of growth hormone secretion (Bielschowsky 1958). The administration of dextrothyroxin may be advisable in some cases, eg, in hypercholesterolemia. This section does not discuss the extensive problem of application of vitamins, particularly nicotinic acid, to raise serotonin concentration in the brain.

Certain Considerations of Prevention and Therapy of Diseases of Compensation

This analysis of drugs already used (or those that should be tested) in the treatment of diseases of compensation points to a wide range of overlapping influences of such drugs, because of the common pathogenic features of this group of diseases. This includes drugs used to treat epilepsy, atherosclerosis, and in clinical oncology.

Let us consider some prospects opened up by application of these drugs for prevention and therapy of diseases of compensation.

Regarding the climacteric, the main objective should probably consist of maintaining gonadotropin and hormone secretion at levels intrinsic to 20- to 25-year-old women (see Chapters 4 and 10). This will probably delay the loss of oocytes with aging (see Chapter 4). Until this hypothesis is tested experimentally with the aid of sex hormones or sigetin-like pituitary inhibitors, it is desirable to evaluate the hazards and advantages involved in the use of estrogens and progestins in the perimenopausal and menopausal period.

In atherosclerosis, priority should be given to therapy aimed at annulling hyperinsulinemia and elevated blood cortisol level. At present, phenformin (or metformin) (Sirtori et al 1977a, 1977b) and Dilantin are the most effective drugs, provided the disturbances result from age-associated processes rather than random disorders, eg, familial hyperlipidemia. Along with standard checks on lipid levels, it is necessary to monitor cholesterol concentration in lymphocytes, because phenformin decreases, while clofibrate sometimes increases, this index (see Chapter 12). It was reported that a clofibrate-induced rise in LDL-cholesterol was not observed during combined treatment with phenformin (Vogelberg 1976).

Our methods of prevention and therapy of cancer will probably improve, if standard oncologic procedures are supplemented with administration of drugs that bring metabolism to normal. It should be kept in mind that, first, body condition is a vital factor determining the fate of a cancer patient. For instance, recurrence of breast carcinoma after radical mastectomy correlates with preoperative body weight among patients observed for up to 24 years (Donegan et al 1978). Moreover, our observations show that the five-year survival rates were lower in women aged 50 years and older who had given birth to large babies (4 kg and more), than in mothers of babies weighing less than 4 kg, 53.8% ± 9.6% and 76.3% ± 6.9%, respectively. Therefore, I suggested that phenformin be studied with regard to its ability to suppress the development not only of atherosclerosis but of tumors as well (Dilman 1971). The use of diet, clofibrate, cholestyramine, and other hypocholesterolemic drugs offers some advantages in this respect.[1] Tumor cells vigorously synthesize cholesterol from fatty acids. Therefore, it is necessary not only to lower cholesterol levels, but also to eliminate the cancer susceptibility syndrome (see Chapter 17). Also, it is desirable to study 25-hydroxycholecalciferol (vitamin D_3) or 25-hydroxycholesterol, which inhibit cholesterol synthesis in normal and, probably, tumor cells (Philipott et al 1977).

Elimination of metabolic immunodepression is important as a feasible means of prevention of both cancer and some autoimmune disturbances (see Chapter 16). As far as cancer prevention is concerned, remember that if radical methods of cancer therapy are employed, prophylactic measures will always be important because the efficacy of

---

[1]Administration of cholestyramine resulted in a dramatic reduction in cholesterol level and stabilization of the tumor process in three patients with prostatic cancer (Addellman 1972). It should be taken into account that cholestyramine raises cholesterol excretion in the intestine, leading to an increased yield of experimental tumors (Nigro et al 1977).

diagnostic tests is still very limited. For instance, trophoblastic tumors, producing chorionic gonadotropin as a marker, cannot be detected unless 200,000 cells have formed. However, this tumor produces a level of the marker uncharacteristic of other types of tumors.

Stimulation of high density lipoprotein production, for example, by estrogens (Barclay and Skipski 1975) in cases of tumors other than those of the reproductive system, may yield good results. Administration of immunostimulators, eg, levamisole, perhaps will be more effective, if preceded by elimination of metabolic immunodepression.

Finally, there is evidence suggesting more profound studies of preparations, which reduce glucocorticoid production (Dilantin, ACTH anahormones, and pantothenic acid antagonists).

These general objectives of therapy may be summarized as follows: to counteract aging and the acceleration of development; to reduce the incidence of age-specific pathology, by administering drugs capable of restoring the rhythmic function of the main homeostatic systems, and by shifting metabolism toward the predominant utilization of glucose rather than free fatty acids as an energy source.

Table 24-7 shows the range of possible therapeutic effects of some drugs administered for diseases of compensation.

Table 24-7
Range of Possible Therapeutic Effects of Drugs Administered for Diseases of Compensation*

	A	B	C	D	E	F	G	H	I
Phenformin or metformin	+	+	+	±	+	?	±		?
Dilantin or aminoglutethimide	+	+	+	±	+	+	+	+	?
Clofibrate	?	+	±	±	+	±	?	?	?
Estrogens, progestins, sigetin	±	+	+	±	±	±	+	?+	?
Triiodothyronine	+	?	+	±	?+	±	+	+	?
Restricted food intake	+	+	+	+	+	+	+	+	+
Insulin	−	−	−	−	±	−	?	−	?−

*Diseases are as follows:
A Obesity
B Maturity-onset diabetes mellitus
C Atherosclerosis
D Cancer
E Metabolic immunodepression
F Essential hypertension
G Climacteric
H Aging
I Autoimmune disorders

Symbols are as follows:
+ beneficial effect
− pernicious effect
? data not available

25 Conclusion: A Model of the Elevational Mechanism of Human Development, Aging, and Age-Specific Pathology

It is easy to see that all diseases of aging are so much alike that we should suggest the existence of one major disease with ten symptoms rather than ten main diseases of aging.

Before we proceed further, let us reconsider the situation of a patient suffering from endometrial carcinoma (see Table 1-1). This typical case reveals ten diseases at the same time.[1] On the basis of the different data in this book, it is now possible to try to disclose an integral mechanism responsible for formation of a specific group of diseases which claim 85 out of every 100 deaths. If we take into account that the incidence rates of these diseases increase with advancing age, the hypothesis of the existence of a definite correlation between aging and the formation of a specific group of diseases of aging provides a basis for

[1] It should be recalled that the physicians diagnosed ten diseases in this patient. Therefore, the main aim of this book was to demonstrate the mechanism of interrelationship between these diseases, the mechanism that caused all of them to occur in one patient. But since in my story each specialist is an expert in his field and lacks knowledge in the other fields, it seemed impossible to present any substantial arguments in favor of the integrated approach unless the state-of-the-art pertaining to each of the ten diseases was considered. This has inevitably enlarged this book, but I hope it will enable each specialist to form his own idea of the problem of integrated clinical medicine.

development of measures of prevention of premature age-specific pathology. Finally, once we accept the fact that acceleration of development contributes to that of aging, and that acceleration of aging of the maternal organism may promote that of infant development, attempts to outline an integral mechanism of development, aging, and age-specific pathology become still more justified and urgent. Initially, however, it is necessary to discuss some factors related to the mechanism of organism development and then to consider the manner in which this mechanism causes such manifestations of age-specific pathology as obesity, dysadaptosis, prediabetes and maturity-onset diabetes, premyxedema, atherosclerosis, hypertension, mental depression, metabolic immunodepression, autoimmune disturbances, climacteric, and cancer.

In order for an organism to survive it must experience only a very narrow range of variation in the parameters of its internal environment. The range of these variations is restricted, particularly in unicellular organisms, but death here is caused mainly, if not always, by external environmental factors. The process of cell division appears not to be limited by any internal causes, and immortality seems at least theoretically possible.

Highly specialized organisms, on the other hand, have become more independent of environmental factors by developing systems to maintain a stable internal environment. It appears, however, that these same stabilizing systems, the homeostats, have a mechanism that leads inevitably to an instability of the internal environment, and eventually to death caused by this internal instability. An organism cannot develop from a zygote to a specialized multitissue system unless the vigor of its main homeostatic systems is also increased. The stabilizing system must keep pace with the rest of the organism in order to cope with the constantly increasing demands placed on it by the growing organism. Although homeostatic systems in complex growing organisms operate as cybernetic systems, maintaining permanent, fixed parameters, the main three homeostatic systems undergo constant changes in order to keep pace with the growth of the organism.

Following completion of the organism's growth, however, these homeostatic systems do not become stabilized along with the rest of the organism. Instead, they continue to grow and influence the parameters of internal environment. Eventually they cause the death of the organism because their continual shift provides in the end for an internal environment incompatible with life. So the internal causes of natural death are determined not by a decline in homeostatic function, but by the relentless intensification of these functions. Hence, it is precisely the formation of systems to ensure relative freedom from external environmental factors that has given rise to the phenomenon of death from internal causes.

Figuratively speaking, in choosing between the internal and external causes of death in the course of complex homeostatic system development, evolution has provided that higher organisms should have an opportunity to complete the species-specific life span, to suffer from diseases, and to die in old age rather than risk death at any moment as an individual free from programmed diseases, solely because of factors of the external environment. The concept of an elevating mechanism of development, aging, and death may be tested further by the consideration of concrete data on which the proposed model is based.

There are three functions indispensable for a living organism: energy metabolism, adaptation to changes in the internal and external environment, and reproduction. Accordingly, there are three main homeostatic systems: energy, adaptive, and reproductive homeostats. Figure 25-1 illustrates interactions between the main homeostats of the body. The interrelations between the reproductive, adaptive, immunologic, and energy homeostats is evident. Stable functioning of these systems is maintained chiefly by negative feedback mechanisms that connect the periphery of each system with the central level; this is the hypothalamic-pituitary complex in higher organisms.

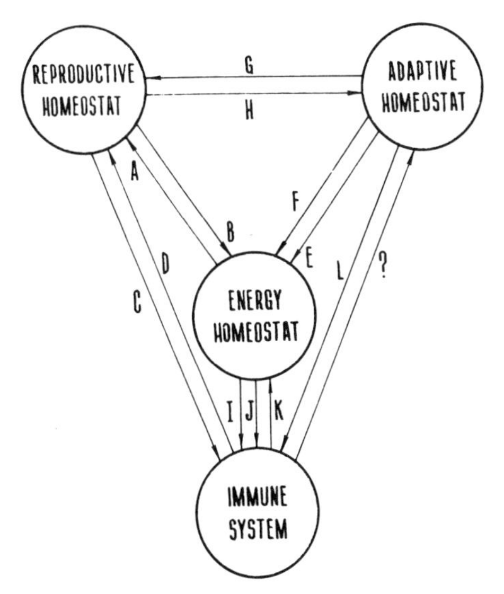

Figure 25-1 Scheme of interaction of the main homeostatic systems in ontogenesis. A: Switching-on of reproductive function upon reaching "critical body weight"; B: Estrogen-induced increases of growth hormone levels; C: Inhibition of cellular immunity by estrogens; D: Thymic control mechanism in ovarian development (Pierpaoli and Besedowsky 1975); E: Cortisol-induced decrease in glucose tolerance; F: Stress-induced intensification of lipolysis; G: Inhibition of reproductive function by stress; H: Compensatory hypertrophy of adrenal cortex in postmenopausal women; I: Metabolic immunodepression; J: Antagonistic effect of brown adipose tissue on cellular immunity (Jankovic et al 1975); K: FFA-induced lysis of lymphocytes; L: Suppression of immune system by stress.

In order for the organism to grow, the activities of the main homeostatic systems must be increased. Yet this, increase of activity in a negative feedback system may not be ensured unless the resistance of the hypothalamic-pituitary complex or the sensitivity threshold of the hypothalamus to homeostatic suppression is also elevated. Indeed, in the adaptive and reproductive homeostats the hypothalamic set point of sensitivity is elevated with aging (see Chapters 3 and 4). The age-connected changes in the energy homeostat are characterized by the elevation of the hypothalamic threshold of sensitivity to the suppressive action of glucose (see Chapters 5 and 6) and the decrease to inhibitory action of free fatty acids (see Chapter 6). In the final analysis, because of the interrelationship between the main homeostatic systems in postnatal ontogenesis, it is possible to distinguish four stages in this process. Here, we shall limit our discussion to the consideration of certain energy aspects of this problem (see Chapters 8 and 9).

There are data that show that the blood fatty acid level is much higher in immature children than after the switching-on of the reproductive cycle (Heald et al 1967); accordingly, glucose utilization is decreased. Such a metabolic pattern has much in common with that of aging, as we can see when we consider the role of hypercholesterolemia in growth processes in light of the elevational model of development. According to this model, enhanced cholesterol synthesis is brought about by a shift toward predominant utilization of free fatty acids. It is likely that this, in turn, is caused in children by an increased secretion of growth hormone and relative hyperproduction of glucocorticoids (with reference to body surface area, see Okuno 1972). Therefore, considering the metabolic features it has in common with prediabetes, which occurs in normal aging, this stage of intensive growth may be considered a stage of pre-prediabetes (see Chapter 8). On the other hand, age-associated switching-on of reproductive function is accompanied by a decrease in fatty acid and cholesterol levels, and a trend toward "ideal" body weight. This is typical of the transition stage from pre-prediabetes to stabilization. Chapter 8 contains some evidence supporting the view that the stage of metabolic stabilization is influenced by estrogens that counteract the lipolytic effect of growth hormone and thus create optimal conditions for reproduction.

However, elevation of the hypothalamic threshold in the reproductive homeostat leads further to switching-off of the reproductive cycle. The period of stabilization ends with a decrease in classic estrogens output and, as a result, changes appear in the energy and adaptive homeostats, which manifest metabolic features characteristic of prediabetes. At this time the process of formation of diseases of aging becomes particularly active. If these diseases do not terminate in death, however, the advancement of pathologic processes in such individuals appears to be delayed because of involutional changes that develop in the system responsible for formation of the diseases of compensation. For example, this phenomenon may result in a decrease in blood cholesterol after age 70, thus increasing the likelihood of a longer-than-average life span.

Owing to age-associated deviation of the hypothalamic threshold, and the normal interaction of the main homeostatic systems, metabolic development in normal ontogenesis passes through the following four stages: pre-prediabetes or growth; stabilization; prediabetes or age-specific pathology; and involution or senescence. The respective lengths of these periods are genetically predetermined. The stabilization phase is lacking in males, since the male reproductive homeostat functions continually, rather than cyclically. This results in an earlier onset of prediabetes in the male organism and therefore a lower life expectancy because of the subsequent earlier onset of atherosclerosis (see Chapter 9). Many regularities associated with assuring energy supply of postnatal ontogenesis may be established with the aid of studies of ontogenesis in the prenatal period. Of particular interest in this connection is a comparison of the mechanisms responsible for energy supply during pregnancy and the postnatal period.

Pregnancy features a metabolic shift toward the increased utilization of free fatty acids and, therefore, an increased production of cholesterol. The latter is indispensable for an intense "synthesis of cells" in the fetal organism. During pregnancy, however, chorionic somatomammotropin becomes the main insulin antagonistic factor, rather than growth hormone. In conjunction with some other factors, chorionic somatomammotropin reduces tolerance to carbohydrates and, therefore, increases free fatty acid utilization. Such a metabolic shift causes cholesterol synthesis in the maternal organism to increase according to the mechanism discussed in Chapters 6 and 15. If certain age-associated disturbances occur in the maternal organism during pregnancy, a higher-than-normal level of hyperglycemia stimulates excessive secretion of insulin in the fetus. As a consequence, the quantity of adipose tissue increases and excessive fat is accumulated in these cells. The development of a large baby (4 kg and heavier on delivery) indicates hyperinsulinemia in the fetus. This indicates an increased likelihood of not only diabetes mellitus in the maternal organism, but tumor processes as well (see Table 17-4). According to some observations, the age at which reproductive function is switched on is determined by the stage at which a critical level of body weight is reached, rather than chronologically (Frisch and Revelle 1970), and an infant with an excess of fat reaches that critical body weight at an earlier age. This excess of fat mass remains a factor in a further intensified accumulation of fat in the subsequent development of the organism, and leads to an earlier onset of age-specific pathology in the male organism (see Chapter 9).

Considering the changes in ontogenesis, it is possible to summarize certain data concerning the limits of age-related norms. The traditional assertion, deep-rooted in present-day gerontology, that each age has its own norms, ie, is characterized by specific limits of normal age-associated shifts, is misleading (see Chapter 10). Instead of establishing successive norms as age advances, the individual's hormonal-metabolic status should be assessed at the age of 20 to 25 years, and should remain the basis for determining further deviations of physiologic parameters in subsequent ontogenesis. The norm recedes inevitably with advancing age in conformity with the elevating mechanism of the genetic program of development. In this context, the clinical conclusion that a state of health exists even when the hormonal-metabolic pattern has deviated from the pattern of the stabilization stage is a dangerous myth. It follows from the concept of a stable norm that the pattern observed in each individual at the stage of stabilization of normal ontogenesis should be established as the criterion of the norm. The state of the norm inevitably is lost in the course of normal aging; accordingly, aging should be considered a disease or a confluence of diseases of compensation (see Chapter 18).

At this stage, having summarized the data related to the role played by the Law of Deviation of Homeostasis in the implementation of organism development (see Chapters 1 through 10), it is possible to consider the relationship between the changes taking place in the course of development and the formation of age-specific pathology. The following analysis is based mainly on the data pertinent to the age-associated disturbances in energy homeostat functioning.

The energy homeostat is a system of interrelationships between glucose and fatty acid utilization, and growth hormone and insulin (see Chapter 6). Normally, when food is ingested, glucose provides the main source of energy. Therefore, the secretion of growth hormone, which exerts insulin antagonistic and lipolytic effects, is inhibited by hyperglycemia via the hypothalamic glucoreceptors, creating optimal conditions for the uptake of glucose by muscle tissue. Conversely, in fasting, growth hormone secretion is increased, thus stimulating lipolysis. Free fatty acids become the main source of energy. Glucose uptake by muscle tissue is suppressed, and glucose is thus saved for uptake by the nervous tissue. Hence, there are two alternative modes of energy supply, a predominant utilization of glucose or a predominant utilization of fatty acids. The latter shift is a typical feature of aging. Hence, although different chapters of the present book cite different data on the pathogenesis of the main diseases of aging, this pathogenesis may be regarded as the confluence of interrelated events caused by disturbances in the energy homeostat.

Prediabetes

Aging inevitably involves a decrease in glucose utilization (see Chapter 6). This is accompanied by a rise in the level of reactive insulinemia. These data make it likely that aging entails a decline in the sensitivity of muscle tissue to insulin action, as suggested earlier by Himsworth and Kerr (1939). My approach to the problem is that age-associated insulin resistance is caused by such factors as inadequate decrease in blood growth hormone level in response to postprandial hyperglycemia (see Chapter 6), disturbances in the sensitivity of adaptive homeostat functioning (see Chapter 3), and the hypothalamic disregulation of appetite (see Chapter 5), which in conjunction with these factors brings about an increased utilization of FFA.

If we proceed from the postulate of age-associated changes in hypothalamic sensitivity threshold, the entire system of age-associated shifts may be given the following interpretation as a physiologically inevitable sequence of interrelated events.

The inadequate suppression of growth hormone secretion by glucose is conducive to relative hypersomatotropism, which leads to the simultaneous functioning of the two antagonistic mechanisms, nonutilization of glucose and utilization of fatty acids. Under these circumstances, the sequence of hormonal-metabolic changes responsible for disturbances in the energy homeostat are as follows (Figure 25-2, cycle I).

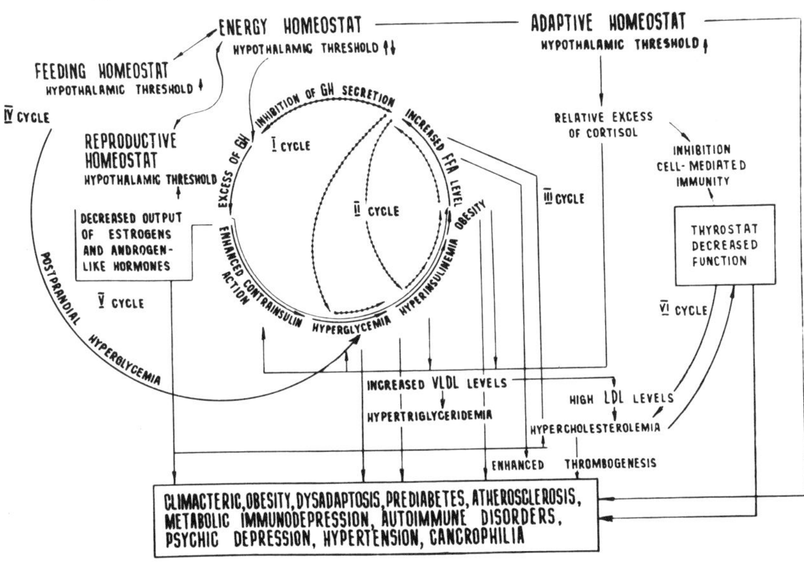

Figure 25-2 Integral scheme of the hypothalamic mechanism of development, aging, and age-specific pathology formation.

Excessive growth hormone exerts an insulin antagonistic effect, partially caused by the diminished sensitivity of muscle tissue to insulin action. This results in hyperinsulinemia, which normally exerts a compensatory effect intended to counteract the insulin antagonistic action of growth hormone. However, as seen from the findings on the age-associated rise in postprandial hyperglycemia, compensatory hyperinsulinemia does not prevent a decrease in glucose utilization. This results in the age-associated decline in glucose tolerance, ie, a state that reveals the features of prediabetes, chemical diabetes, or maturity-onset diabetes mellitus, depending on the degree (see Chapter 11).

Obesity

Excess glucose unutilized by muscle tissue is taken up by the adipose tissue for triglyceride synthesis. Consequently, body weight, or to be more precise, body fat content, increases with aging (Dudl and Ensinck 1977). This leads to the formation of age-associated metabolic obesity stemming from prediabetes typical of normal aging (see Chapter 6). This process is accompanied by the development of regulatory obesity caused by disturbances in the function of hypothalamic systems that regulate appetite and body fat level (see Chapter 5). It should be pointed out in this connection that food intake is regulated chiefly through the mediation of glucose which binds to the glucoreceptors of the hypothalamic center of satiety. It was suggested that postprandial hyperglycemia and hyperinsulinemia activate the satiety center, the latter inhibiting the feeding center (Mayer 1965). I suggested earlier (before these two hypothalamic centers of food intake regulation were distinguished) that the increased food intake concomitant with advancing age is caused by the elevation of the sensitivity threshold in the system of hypothalamic regulation of appetite, because postprandial hyperglycemia increases with aging, while food intake does not decrease (Dilman 1958). On the basis of present knowledge it is possible to relate the elevation of the sensitivity threshold of the satiety center to the age-associated decline in the levels of noradrenaline (Saller and Stricker 1976) and serotonin (Breisch et al 1976) in the hypothalamus. Finally, increased food intake leads to the accumulation of fat, which brings about the whole complex of the hormonal-metabolic disturbances inherent in aging.

According to the hypothesis of Woods and Porte (1978), there is a hypothalamic control mechanism, which regulates body fat content via the basal level of insulin in cerebrospinal fluid. Since this mechanism fails to maintain optimal fat content during aging, it may be suggested that the sensitivity threshold to insulin action is elevated in this hypothalamic system. It may also be supposed that the elevation of threshold sensitivity in turn is caused by diminution of the concentration of insulin receptors produced by the age-related rise in blood insulin levels. Bearing this in mind, it may be suggested that obesity itself creates a mechanism that maintains obesity, with hyperinsulinemia as a key factor that causes and maintains obesity at the same time. Moreover, hyperinsulinemia is directly responsible for the enhancement of triglyceride synthesis in the liver (Bagdade et al 1971), thus leading to age-associated hypertriglyceridemia. As fat cells grow in size because of fat accumulation, the sensitivity of these cells to lipolytic factors increases (Jacobsson et al 1976), thus stimulating lipolysis. But, simultaneously, hyperinsulinemia exerts an antilipolytic effect. Consequently, the initial stages of age-associated metabolic disturbances are not accompanied by a marked increase in blood free fatty acids. However, since less glucose is taken up by muscle tissue, because of an intensified insulin antagonistic action, it may be that the deficient supply of energy from glucose stores is compensated for by an increased utilization of fatty acids, characterized by the high rates of metabolic turnover. In this manner metabolic shifts intrinsic to normal aging, decreased glucose tolerance, obesity, and intensified utilization of free fatty acids, take place as a result of the formation of the central type of homeostatic failure.

Dysadaptosis[1]

As a consequence of the above metabolic disturbances, FFA become the main source of energy supply. This factor causes important changes in the basic mechanism of the age-associated alterations in the energy homeostat. The rise in blood FFA level suppresses the secretion of growth hormone (see Chapter 6), thus eliminating one of the primary disturbances which are responsible for the age-related shift of metabolism. However, the inhibition of growth hormone secretion does not lead at this stage to normalization of metabolism, because hyperlipidemia triggers cycles of metabolic disturbances that form the following lipid shunt (see Figure 25-2, cycle II): an increased utilization of FFA inhibits the glucose uptake by muscle tissue; hyperglycemia stimulates an enhanced secretion of insulin, leading to an intensification of lipogenesis, thus maintaining obesity despite the increased lipolysis; simultaneously, obesity maintains spontaneous lipolysis at a high level; and then all these events recycle. In obese humans the four-component energy homeostat functions essentially as a three-component system, with growth hormone secretion being inhibited. Figuratively speaking, an obese individual may

[1]Here only the network of metabolic disturbances is considered, while the hypothalamic mechanisms of normal diseases are presented in corresponding chapters.

be likened to a decerebrated organism with an intensified fat metabolism. At this stage, obesity plays a key role in the development of the main diseases of aging. Following are some of the consequences of increased body fat mass.

First, since the uptake of FFA by most tissues is proportional to the FFA concentration in blood, the utilization of FFA by muscle tissue, which is the main consumer of this energy-producing substrate, is increased. Finally, FFA lowers glucose uptake and reduces its oxidation by muscle tissue, in keeping with the mechanism of the glucose fatty acid cycle (Randle 1965). This factor reduces glucose tolerance, which falls still more with aging. Thus, obesity and diminished uptake of glucose by muscle tissue stimulate the glucocorticoid function of the adrenal gland, which intensifies gluconeogenesis and produces a compensatory effect as glucose uptake by muscle tissue is decreased. This process triggers cycle III of metabolic disturbances (see Figure 25-2), which are further stimulated by the independent age-associated elevation of the hypothalamic threshold to suppression in the adaptive system. Finally, one of the normal diseases of aging, dysadaptosis, develops.

In addition, FFA is known to activate glucoeogenesis (Weber et al 1966). One of its consequences is the increased lysis of T-dependent lymphocytes, which leads to the development of metabolic immunodepression. Suffice it to say that the intensification of gluconeogenesis caused by the disturbed feedback control of functioning of the adaptive homeostat adds to the changes that occur in the energy homeostat.

Atherosclerosis

Second, the excessive utilization of FFA results in an enhanced synthesis of triglycerides and very low density lipoproteins (VLDL) in the liver. It is likely to involve an intensification of synthesis of cholesterol, which is a component of LDL. Low density lipoproteins are delivered from VLDL in the circulation. As a result, aging is concomitant with a rise in the blood levels of both VLDL and LDL. Therefore, the levels of triglycerides and cholesterol rise, though that of HDL-cholesterol does not (Mjøs et al 1977), contributing to atherosclerosis because the lipids of the atheromatous plaque are derived from the plasma lipoproteins.

Evidence has been presented that each plaque contains a single clone of smooth muscle cells (Benditt and Benditt 1973). Now it is known that certain lipoproteins exert growth-promoting action on the smooth muscle cells (Chen et al 1977a, Bierman and Albers 1975). As to the role of autoimmune disturbances in the pathogenesis of atherosclerosis (Beaumont 1970, Klimov 1973), the enhanced synthesis of triglycerides and cholesterol (or their enhanced transport from the liver) seems to stimulate the synthesis of VLDL (Björntorp et al 1970). Such a hyperstimulation was suggested to cause qualitative changes to take place in the structure of apoproteins, thus giving a clue to the induction of antibodies against endogenous serum lipoproteins (Dilman 1974a, p 137). This hypothesis is in agreement with the results of Sirtori and coworkers (Sirtori et al 1977a, Rodriguez et al 1976). Finally, hyperlipidemia promotes the aggregation of platelets (see Chapter 12). Moreover, in tissue culture the proliferation of arterial smooth muscle cells is stimulated by a factor released by aggregating platelets (Rutherford and Ross 1976). Metabolic immunodepression also can contribute to atherosclerosis (see Chapter 12). In such manner, basic data available on the pathogenesis of atherosclerosis may be accounted for on the basis of the elevational model.

Metabolic Immunodepression

The rise in the blood levels of FFA, cholesterol, and probably insulin inhibits cell-mediated immunity, ie, it forms a phenomenon designated by me as metabolic immunodepression (Dilman 1978a). FFA were found to inhibit the blastogenic reaction of lymphocytes considerably (Mertin and Hunt 1976). FFA suppresses the functional activity of the reticuloendothelial system (Di Lusio and Wooles 1975) and macrophages (Dianzani et al 1976). The high level of FFA has a cytotoxic effect on lymphoid cells (Kigoshi and Ito 1973). FFA are likely to participate in the glucocorticoid-induced lysis of lymphocytes (Turnell et al 1973). It was shown by our staff that intravenous injection of fat emulsion-intralipid inhibits the blastogenic reaction of lymphocytes.

Concerning hypercholesterolemia, it should be stressed that the saturation of lymphocyte membranes with cholesterol inhibits the reaction of blast transformation (Alderson and Green 1975). Also, there is a direct correlation between blood LDL level and cholesterol content of the plasma membrane of cells (Goldstein and Brown 1975).

Finally, it is likely that the rise in blood insulin level also contributes to the formation of metabolic immunodepression. Hyperinsulinemia is responsible for the decrease in the concentration of insulin receptors on the plasma membrane of lymphocytes and/or monocytes (Gavin et al 1974, Schwartz et al 1975). This may cause disturbances in the transport of glucose to these cells. This factor may, in turn, raise the utilization of FFA and, therefore, have a toxic effect of FFA on lymphocytes. Besides, antigens induce the emergence of insulin receptors on T cells (Helderman and Strom 1977) and, therefore, hyperinsulinemia probably inhibits this process. Also, some data show that hyperinsulinemia inhibits the phagocytic activity of macrophages (Bar et al 1976). Moreover, it should be stressed that the increase in FFA blood levels suppresses growth hormone secretion, whereas hypercholesterolemia lowers the function of the thyroid gland (see Chapter 7). These disturbances can cause a decline in immune activity, because growth hormone and thyroid hormones stimulate the function of the thymus (Pierpaoli et al 1970, Fabris et al 1972).

Autoimmune Disorders

Previously, I suggested that if metabolic immunodepression affects T suppressor cells, disturbances in their function may be accompanied by an increase in the response of B lymphocytes, thus promoting the development of autoimmune disorders (Dilman et al 1977a, Dilman 1978a). A relationship between the metabolic pattern intrinsic to aging and the immune response is suggested by the data indicating that immunization is followed by a rise in blood cortisol (Besedovsky and Sorkin 1977) and LDL and cholesterol levels (Di Perri 1975). It may be supposed that these shifts participate in the formation of an immune response and, in particular, potentiate humoral immunity (see chapter 16). This gives a clue to the data that show that calorie restriction inhibits autoimmune disorder development (Fernandes et al 1978). On the other hand, autoimmune disorders occur frequently in patients with diabetes mellitus, who generally reveal a metabolic pattern typical of metabolic immunodepression (Lender et al 1977). Our findings also show that the elimination of metabolic immunodepression by phenformin treatment results in a decrease in the number of B-lymphocytes. It is known that hyperlipidemia is often concomitant with autoimmune diseases (Beaumont 1970). This phenomenon is likely to be associated with the mechanism of metabolic immunodepression. This suggestion is consistent with the observations on the age-related increase in the incidence of autoimmune diseases (Blumenthal 1967).

Cancer Susceptibility

The shift toward an enhanced utilization of FFA for energy supply lowers the efficiency of cellular immunity (see Chapter 15). There is substantial evidence to suppose that it is the metabolic pattern leading to metabolic immunodepression development that stimulates the division of nonlymphoid somatic cells (Dilman 1978a). I think that such an opposite-directed influence of the same metabolic pattern on somatic nonlymphoid cells, on the one hand, and T-dependent lymphocytes and macrophages, on the other, is responsible for the formation of the syndrome of metabolic cancer susceptibility (Dilman 1978a).

This hypothesis may be supported both by experimental findings and theoretical conclusions. For example, hyperlipidemic serum stimulates the division of smooth muscle cells of the arterial wall (Chen et al 1977a, Bierman and Albers 1975). A similar effect is exhibited by serum from diabetic patients (Ledet 1977). It is well known that cell division is impossible, unless cholesterol supply to cells is assured (Chen et al 1978). It is particularly important that cells do not divide at all if cholesterol accumulation in these cells is inhibited. The key importance of cholesterol in cell division is illustrated by the role played by it as a structural component of the plasma membranes of cells. There are abundant data that demonstrate that cholesterol synthesis is enhanced in nonlymphoid tumors (Howard and Kritchevsky 1969, Hilf et al 1970, Chen et al 1978), and that drugs administered to lower cholesterol levels inhibit the growth of solid tumors (Szepsenwol 1966). Moreover, hyperinsulinemia promotes cell division (Temin 1969), chiefly by exerting its effects on glucose transport and metabolism directly, and by raising the level of somatomedin (Daughaday et al 1976). The data obtained at our laboratory showed that blood somatomedin level increases with advancing age and in some age-connected diseases (obesity, maturity-onset diabetes mellitus, and atherosclerosis), ie, in states characterized by elevated blood levels of insulin and FFA (see Table 6-8). FFA also stimulates cell division, particularly in tumor cells (Spector 1975, Holley et al 1974).

Although most data show that the proliferative pool in different tissues decreases with aging, it cannot be ruled out that metabolic shifts inherent to aging may obviate this limitation at some stage, thus contributing to the age-associated increase in cancer incidence. This point is supported first of all by the evidence demonstrating that an improvement in metabolic pattern achieved by treatment with phenformin, epithalamin or a calorie-restricted diet is followed by a drop in cancer incidence rates (see Chapter 17). It is also likely that the metabolic pattern intrinsic to cancer susceptibility syndrome is favorable for the survival of tumor cells; perhaps it even stimulates their division as is the case with Ehrlich carcinoma (Brennerman et al 1974).

The conclusion can be drawn that until the actual factors responsible for malignant transformation are established and relevant methods of prevention and suppression are identified, the elimination of the hormonal-metabolic pattern that promotes cancer susceptibility should be regarded as an effective means of lowering the cancer rate.

Essential Hypertension

As far as hypertension is concerned, it should be emphasized that patients with essential hypertension frequently reveal obesity, decreased glucose tolerance (Lang 1950), and hyperinsulinemia (Welborn et al 1966). It is also reported that such patients exhibit an elevated level of blood prolactin. Thus, all these data suggest that hypothalamic mechanisms are implicated in the age-associated rise in the frequency of essential hypertension. Therefore, it may be supposed that the rise in arterial blood pressure generally concomitant with aging is related to the elevation of the sensitivity threshold of the hypothalamic centers, which control blood pressure, to homeostatic stimuli.

Psychic Depression

Age-associated rise in the incidence of mental depression may be accounted for as a by-product of the mechanism of implementation of the program of organism development. In actual fact, if the deviation of set point of the hypothalamic sensitivity threshold to feedback control in the main homeostatic systems is caused by the decline in the levels of biogenic amines (see Chapter 18), the same phenomenon should pave the way to mental depression by lowering the level of biogenic amines in the brain. Consequently, an elevation of the hypothalamic threshold of sensitivity to suppression by dexamethasone both in mentally depressed patients and normal aging subjects (see Chapter 14) is a manifestation of these relationships.

Premyxedema

The age-associated decline in thyroid function seems to be due to a group of factors, including an enhanced body fat content. It is possible that the relationship between adiposity and thyroid function is mediated by the rise in blood LDL levels, since β-lipoproteins and cholesterol inhibit ^{131}I uptake by the thyroid (see Chapter 7). The changes in the threshold of thyrostat sensitivity caused by the age-connected dynamics of the biogenic amine level of CNS also may make a certain contribution to the alterations that occur with advancing age in thyroid function.

Climacteric

The elevation of the sensitivity threshold in the reproductive homeostat brings about the age-associated switching-off of reproductive function in women (see Chapter 4). Some of the consequences of this process may make their contributions to age pathology. For example, the level of gonadotropin secretion increases severalfold in women with a normal menstrual cycle between 25 and 45 years of age. Therefore, ovaries become subjected to constant hyperstimulation with advancing age. Meanwhile, such hyperstimulation is known to provide a carcinogenic factor (see Chapter 17). Since the androgens produced by postmenopausal ovaries are biotransformed to estrogens in adipose tissue, a factor like obesity in the climacteric period promotes the development of endometrial carcinoma and breast cancer. On the other hand, decreased output of classic estrogens contributes to the development of atherosclerosis and osteoporosis, at the same time.

Therefore, changes in the hypothalamic sensitivity threshold to homeostatic regulatory stimuli in the energy, adaptive, reproductive, and thyroid homeostats may trigger a string of such hormonal-metabolic shifts typical of age-specific pathology as obesity, maturity-onset diabetes mellitus, premyxedema, atherosclerosis, metabolic immunodepression, autoimmune disorders, mental depression, essential hypertension, climacteric, and cancer susceptibility. Since this hypothalamic phenomenon is an indispensable component of the program of organism development, it would be wrong to suggest the existence of a special program of diseases of aging and natural death. We should rather speak of the transformation of the program of development to the mechanism of age-specific pathology. Moreover, relationships between the changes that ensure the implementation of the program of body development and those inherent in the diseases of aging are incompatible with the view that the latter are caused primarily by external environmental factors or accidental breakdowns at different levels of the system. The latent period of nearly all main diseases should be sought in the course of normal aging; provided the organism develops precisely as it was programmed, these diseases should inevitably occur. If we stick to such reasoning, it is easy to explain why the specific diseases of aging occur in one patient as a single syndrome, as is the case with 50% to 70% of endometrial carcinoma patients (Dilman 1974a). However, if the key components of these diseases are compared (Table 25-1), it becomes apparent that the hormonal-metabolic patterns of the main diseases of aging are identical. This points to common pathogenetic features of special diseases of aging, thus validating an approach that considers all of them to be different manifestations of a single superdisease that inevitably develops according to the Law of Deviation of Homeostasis (see Chapters 11 through 18).

We have designated these certain age-specific diseases, by virtue of the mechanism of their formation, as diseases of compensation, or normal diseases. All these diseases show uniform mechanisms based on the cardinal elements: a shift of set point of the hypothalamic threshold of sensitivity to feedback control; a compensatory increase of peripheral en-

Table 25-1
Comparison of Hormonal-Metabolic Patterns of Pregnancy, Acceleration of Development, Aging, Stress, Cancer, and Atherosclerosis

	Physiologic and Pathophysiologic Disorders*							
	A	*B*	*C*	*D*	*E*	*F*	*G*	*H*
Relative excess or lack of GH suppression after glucose load	+[†]	+	+	+[‡]	+	+[‡]	+[‡]	+[‡]
Insulin resistance	+	+	+	+	+	+	+	+
Hyperinsulinemia	+	+[ǂ]	+	+	−[§]	+	+[ǂ]	
Decreased glucose tolerance	+	+	+	+	+	+	+	+
Excess body weight	+	+	+	+	−	+	+	+
Relative increase of glucocorticoids	+	+	+	+	+	+	+	+
Suppression of cell-mediated immunity	+	+	+	+	+	+	±[//]	+
Predominant utilization of FFA as energy source	+	+	+	+	+	+	+	+
Decreased thyroid activity	−	−	−	±	±	+[¶]	±[#]	+
Shift in spectrum of secreted hormones, ectopic production of hormones	+[⨍]	? +	? +	+	+[∮]	+	+[∯]	+[⨍⊕]
Output of anabolic steroids, classic estrogens, and androgens	+	+	+	−	−	+	+	−

*A Pregnancy
B Acceleration of development
C Growth and development (latent diabetes)
D Aging (prediabetes)
E Stress
F Maturity-onset diabetes mellitus
G Atherosclerosis
H Cancer (cancer susceptibility)

†High level of output of growth hormone analog, somatomammotropin, in pregnancy.

‡Suppression of growth hormone secretion in obesity; however, metabolic disturbances recycle on their own.

ǂBirth of large babies.

§As far as stress is concerned, hyperadrenalinemia-induced suppression of insulin secretion assures an overintensified lipolysis.

//Breakdown of natural tolerance to lipoproteins.

¶Decrease as a result of autoantibody accumulation (Blumenthal 1967).

#Frequent premyxedema.

⨍Increased level of nonclassic phenolsteroids and predominance of estriol. Production of embryonal antigens in pregnancy; production of carcinoembryonal antigens in cancer.

∮Shift in the spectrum of secreted hormones (Wexler and Kittinger 1965).

∯Hyperlipidemia-induced shift in the spectrum of secreted lipoproteins may occur (see Chapter 12).

⊕Ectopic production of hormones, including ACTH and chorionic gonadotropin. Presence of tumor-specific antigens (Hollinshead et al 1972).

docrine gland function (pituitary included); and a rise in the blood levels of the energy-producing substrates, glucose, and free fatty acids.

On the other hand, external environmental factors, which can influence the internal factors of the pathogenesis of this superdisease, inhibit or accelerate the formation of natural diseases (see Chapter 19 through 22). The chief villain here is stress. According to the proposed elevational model of aging and age-specific pathology, these external factors accelerate the aging process by switching on the adaptational mechanism that counteracts the influence of external factors by further raising the hypothalamic set point. The changes in metabolism brought about by this phenomenon, though indispensable for defense, also upset the stability of its internal environment, thus providing causes for the formation of diseases both of adaptation and of compensation. It should be emphasized that, in situations of stress, energy is provided chiefly by free fatty acid utilization, ie, in the mode characteristic of aging and diseases of compensation. It should be noted also that the primary stimulator of lipolysis in stress is the adrenaline-induced inhibition of insulin secretion. This reduces antilipolytic action, promotes adaptational mechanisms and, as a result of increased lipolysis, is conducive to considerable pathologic shifts. For instance, thrombogenesis is stimulated by high levels of fatty acids, and thrombosis may enhance the development of cancer metastases. Thus, stress intensifies metabolic shifts as well as age-associated metabolic disturbances intrinsic to diseases of compensation.

Populational stress also activates the adaptive homeostat, thus leading to inhibition of reproductive function and to a higher mortality from infectious diseases (Christian 1968, 1976). Intensification of the elevating mechanism also may take place under other conditions (see Chapter 19). The pathogenicity of overfeeding, often determined by social factors which govern feeding behavior, should be mentioned here. Exposure to intense artificial and natural light inhibits pineal gland activity and, as a result, the functions of systems governed by stimulating releasing hormones are increased. Again, these effects are produced through an intensification of the elevating mechanism (Hoffman 1973).

Many carcinogens also are capable of raising the hypothalamic threshold and causing a shift in fat-carbohydrate metabolism toward a decreased utilization of glucose with unfavorable consquences (see Chapter 20). It should be mentioned that the mean age of menopause is 47.4 years in smokers and 49.4 in nonsmokers (Daniele 1978). There is a consistent inverse correlation between cigarette smoking and blood HDL level (Garrison et al 1978). Still, all the external environmental factors that promote age-specific pathology serve to increase the likelihood that the mechanism of acceleration is switched on. These factors include stress, obesity, exposure to intense lighting, and pregnancy at an advanced age. Even pregnancy involves certain changes that may be justifiably referred to as a syndrome of the "normal disease of the pregnant organism." Excessive development of this disease because of external environmental factors is actually the disease leading to acceleration of development. Hence, when relevant internal and external environmental factors come into play, the interrelationships of these factors are manifested in a phenomenon of "acceleration of development" (see Chapter 21). Because of its nature, particularly the accumulation and utilization of more-than-normal fat reserves, acceleration of body development is simultaneously the acceleration of formation of diseases of aging.

Among the consequences of an acceleration in the female organism are a prolonged reproductive period, which decelerates the development of atherosclerosis, but increases the rate of cancer incidence in the reproductive system. This accounts for a positive correlation between "late-onset menopause" and frequency of endometrial and breast cancer (McMahon et al 1973), as well as the increased incidence of these tumors within recent decades.

The process of acceleration of development passes through the same stages as diseases of compensation. Consequently, the accelerational power, the number of accelerates in certain populations, and the frequency of premature age-specific pathology increase. Thus, accelerated development should be regarded as the acceleration of aging and age-specific pathology as well, since all of these physiologic and pathologic processes occur by the same mechanism. This similarity becomes almost an identity, however, when the metabolic patterns of the most typical diseases of compensation are compared in greater detail with pregnancy, acceleration of development, and aging (see Table 25-1). This throws some light on all those problems that confront physicians whenever they examine a case exhibiting a complex of diseases caused by internal and certain external factors (see Chapter 1).

Again, it is important to emphasize that free fatty acids are utilized as the predominant source of energy in pregnancy, acceleration of development, and all diseases of aging and stress. On the basis of an analysis of the hormonal-metabolic patterns in all of these seemingly different states, it may be said that we are consumed in a flame of fats (Figure 25-3). As these physiologic and pathologic processes progress, they feed more fatty acids into the furnace, stepping up the rates of aging and age-specific pathology.

Chapter 22 lists 12 distinguishing features of diseases of compensation as regular manifestations of the elevating mechanism of development and aging. A peculiar trait of these normal diseases is that the activation of one element of the elevating mechanism increases the likelihood of triggering other disturbances. To illustrate, hyperinsulinemia and obesity are risk factors in late-onset diabetes mellitus, atherosclerosis, and cancer (see Chapter 18). Moreover, there is a relationship of these factors (primarily hyperinsulinemia) to implementation of the program of normal development, including acceleration of development and age-specific pathology (see Chapter 21). Taking account of the significance of these risk factors in diabetes, atherosclerosis, and cancer provides a basis for the elaboration of methods of the metabolic epidemiology of diseases of aging. It may be inferred from some theoretical conclusions and available experimental findings that enhanced body fat content, high level of glycemia after glucose loading, raised concentration of triglycerides in blood, and giving birth to large babies are risk factors in cancer (see Chapter 17); these changes are the manifestations of different facets of the elevating mechanism of formation of diseases of aging. Accordingly, the antirisk factors of accelerated formation of age pathology also prove to be of the same nature. For instance, the increase in high density lipoprotein levels corresponds to the decrease in the likelihood of development of atherosclerosis, cancer, and probably metabolic immunodepression (Barclay and Skipski 1975; see Chapter 15), and is one of the main characteristics of the syndrome of longevity (Glueck et al 1977).

Figure 25-4 attempts to integrate the main physiologic processes included in the elevating mechanism from conception to death. These take place in the course of implementation of the genetic program of development of the organism, exposed to innumerable adverse influences of the external environment, in a single scheme of the interrelationships of

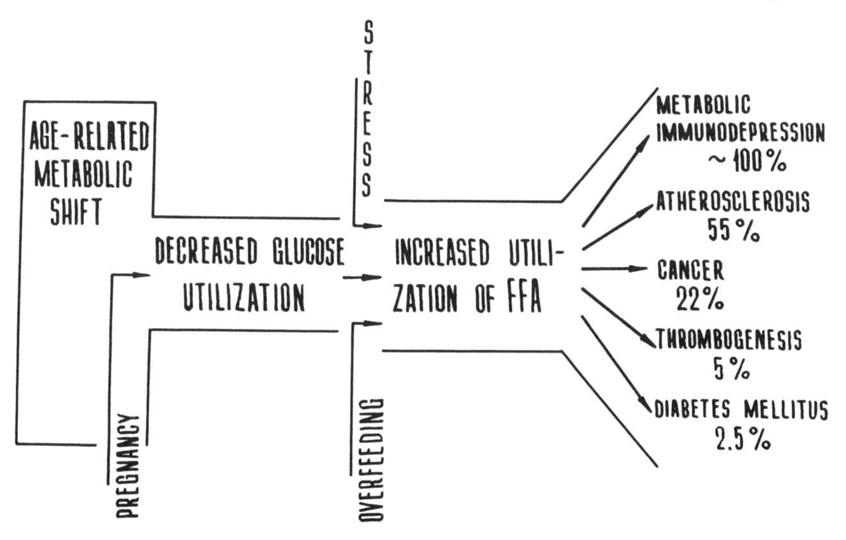

Figure 25-3 Excessive utilization of fats and age-specific pathology.

causes and consequences. The elevating mechanism includes: 1) the metabolic pattern of pregnancy, 2) acceleration of development, 3) the metabolic pattern involved in growth and development of the organism in the postnatal period (pre-prediabetes), 4) age-associated switching-on of reproductive function, 5) the phase of stabilization, 6) age-associated switching-off of reproductive function, 7) prediabetes and intensification of age-specific pathology and diseases of compensation, 8) climacteric, 9) obesity, 10) dysadaptosis, 11) maturity-onset diabetes mellitus, 12) essential hypertension, 13) atherosclerosis, 14) metabolic immunodepression, 15) autoimmune normal disorders, 16) mental depression, 17) cancer susceptibility, 18) the phase of involution at which age-specific pathology is decelerated; processes which promote development, aging, and age-specific pathology, and are modified by external environmental factors, including: 19) acute stress, 20) chronic (populational) stress, 21) overfeeding, 22) exposure to excessive lighting, 23) the influence of ionizing irradiation, 24) the influence of some carcinogens, 25) interaction of diseases of compensation, including such processes as tumor-induced stimulation of secondary cancer susceptibility, 26) accumulation of accelerational power resulting in increased frequency of secondary accelerates in a population characterized by 27) premature age-specific pathology, leading to 28) natural death at the 30) cellular level and 31) tissue level. Finally, 29) the rate of progression of the elevating

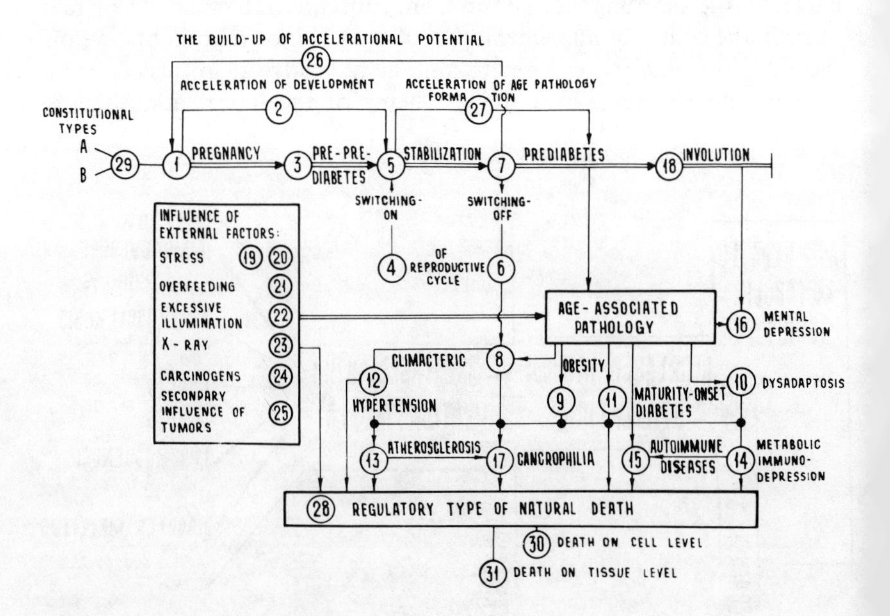

Figure 25-4 Integral diagram of the action of the Law of Deviation of Homeostasis. See text for explanation.

mechanism of development, aging, and death in time is shown to be correlated with certain properties inherent in different constitutional types of man.

It would be superfluous to analyze each of the 31 elements of the elevating mechanism and its relationships with external environmental factors, since this has already been presented in the relevant chapters of this book and, partially, in this conclusion. I think it is necessary to dwell only on three items of this diagram.

Item 29 This may be interpreted in terms of two constitutional types, A and B. Atherosclerosis-prone type A is characterized by a high blood cortisol level (Friedman et al 1972b). A relationship between the constitutional type and individual "choice" of the main disease from the group of diseases of compensation may be assumed to exist.

Item 30 According to Hayflick (1976), aging may be regarded as a specific case of morphogenesis: cells may be simply programmed to run out the program. Some authors believe that the Hayflick phenomenon sets limits on the life span of every species, and may be responsible for the age-associated exhaustion of immunologic defense mechanisms (Burnet 1970). It may also account for the cell-mediated implementation of the program of death. It is not yet clear which factors influence the rate at which Hayflick's limit is reached. If, for example, the conditions imposed by the limit of Hayflick are considered as one of the possible mechanisms of aging, the rate of exhaustion of the genetic limit of cell division, eg, in fibroblasts, may be controlled by such factors as the blood levels of LDL-cholesterol (Brown et al 1975) and insulin (Morell and Froesch 1973), or somatomedin (Temin 1969).

Item 31 The relation of the processes of aging on the tissue level to the elevating mechanism has not yet been established reliably. The cross-linking of collagen may serve as an example. Under experimental conditions, the rate of this process is in distinct correlation with calendar age (Verzár 1953), and is frequently regarded as an indication of aging on the tissue level. However, reduced food intake and hypophysectomy retard the cross-linking of collagen, too (Delbridge and Everitt 1972, Everitt 1973). This indicates that the so-called local or tissue phenomena of aging actually may be controlled by regulation of the elevating mechanism. This also applies to the age-dependent control of enzyme adaptation (Adelman 1976).

Finally, Part IV of this book deals with the problems chiefly related to therapeutic and prophylactic measures aimed at retarding the rate of progression of diseases of aging. The choice of such measures is determined to a considerable extent by current concepts of the mechanism of aging (see Chapter 23) and key mechanisms of diseases of compensation. It should be recalled that Chapter 18 lists the following factors that provide for an age-associated deviation of the hypothalamic threshold:

reduced levels of neurotransmitters (catecholamines and serotonin in particular) in the hypothalamus; reduced quantity of hypothalamic receptors of hormones, which may be caused partially by the drop in biogenic amine concentration; decline in the secretion of pineal gland hormones, primarily pineal polypeptide hormones; accumulation of fat mass in the organism; and reduced utilization of glucose, which according to Laborit (1965) determines the efficiency of the so-called potassium pump.

The above data suggest the conclusion that the program of development, aging, and age-specific pathology is open to therapeutic intervention. Proceeding from the concept of the elevating mechanism of implementation of this program, it is possible to suggest measures aimed at improvement of the hypothalamic threshold of sensitivity to feedback control; reduction of hypothalamic-pituitary activity; inhibition of the compensatory and intensified function of peripheral endocrine glands including the pituitary; inhibition of compensation-induced metabolic changes, particularly the increased utilization of free fatty acids; counteraction of untoward effects of excessive hormones on the target tissues; and substitution therapy (see Chapter 24).

In other words, age-specific pathology should be forestalled chiefly by inhibiting the activity of the main homeostatic systems and, to be more precise, by causing them to resume their normal rhythm rather than simply by stimulating them. Chapter 24 deals with the following examples of therapeutic intervention: pineal polypeptide extracts, phenformin, Dilantin, L-dopa, and L-tryptophan, as well as other neurotropic preparations that can normalize the hypothalamic threshold of sensitivity to homeostatic stimuli, particularly various hormones and anahormones, although theoretically, therapeutic measures need not be confined to the use of drugs. Since the elevating program of diseases of compensation may ultimately determine life span limits, it is possible that therapeutic intervention in these diseases might prolong the life span of human beings. The functional nature of diseases of compensation offers unprecedented possibilities for the control of development, aging, and age-specific pathology. Thus, this book points to a regulatory origin as the principal cause of death in humans today. Further studies may disclose, however, that the so-called mechanism of regulatory death is actually a more complex phenomenon involving interaction of regulatory mechanisms. It is probable that the mechanism of the regulatory type of diseases of aging and natural death is merely a superstructure of some ancient mechanism of properties and manifestations of diseases, which we have not yet discovered, since the regulatory type of death ends the existence of an individual organism before this ancient mechanism has time to become manifest. Not until control over the regulatory mechanism of natural death is achieved, will it be possible to learn what contribution to natural death in higher organisms is made by some primordial mechanism operating on cellular and tissue levels. But the importance of the control over the regulatory mechanism of development, aging, and age pathology formation is also determined by other factors. Actually this is a multipurpose control. For example, it is intended to curb acceleration of development. As far as aging is concerned, three objectives have to be achieved at the same time: a) to prevent premature formation of age pathology, b) to ensure the completion of the specific life span in each individual, and c) to extend the specific life span of humans. The general problem will not be solved unless fundamental cellular mechanisms of aging are controlled, because the formation of specific diseases of aging is determined primarily by regulatory processes.

Thus, the identity of the mechanisms of development and aging and those of diseases of compensation, stress, pregnancy, and acceleration of development as well as processes leading to greater numbers of accelerates in a population; the common factors of risk and antirisk of diseases of compensation; the type of metabolic epidemiology common to all of them; the ability of one disease to promote the development of others or, conversely, the ability of the same therapeutic means to influence several diseases of compensation as well as processes of development and aging—all these point to the limitations of an approach based on the principle of strict specialization and differentiation in medical science.

At the same time, the above shows that application of the approach based on the Law of Deviation of Homeostasis, which covers both internal and external environmental factors responsible for the above phenomena, validates an attempt to outline a mechanism of a more integral nature than is feasible at present.

In conclusion, I have endeavored to show that the main processes of development, aging, and death depend on a single principle: the principle of self-development of homeostatic systems, which depend on a single mechanism, the deviation of activity of these systems or, in other words, on the Law of Deviation of Homeostasis. The model of an elevating mechanism encompasses in a single process the main biologic developments from pregnancy to natural death. In my opinion this is what determines the importance of the proposed model; although many of its details are still missing, and some aspects require greater precision, it provides a basis for establishing deviations from the ideal norm and seeking further means to retard the rate of development of the main diseases of man.

time to become manifest. Not until control over the regulatory mechanism of natural death is achieved, will it be possible to learn what contribution to natural death in higher organisms is made by some primordial mechanism operating on cellular and tissue levels. But the importance of the control over the regulatory mechanism of development, aging, and age pathology formation is also determined by other factors. Actually this is a multipurpose control. For example, it is intended to curb acceleration of development. As far as aging is concerned, three objectives have to be achieved at the same time: a) to prevent premature formation of age pathology, b) to ensure the completion of the specific life span in each individual, and c) to extend the specific life span of humans. The general problem will not be solved unless fundamental cellular mechanisms of aging are controlled, because the formation of specific diseases of aging is determined primarily by regulatory processes.

Thus, the identity of the mechanisms of development and aging and those of diseases of compensation, stress, pregnancy, and acceleration of development as well as processes leading to greater numbers of accelerates in a population; the common factors of risk and antirisk of diseases of compensation; the type of metabolic epidemiology common to all of them; the ability of one disease to promote the development of others or, conversely, the ability of the same therapeutic means to influence several diseases of compensation as well as processes of development and aging—all these point to the limitations of an approach based on the principle of strict specialization and differentiation in medical science.

At the same time, the above shows that application of the approach based on the Law of Deviation of Homeostasis, which covers both internal and external environmental factors responsible for the above phenomena, validates an attempt to outline a mechanism of a more integral nature than is feasible at present.

In conclusion, I have endeavored to show that the main processes of development, aging, and death depend on a single principle: the principle of self-development of homeostatic systems, which depend on a single mechanism, the deviation of activity of these systems or, in other words, on the Law of Deviation of Homeostasis. The model of an elevating mechanism encompasses in a single process the main biologic developments from pregnancy to natural death. In my opinion this is what determines the importance of the proposed model; although many of its details are still missing, and some aspects require greater precision, it provides a basis for establishing deviations from the ideal norm and seeking further means to retard the rate of development of the main diseases of man.

EPILOGUE

> "We shall never have a science of medicine as long as we separate the explanation of the pathological from the explanation of normal vital phenomena" (Bernard, 1865).
>
> "The textural changes which old age induce in the organism sometimes attain such a point that the physiological and pathological states seem to mingle by an imperceptible transition, and to be no longer sharply distinguishable" (Charcot, 1881).
>
> "...man will never die of old age alone but always from disease. However, terminal disease of the future will be different from that we are faced with now and presumably more diversified" (Ludwig, 1980).
>
> "It remains possible that the major reason for the predominance of older individuals in the cancer population is the time lag between the events initiating oncogenesis and the appearance of disease in a clinically recognizable form. However, as of now there is a considerable body of evidence arrayed against this rather simplistic hypothesis" (Good, 1980).

The central thesis of this volume is that the mammalian organism possesses three groups of homeostats—energy, reproductive, and adaptive, and that many of the phenomena considered to represent normal aging, as well as the diseases prevalent in middle and old age, derive from the same genetic program and from the same developmental changes in these homeostats. Thus, the principal difference between biologic aging and the diseases of aging is a quantitative, rather than a qualitative one, and Dilman designates that latter are "normal" diseases of aging. Moreover, Dilman argues persuasively that both biologic aging and these diseases are intrinsic, and that certain environmental factors may produce changes in the same direction and should be regarded as accelerators or intensifiers of aging and the diseases of aging rather than as separate causes.

This concept confronts and challenges the commonly held view regarding the relationship between so-called biologic and pathologic aging, particularly the view that the former is genetically programmed, while the latter derives from environmental factors which act over several decades before their effects become manifest. In the latter, aging is incidental to the long latent period required by a causal environmental agent. This separatist concept enjoys such popularity that some time-honored views have largely been ignored. The first two quotations presented at the beginning of this epilogue exemplify views held by some luminaries about a century ago, while the following two provide evidence that the older concept still enjoys some support. Dilman makes the point that optimal function occurs during the first half of the third decade of life (ages 20 to 25), and that this should be the frame of reference against which deviations should be measured. In this regard, the use of a sliding scale of "norms" adjusted for each decade may be as simplistic as the concept of a time lag of decades between the events initiating a disease and its appearance in clinically recognizable form. One might even regard Dilamn's concept as an old idea whose time is finally coming.

Even so, the detailed, integrated concept which is presented in this book could not possibly have been foreseen, even by men of such great vision and foresight as Bernard and Charcot. To an important degree, the content of this book is a product of modern technology and the revolution in biology which has taken place over the past four decades. Stoker (News Item, 1980), in this second Fraser lecture of the British Postgraduate Medical Federation, has pointed out that this expansion of biological knowledge has been greatest with respect to phenomena at the subcellular and cellular levels, but that similar solutions to the complexities of tissue, organ, and whole animal are still to come. He concludes that the impact of the new biology in the prevention and cure of disease has been minimal, although the potential for such impact is great. On the other hand, this book deals largely with the complexities at the tissue, organ, and whole animal levels and even proposes methods for prevention and cure of disease based on the new biology.

Early in this volume Dilman presents a hypothetical patient examined by a number of specialists each of whom makes a diagnosis relevant to his/her specialty. The result is a number of different diagnoses equal to the number of specialists. This exemplifies what is commonly referred to as the polypathy of aging—the reality that many aged patients concomitantly manifest two or more disease entities. The traditional strategy of clinicians in arriving at a definitive diagnosis is to practice a process of exclusion in order to arrive at a single diagnosis, ie, one disease. However, Stoddard (1980) points out that "as biotechnical data have multiplied, crossover similarities among cases in different disease classes have become troublesomely frequent," and that there is a need to construct new classes of disease which take into account the overlap in abnormalities rather than the differences between disease categories. One might argue that this overlap also derives from the fact that the extension of life expectancy has resulted in an increasing frequency of the various diseases of aging, and that the overlap stems from a common substrate, the various manifestations of aging discussed by Dilman.

Perhaps the most important contribution this book makes is its display and documentation of a new medical model. As Ludwig (1980) points out, medicine's current model is, in principle, ecological. It derives from the era of discovery that identifiable microorganisms or dietary deficiencies cause specific diseases. "Contemporary medicine, [therefore] attempts to cure or prevent damage wrought by the environment. It achieves this by neutralizing pathogens or by compensating for the lack of something the environment normally supplies." The new model regards the diseases of aging to be basically intrinsic in origin, and the strategy for preventing or retarding the onset of these diseases to be that of regarding or modifying biologic aging. Unlike the current model which attempts to deal with selected environmental factors relevant to particular disease entities, the new model regards the modification of biologic aging as potentially capable of affecting a number of diseases of aging concomitantly.

In editing this volume an attempt has been made to retain, to the maximum extent possible, Professor Dilman's style in order to retain the fidelity of the concepts by which he has reached his conclusions. Therefore, the reader may encounter expressions which are at some variance with those common in the American literature. Nevertheless, the text contains a unique amalgamation of Soviet and Western research supporting my contention in the introduction that the author is remarkably well informed regarding ongoing biomedical research in the western hemisphere.

Herman T. Blumenthal, PhD, MD

SELECTED READINGS

Bernard C: *An Introduction to the Study of Experimental Medicine.* Translated by Greene HE, New York, Henry Ackerman Inc, 1949.

Charcot JM: *Clinical Lectures on the Diseases of Old Age.* Translated by Hunt LH, New York, Wood, 1881.

Good RA: Editorial: Cancer and aging. *Hosp Prac* 15:10–15, 1980.

Ludwig FC: Editorial: What to expect from gerontological research. *Science* 209:1071, 1980.

News Item: New medicine and new biology. *Lancet* 2:21–23, 1980.

Stoddard LD: Toward a new human pathology. I. Biopathological populations, or sets: A substitute for the old pathology's diseases. *Hum Path* 11:228–239, 1980.

BIBLIOGRAPHY

Abbo FE: The 17-ketosteroid/17 hydroxycorticosteroid ratio as a useful measure of the physiological age of the human adrenal cortex. *J Gerontol* 21:112–114, 1966.

Acevedo HF, Slifkin M, Pouchet GR, et al: Immunohistochemical localization of a choriogonadotropin-like protein in bacteria isolated from cancer patients. *Cancer* 41:1217–1229, 1978.

Adamopoulos DA, Loraine JA, Dove GA: Endocrinological studies in women approaching the menopause. *Br J Obstet Gynaecol* 78:62–79, 1971.

Addellman W: Cancer, cholesterol, and cholestyramine. *N Engl J Med* 287:1047, 1972.

Adelman RC: An age-dependent modification of enzyme regulation. *J Biol Chem* 245:1032–1035, 1970.

Adelman RC: Age-dependent hormonal regulation of mammalian gene expression, in Everett AV, Burgess JA (eds): *Hypothalamus, Pituitary, and Aging.* Springfield, Ill., Charles C Thomas, 1976, pp 668–675.

Adelman RC: Loss of adaptive mechanisms during aging. *Fed Proc* 38:1968–1971, 1979.

Adlersberg D, Schaefer LE, Steinberg AG, et al: Age, sex, serum lipids, and coronary atherosclerosis. *JAMA* 162:619–622, 1956.

Agid R, Marquie G, Lafontan M: Effects comparatif des sulfamides hypoglycémiants et de biguanides antidiabetiques sur les lèsions vasculaires et les troublees lipidiques entrainés par des règimes athérogénes chez le lapin. *Journées de Diabétologie* Paris: Flammorion et Cie, 1975, pp 259–278.

Ajlouni K, Martinson DA, Hagen ThS: Effect of glucose on the growth hormone response to L-dopa in normal and diabetic subjects. *Diabetes* 24:633–637, 1975.

Albert A: Human urinary gonadotropins. *Recent Prog Horm Res* 12:227–295, 1956.

Albert RE, Vanderlaan M, Burns, FJ, et al: Effect of carcinogens on chicken atherosclerosis. *Cancer Res* 37:2232–2235, 1977.

Albrink MJ, Meigs JW, Granoff MA: Weight gain and serum triglycerides in normal men. *N Engl J Med* 266:484–489, 1962.

Alderson JCE, Green C: Enrichment of lymphocytes with cholesterol and its effect on lymphocyte activation. *FEBS Lett* 52:208–211, 1975.

Alexander P: The functions of the macrophage in malignant disease. *Annu Rev Med* 27:207–224, 1976.

Allison AC: Present concept on mechanism of autoimmunity. *Excerpta Medica* (Series N 414), 49–53, 1977.

Aloia JF, Zanzi I, Cohn SH: Preliminary report: absence of an effect of chronic administration of growth hormone on serum lipids. *Metabolism* 24:795–798, 1975.

Alvarez LC, Dimass CO, Castro A, et al: Growth hormone in malnutrition. *J Clin Endocrinol Metab* 34:400–409, 1972.

Anden NE, Magnusson T: An improved method for the fluorimetric determination of 5-hydroxytryptamine in tissues. *Acta Physiol Scand* 69:87–94, 1967.

Andres R: Aging and diabetes. *Med Clin North Am* 55:835–846, 1971.

Andres R, Tobin JD: Endocrine systems, in Finch CE, Hayflick L (eds): *Handbook of the Biology of Aging.* New York, Van Nostrand Reinhold Company, 1977, pp 357–378.

Anigstein L, Anigstein DM, Rennels EG: Growth inhibition of sarcoma 180 by growth hormone antisera and 5-fluorouracil. *Acta Endocrinol* 42:453–464, 1963.

Anisimov VN: Pharmacological study of adrenergic mechanisms of the ovarian compensatory hypertrophy. *Biull Eksp Biol Med* 79:44–46, 1975.

Anisimov VN, Dilman VM: Carcinogen-induced elevation of threshold of sensitivity of hypothalamus-pituitary system to inhibition by estrogens. *Vopr Onkol* 20:61–66, 1974.

Anisimov VN, Yermoschenkov VS: An increased threshold of sensitivity of the hypothalamic-hypophyseal system to homeostatic action of estrogens in rats with transplantable tumors. *Vopr Onkol* 3:56–60, 1975.

Anisimov VN, Khavinson VH, Morozov VG, et al: Pineal extract-induced decline in sensitivity of hypothalamic-pituitary system to estrogens in old female rats. *Dokl Akad Nauk SSSR* 213:483–485, 1973a.

Anisimov VN, Morozov VG, Khavinson, VH, et al: Comparison of antitumor action of extracts of pineal gland, hypothalamus, melatonin, and sigetin in mice with transplanted breast cancer. *Vopr Onkol* 19:99–101, 1973b.

Anisimov VN, Ostroumova MN, Dilman VM: Age increase in the hypothalamic-hypophyseal threshold to the inhibitory action of estrogens and the effect of pineal extract on this process. *Biull Eksp Biol Med* 77:100–102, 1974.

Anisimov VN, Lvovich EG, Vasiljeva IA, et al: Some hormonal-metabolic disturbances in rats induced by nitrosoamines and 1,2-dimethylhydrazine. Presented at the Second Symposium on Cancerogenic N-nitrosocompounds: Effect, Synthesis, Determination. Tallinn, USSR, 1975, pp 12–14.

Anisimov VN, Pozdeev VK, Dmitrievskaya AU, et al: Age-associated changes of biogenic amines level in the rat brain. *Fiziol Zh SSSR* 63:353–358, 1977.

Anisimov VN, Lvovich EG, Dmitrievskaya AU, et al: 1,2-dimethylhydrazine-induced syndrome of cancrophilia in rats and its treatment with phenformin. Presented at the Third Symposium on Cancerogenic N-nitrosocompounds: Effect, Synthesis, Determination. Tallinn, USSR, 1978, pp. 116–118.

Ansell JB, Beeson MF: A rapid and sensitive procedure for the combined assay of noradrenaline, dopamine and serotonin in a single brain sample. *Anal Biochem* 23:196–206, 1968.

Archer JA, Gordon P, Roth J: Defect in insulin binding to receptors in obese man: amelioration with caloric restriction. *J Clin Invest* 55:166–174, 1975.

Aschheim P: Resultats fournis par la grèffe hètérochrone des ovaries dans l'étude de la regulation hypothalamo-hypophyso-ovarienne de la ratte senile. *Gerontologia* 10:65–75, 1964–65.

Aschheim P: Aging in the hypothalamic-hypophyseal-ovarian axis in the rat, in Everitt AV, Burgess JA (eds): *Hypothalamus, Pituitary, and Aging*. Springfield, Ill., Charles C Thomas, 1976, pp 376–418.

Ash JF, Vogt PK, Singer SJ: Reversion from transformed to normal phenotype by inhibition of protein synthesis in rat kidney cells infected with a temperature-sensitive mutant of Rous sarcoma virus. *Proc Natl Acad Sci USA* 73:3603-3607, 1976.

Astaldi G, Burgio GR, Astaldi A, et al: Growth hormone and lymphocyte activation. *Lancet* 2:709, 1972.

Aubert ML, Gumbach MM, Kaplan SL: Heterologous radioimmunoassay for plasma human prolactin, values in normal subjects, puberty, pregnancy, and pituitary disorders. *Acta Endocrinol* 77:460–476, 1974.

Averbukh ES, Lapin IP: Psychiatric and pharmacologic aspects of some peculiarities of effects of antidepressants in the aged. *Zh Nevropatol Psikhiatr* 2:88–92, 1969.

Axelrod J: The pineal gland: a neurochemical transducer. *Science* 184:1341–1348, 1974.

Azizi F, Gastelli WP, Raben MS, et al: Effect of growth hormone on plasma triglycerides in man. *Proc Soc Exp Biol Med* 143:1187–1190, 1973.

Babichev VN: Characteristics of neurons in the area of the hypothalamus regulating the gonadotropic function of the hypophysis in old female and male rats. *Biull Eksp Biol Med* 75:3–6, 1973.

Bagdade JD, Bierman EL, Porte D: Hyperinsulinism—a metabolic consequence of obesity. *Diabetes* 17(suppl):315, 1968, abst.

Bagdade JD, Bierman EL, Porte D: Influence of obesity on the relationship between insulin and triglyceride levels in endogenous hypertriglyceridemia. *Diabetes* 20:664–672, 1971.

Bagdade JD, Root RK, Bulger RJ: Impaired leukocyte function in patients with poorly controlled diabetes. *Diabetes* 23:9–15, 1974.

Baird JD: Some aspects of carbohydrate metabolism in pregnancy with special reference to the energy metabolism and hormonal status of the infant of the diabetic woman and the diabetogenic effect of pregnancy. *J Endocrinol* 44:139–172, 1969.

Balasse EO, Ooms HA: Role of plasma free fatty acids in the control of insulin secretion in man. *Diabetologia* 9:145–151, 1973.

Balasse EO, Neef MA: Operation of the "glucose fatty acid cycle" during experimental elevations of plasma free fatty acid levels in man. *Eur J Clin Invest* 4:247–252, 1974.

Ball P, Knuppen R, Haupt M, et al: Interaction between estrogens and catecholamines. III. Studies on the methylation of cathechol estrogens, catecholamines and other catechols by the catechol-O-methyltransferase of human liver. *J Clin Endocrinol Metab* 34:736–737, 1972.

Bar RS, Koren H, Roth J: Insulin and macrophage function. *Diabetes* 25:348, 1976, abst.

Baranov VG, Dilman VM: On the so-called climacteric hypertension. *Klin Med* 27:38–45, 1949.

Barclay M, Skipski VP: Lipoproteins in relation to cancer, in Carroll KK (ed): *Progress in Biochemical Pharmacology. Lipids and Tumours.* Basel, S Karger, 1975, pp 76–111.

Barnett JL, Phillips JG: Age-dependent changes in body weight, hematocrit and corticosteroids following sequential castration in rats with a high incidence of spontaneous tumors. *Exp Gerontol* 11:217–230, 1976.

Barnett, RE, Scott RE, Furent LT, et al: Evidence that mitogenic lectines induce changes in lymphocyte membrane fluidity. *Nature* 244:465–466, 1974.

Barr DP: Influence of sex and sex hormones upon the development of atherosclerosis and upon the lipoproteins of the plasma. *J Chronic Dis* 1:63–85, 1955.

Barraclough CA, Haller EW: Positive and negative feedback effects of estrogen on pituitary LH synthesis and release in normal and androgen-sterilized female rats. *Endocrinology* 86:542–551, 1970.

Baserga RL: Cell division and the cell cycle, in Finch CE, Hayflick L (eds): *Handbook of the Biology of Aging.* New York, Van Nostrand Reinhold Company, 1977, pp 101–121.

Baumann EA, Hand AR: Protein kinase activity associated with the D2 hybrid protein related to simian virus 40 T-antigen: some characteristics of the reaction products. *Proc Natl Acad Sci USA* 76:3688–3692, 1979.

Bazzarre TL, Johanson AJ, Huseman CA, et al: Human growth hormone changes with age, in Pecile A, Müller EE (eds): *Growth Hormone and Related Peptides.* Amsterdam, Excerpta Medica, 1976, pp 261–270.

Beaumont JL: Autoimmune hyperlipidemia, in Jones RJ (ed): *Atherosclerosis.* Berlin, Springer-Verlag, 1970, pp 166–176.

Bell ET: Postmortem study of vascular disease in diabetes. *Arch Pathol Lab Med* 53:444–455, 1952.

Belokrylov GA, Morozov VG, Khavinson VH, et al: The action of low molecular extracts from heterological thymus, pineal and hypothalamus on the immune response in mice. *Biull Eksp Biol Med* 81:202–204, 1976.

Ben-David M, Dikstein S, Bismush S, et al: Anti-hypercholesterolemic effect of dehydroepiandrosterone. *Proc Soc Exp Biol Med* 125:1136–1140, 1967.

Benditt EP, Benditt JM: Evidence for a monoclonal origin of human atherosclerotic plaques. *Proc Natl Acad Sci USA* 70:1753–1756, 1973.

Benjamin F: Growth hormone response to insulin hypoglycemia in endometrial carcinoma. *Obstet Gynecol* 43:257–261, 1974.

Benjamin F, Casper DJ, Sherman L, et al: Growth hormone secretion in patients with endometrial carcinoma. *N Engl J Med* 25:1448–1452, 1969.

Benjamin F, Deutsch S: Plasma levels of fractionated estrogens and pituitary hormones in endometrial carcinoma. *Am J Obstet Gynecol* 126:638–647, 1976.

Benson B, Sorrentino S, Evans JS: Increase in serum FSH following unilateral ovariectomy in the rat. *Endocrinology* 84:369–374, 1969.

Benson B, Matthews MJ, Rodin AE: Studies on a nonmelatonin pineal antigonadotropin. *Acta Endocrinol* 69:257–266, 1972.

Bergland RM, Davis SL, Page RB: Pituitary secretion to brain. *Lancet* 2:276–278, 1977.

Berglund G, Larsson B, Andersson O, et al: Body compositions and glucose metabolism in hypertensive middle-aged males. *Acta Med Scand* 200:163–169, 1976.

Bergman W, Engel P: Über den Einfluss von Zirbelextracten auf Tumoren bei weissen Mausen und bei Menschen. *Wien Klin Wochenschr* 62:79–82, 1950.

Bergström S, Carlson LA, Weeks JR: The prostaglandins: a family of biologically active lipids. *Pharmacol Rev* 20:1–48, 1968.

Berken A, Benacerraf B: Depression of the reticuloendothelial system phagocytic function by injected lipids. *Proc Soc Exp Biol Med* 128:793–795, 1968.

Bernard C: *Les Phénoménes de la Vie.* Paris, 1878. Greene HC (trans): *An Introduction to the Study of Experimental Medicine.* New York, Henry Schuman Inc, 1949.

Berns AW, Goldenberg S, Blumenthal HT: Diabetes as an etiologic factor in atherosclerosis, in Blumenthal HT (ed): *Cowdry's Arteriosclerosis,* ed 2. Springfield, Ill., Charles C Thomas, 1967, pp 474–495.

Berstein LM: The excretion of classical estrogens and total phenolsteroids in patients with cancer of uterine body. *Vopr Onkol* 9:48–52, 1967.

Berstein LM: The data on the birth weight of newborns in oncological patients. *Vopr Onkol* 3:48–54, 1973.

Berstein LM: Inhibition by thyroxine of compensatory hypertrophy of thyroid in rats. *Biull Eksp Biol Med* 8:31–33, 1975.

Berstein LM, Vasiljeva IA: On the effect of lipoproteins of serum and tumor tissue on iodine absorption function of thyroid gland. *Proc Conf Young Oncologists. Leningrad, Research Institute of Oncology, USSR Ministry of Health, 1974, pp 11*–12.

Berstein LM, Alexandrov VA: The effect of phenformin on fat-carbohydrate metabolism in pregnant rats. *Biull Eksp Biol Med* 7:825–827, 1976.

Berstein LM, Bochman JV, Mandelstam VA, et al: On the origin and action of nonclassical phenolsteroids of cancer of the corpus uteri in menopausal patients. *Vopr Onkol* 15:42–44, 1969.

Berstein LM, Alexandrov VA, Vasiljeva IA: The effect of phenformin on fat-carbohydrate metabolism and birth weight of fetuses in pregnant rats previously treated with alloxan. *Patol Fiziol Eksp Ter* 2:60–63, 1977.

Besedovsky H, Sorkin E: Network of immune-neuroendocrine interactions. *Clin Exp Immunol* 27:1–12, 1977.

Besser GM, Mortimer CH: Hypothalamic regulatory hormones. *J Clin Pathol* 27:173–184, 1974.

Bielschowsky F: Carcinogenesis in the thyroidectomized rat: the effect of injected growth hormone. *Br J Cancer* 12:231–233, 1958.

Bierman EL, Albers JJ: Lipoprotein uptake by cultured human arterial smooth muscle cells. *Biochim Biophys Acta* 388:198–202, 1975.

Bierman EL, Porte D, Bagdade JD, et al: Lipoprotein lipase and plasma triglyceride, in Jones RJ (ed) *Atherosclerosis.* Berlin, Springer-Verlag, 1970, pp 230–233.

Bishop JS, Marks PA: Studies of carbohydrate metabolism in patients with neoplastic disease. II. Response to insulin administration. *J Clin Invest* 38:668–672, 1959.

Bishop MC, Ross EJ: Adrenocortical activity in disseminated malignant disease in relation to prognosis. *Br J Cancer* 24:719–725, 1970.

Bivens CH, Lebovitz HE, Feldman JM: Inhibition of hypoglycemia-induced growth hormone secretion by the serotonin antagonists cyproheptadine and methysergide. *N Engl J Med* 289:236–239, 1973.

Bjorksten J: The crosslinkage theory of aging. *J Am Geriatr Soc* 16:408–427, 1968.

Björntorp P: Effect of age, sex, and clinical conditions on adipose tissue cellularity in man. *Metabolism* 23:1091–1102, 1974.

Björntorp P, Gustafson A, Tibblin G: Relationship between adipose tissue cellularity and carbohydrate and lipid metabolism in a randomly selected population, in Jones RJ (ed): *Atherosclerosis.* Berlin, Springer-Verlag, 1970, pp 374–377.

Björntorp P, Gustafson A, Persson B: Adipose tissue fat cell size and number in relation to metabolism in endogenous hypertriglyceridemia. *Acta Med Scand* 190:363–367, 1971.

Björntorp P, Fahlen M, Brimby G, et al: Carbohydrate and lipid metabolism in middle-aged physically well-trained men. *Metabolism* 71:1037–1044, 1972.

Björntorp P, De Jounge K, Krotkiewski M, et al: Physical training in human obesity. III. Effect of long-term physical training on body composition. *Metabolism* 22:1467–1475, 1973.

Blackard WG, Boglen CT, Hinson TC, et al: Effect of lipid and ketone infusion on insulin-induced growth hormone elevations in Rhesus monkeys. *Endocrinology* 85:1180–1185, 1969.

Blagosklonnaya JV: Effect of sex hormone preparation on hypercholesterolemia. *Probl Endokrinol* 6:43–47, 1959.

Blagosklonnaya JV: Effect of sex hormone preparation on certain disturbances in carbohydrate metabolism in ischemic heart patients. *Klin Med* 1:67–71, 1968.

Blichert-Toft M: Secretion of corticotropin and somatotropin by the senescent adenohypophysis in man. *Acta Endocrinol* 195(suppl):1–157, 1975.

Blichert-Toft M: The adrenal glands in old age, in Greenblatt RB (ed): *Geriatric Endocrinology,* vol 5. New York, Raven Press, 1978, pp 81–102.

Bloch GJ, Masken J, Kragt CL, et al: Effect of testosterone on plasma LH in male rats of various ages. *Endocrinology* 94:947–951, 1974.

Bloch K, Borek E, Rittenberg D: Synthesis of cholesterol in surviving liver. *J Biol Chem* 162:441–449, 1946.

Block E: Quantitative morphological investigations of the follicular system in newborn female infants. *Acta Anat* 17:201–206, 1953.

Blumenthal HT: Relation of age to the hormonal content of the human anterior hypophysis. *Arch Pathol Lab Med* 54:481–494, 1954.

Blumenthal HT: Age related autoimmune phenomena of the endocrine glands, in Gitman L (ed): *Endocrines and Aging*. Springfield, Ill., Charles C Thomas, 1967, pp 51–65.

Blumenthal HT: Aging and disease—a casual or causal relationship? With special reference to the genesis of athero-arteriosclerosis, in *Criteria for Determination of Biological Age in Man*. Leningrad, Nauka, 1974, pp 99–101, abst.

Bobrov YF, Patokin SV, and Dilman VM: The resistance to inhibition of the growth hormone and free fatty acids with glucose in patients with cancer of the mammary gland and uterine body. *Vopr Onkol* 17:40–44, 1971.

Boden GJ, Soeldner S, Gleason RW, et al: Elevated serum growth hormone and decreased serum insulin in prediabetic males after intravenous tolbutamide and glucose. *J Clin Invest* 47:729–739, 1968.

Bolton CH, Ellwood M, Hartog M, et al: Comparison of the effects of ethinyl oestradiol and conjugated equine oestrogens in oophorectomized women. *Clin Endocrinol* 4:131–138, 1975.

Borth R, Linder A, Riondel A: Urinary excretion of 17-hydroxycorticosteroids and 17-ketosteroids in healthy subjects: in relation to sex, age, body weight and height. *Acta Endocrinol,* (Kbh) 25:15–74, 1957.

Bortz WM: On the control of cholesterol synthesis. *Metabolism* 22:1507–1524, 1973.

Boudjers G, Bjørkern S: HDL-dependent elimination of cholesterol from human arterial tissue. *Proc Eur Soc Clin Invest* 9:51, 1975, abst.

Boyd GS: Endocrines in lipid metabolism. *Fed Proc* 20(suppl):152–160, 1961.

Boyle E: Biological patterns in hypertension by race, sex, body weight, and skin color. *JAMA* 213:1637–1643, 1970.

Bray GA, Glennon JA, Salans LR, et al: Spontaneous and experimental human obesity: effect of diet and adipose cell size on lipolysis and lipogenesis. *Metabolism* 26:739–748, 1977.

Breisch ST, Zendan F, Holbel B: Hyperphagia and obesity following serotonin depletion by intraventricular p-chlorphenylalanine. *Science* 192:385–385, 1976.

Brennerman DE, McGee R, Spector AA: Cholesterol metabolism in the Ehrlich ascites tumor. *Cancer Res* 34:2605–2611, 1974.

Brodish A: Tissue corticotropin releasing factors. *Fed Proc* 36:2088–2093, 1977.

Brody JS, Buhain WJ: Hormone-induced growth of the adult lung. *Amer J Physiol* 223:1444–1450, 1972.

Brody H, Vijayashankar N: Anatomical changes in the nervous system, in Finch CE, Hayflick L (eds): *Handbook of the Biology of Aging*. New York, Van Nostrand Reinhold Company, 1977, pp 241–261.

Brook CG, Lloyd JK, Wolff OH: Relation between age of onset of obesity and size and number of adipose cells. *Br Med J* 2:25–27, 1972.

Brown M, Faust JR, Goldstein JL: Role of the low density lipoprotein receptor in regulating the content of free and esterified cholesterol in human fibroblasts. *J Clin Invest* 55:783–793, 1975.

Brunelle P, Bohuon C: Baisse de la triiodothyronine serique avec l'âge. *Clin Chim Acta* 42:201–208, 1972.

Brunzell JD, Lerner BL, Hazzard WR, et al: Improved glucose tolerance with high carbohydrate feeding in mild diabetes. *N Engl J Med* 284:521–524, 1971.

Brunzell JD, Chait A, Bierman EL: Pathophysiology of lipoprotein transport. *Metabolism* 27:1109–1127, 1978.

Bulbrook RD: Urinary androgen excretion and the etiology of breast cancer. *J Natl Cancer Inst* 48:1039–1042, 1972.

Bulbrook RD, Hayward JL, Spicer CC: Relation between urinary androgen and corticoid excretion and subsequent breast cancer. *Lancet* 2:395–398, 1971.

Burch PRJ: Coronary heart disease: risk factors and aging. *Gerontology* 24:123–155, 1978.

Burnet FM: *Cellular Immunology.* London, Cambridge University Press, 1969.

Burnet FM: An immunological approach to aging. *Lancet* 2:358–360, 1970.

Burnet FM: *Immunology, Aging, and Cancer. Medical Aspects of Mutation and Selection.* San Francisco, WH Freeman and Company, 1976.

Burstein R, Frankel S, Soule SD, et al: Aging of the placenta: autoimmune theory of senescence. *Am J Obstet Gynecol* 116:271–276, 1973.

Burstein RH, Blumenthal HT: Immune reactions of normal pregnancy. *Am J Obstet Gynecol* 104:671–678, 1969.

Buswell RC: The pineal gland and neoplasia. *Lancet* 1:34–35, 1976.

Butcher RL: Changes in gonadotropins and steroids associated with unilateral ovariectomy of the rat. *Endocrinology* 101:830–840, 1977.

Byers SO, Friedman M, Elek SR, et al: Neurogenic hypercholesterolemia. Influence of autonomic drugs. *Atherosclerosis* 24:189–198, 1976.

Byrnes WW, Meyer KK: Effect of physiological amounts of estrogen on the secretion of follicle-stimulating and luteinizing hormones. *Endocrinology* 49:449–460, 1951.

Cahill GF, Herrera MG, Morgan AP, et al: Hormone-fuel interrelationships during fasting. *J Clin Invest* 45:1751–1769, 1966.

Cannon WB: Organization for physiological homeostasis. *Physiol Rev* 9:399–431, 1929.

Cannon WB: Ageing of homeostatic mechanisms, in Cowdry EV (ed): *Problems of Ageing.* Baltimore, Williams and Wilkins, 1942, pp 567–582.

Caraceni T, Poneroi AE, Paroti EA, et al: Altered growth hormone and prolactin responses to dopaminergic stimulation in Huntington's chorea. *J Clin Endocrinol Metab* 44:870–875, 1977.

Cardinali DP, Nagle CA, Gomez E, et al: The norepinephrine turnover in the rat pineal gland: acceleration by estradiol and testosterone. *Life Sci* 16:1717–1724, 1975.

Carey RW, Pretlow TG, Erdinii EZ, et al: Studies on the mechanism of hypoglycemia in a patient with massive intraperitoneal leiomyosarcoma. *Am J Med* 40:458–469, 1966.

Carlson LA, Fröberg SO, Nye ER: Effect of age on blood and tissue lipid levels in the male rat. *Gerontology* 14:65–79, 1968.

Carroll BJ, Curtis GC, Mendels J: Neuroendocrine regulation in depression: limbic system adrenocortical dysfunction. *Arch Gen Psychiat* 33:1039–1044, 1976.

Carter AC, Lefkon BW, Farlin M, et al: Metabolic parameters in women with metastatic breast cancer. *J Clin Endocrinol* 40:260–264, 1975, abst.

Carter AC, Feldman EB, Lefkon E: The glucose fatty acid cycle in women with metastatic breast carcinoma. *Excerpta Medica* (ICS) 140:179, 1967.

Carvalho, ACA, Colman RW, Lees RS: Platelet function in hyperlipoproteinemia. *N Engl J Med* 290:434–438, 1974.

Cavagnini F, Peracchi M, Raggi U, et al: Impairment of growth hormone and insulin secretion in hyperthyroidism. *Eur J Clin Invest* 4:71–77, 1974.

Ceresa F, Angeli A, Boccuzzi G, et al: Impulsive and basal ACTH secretion phases in normal subjects, in obese subjects with signs of adrenocortical hyperfunction and in hyperthyroid patients. *J Clin Endocrinol Metab* 31:491–501, 1970.

Ceresa F, Angeli A, Boccuzzi G: Cortisol circadian rhythm in obese subjects with signs of hyperadrenocorticism. *Excerpta Medica* (ICS) 256:83, 1972, abst.

Charles D, Bell E, Loraine I: Endometrial carcinoma—endocrinological and clinical studies. *Am J Obstet Gynecol* 91:1050–1059, 1965.

Chatterton RT, Murray CL, Hellman L: Endocrine effect on leukocytopoiesis in the rat. I. Evidence for growth hormone secretion as the leukocytopoietic stimulus following acute cortisol-induced lymphopenia. *Endocrinology,* 92:775–788, 1973.

Chazov EI, Isachenkov VA: *The Pineal Gland.* Moscow, Nauka, 1974.

Chazov EI, Isachenkov VA, Kryvosheev OG, et al: Biosynthesis of pituitary hormones. III. Effect of pineal extracts and melatonin on biosynthesis of growth hormone and prolactin in rats' pituitary. *Vopr Med Khim* 17:3–7, 1972.

Cheesman DN, Forsham PH: Inhibition of induced ovulation by a highly purified extract of the bovine pineal gland. *Proc Soc Exp Biol Med* 146:722–724, 1974.

Chen HJ, Meites J: Effects of biogenic amines and TRH on release of prolactin and TSH in the rat. *Endocrinology* 96:10–14, 1975.

Chen HW, Heiniger HJ, Kàndutsch AA: Relationship between sterol synthesis and DNA synthesis in phytohemagglutinin-stimulated mouse lymphocytes. *Proc Natl Acad Sci USA* 72:1950–1954, 1975.

Chen HW, Heiniger HJ, Kandutsch AA: Stimulation of sterol and DNA synthesis in leukemic cells by low concentrations of phytohemagglutinin. *Exp Cell Res* 109:253–262, 1977b.

Chen RM, Getz GS, Fischer-Dzoga K, et al: The role of hyperlipidemic serum in the proliferation and necrosis of aortic medial cells in vitro. *Exp Mol Path* 26:359–368, 1977a.

Chen S-H, Keenan RM: Effect of phosphatidylcholine liposomes on the mitogen stimulated lymphocyte activation. *Biochem Biophys Res Commun* 79:852–858, 1977.

Cheraskin E, Ringsdorf WM, Setyaadmadja ATSH, et al: Cancer proneness profile: a study in weight and blood glucose. *Geriatrics* 23:134–137, 1968.

Chlouverakis C, Jarrett RJ, Keen H: Glucose tolerance, age, and circulating insulin. *Lancet* 1:806–809, 1967.

Christian JJ: Endocrine behavioral negative feedback response to the increased population density. *Colloq Internat Centr Nation Réchèrche Scientif* (Paris) 173:289, 1968.

Christian JJ: Anterior pituitary in relation to renal disease, in Everitt AV, Burgess JA (eds): *Hypothalamic Pituitary and Aging.* Springfield, Ill., Charles C Thomas, 1976, pp 297–332.

Christiansen P: Urinary follicle stimulating hormone and luteinizing hormone in normal adult women. *Acta Endocrinol* 71:1–6, 1972.

Chung AC: The influence of Dilantin on the development of atherosclerosis in rabbits. *Atherosclerosis Res* 7:373–379, 1967.

Ciswicka-Sznejderman M, Berent H, Rymaszewski Z: The effect of combined treatment with phenformin and stanazolol on blood lipids and fibrinolytic activity in patients with hypertriglyceridemia. *Atherosclerosis* 19:153–159, 1974.

Claeys-DeClerg P, Levin S, Borkowski H: Study of growth hormone secretion in lung carcinoma. *Eur J Cancer* 11:565–569, 1975.

Clemens JA, Meites J: Hypothalamic control of prolactin secretion, in Stoll BA (ed): *Mammary Cancer and Nevroendocrine Therapy*. London, Butterworth & Co, 1974, pp 160–178.

Clemensen J, Fredriksen V, Plum CM: Are anticonvulsants oncogenic? *Lancet* 1:705–707, 1974.

Cohen MS, Strauss BL: Enhancement of the antitumor effect of 1,3-bis-(2-chloroethyl)-1-Nitrosourea (BCNU) by phenformin. *Oncology* 33:257–259, 1976.

Cohen MS, Bower RH, Fidler SM, et al: Inhibition of insulin release by diphenylhydantoin and diazoxide in a patient with benign insulinoma. *Lancet* 1:40–41, 1973.

Cohen MS, Lippman M, Chabner B: Role of pineal gland in etiology and treatment of breast cancer. *Lancet* 2:814–816, 1978.

Cohen ND, Hilf R: Influence of insulin on growth and metabolism of 4,12-dimethylbenz(a)anthracene-induced mammary tumors. *Cancer Res* 34:3245–3252, 1974.

Coleman JE: Metabolic interrelationships between carbohydrates, lipids and proteins, in Bondy PK (ed): *Duncan's Diseases of Metabolism*. Philadelphia, WB Saunders, 1969, pp 161–274.

Coleman JR, Lederis K: Urinary gonadotropins in patients with advanced mammary carcinoma. *Acta Endocrinol* 100(suppl):195, 1965, abst.

Collett MS, Erikson RL, Purchio AF, et al: A normal cell protein similar in structure and function to the avian sarcoma virus transforming gene product. *Proc Natl Acad Sci USA* 76:3159–3163, 1979.

Colman RW: Platelet function in hyperbetalipoproteinemia. *Thromb Haemost* 39:284–293, 1978.

Colucci CF, D'Alessandro B, Bellastella A, et al: Circadian rhythm of plasma cortisol in the aged (Cosinor method). *Geront Clin,* Basel, 17:89–95, 1975.

Comfort A: *Aging, the Biology of Senescence.* New York, Holt, Rinehart and Winston Inc, 1964.

Comfort A: Test-battery to measure aging-rate in man. *Lancet* 2:1411–1414, 1969.

Comfort A: Measurement of the human aging rate. *Mech Ageing Dev* 1:101–110, 1972.

Contractor SF, Davies H: Effect of human chorionic somatomammotropin and HCG on PHA lymphocyte transformation. *Nature (New Biology)* 243:284–286, 1973.

Cornblath M, Parker ML, Reisner SH, et al: Secretion and metabolism of growth hormone in premature and full-term infants. *J Clin Endocrinol Metab* 25:209–218, 1965.

Corvilain J, Loeb H, Champenois A, et al: Effect of fasting on levels of plasma-nonesterified fatty acids in normal children, normal adults, and obese adults. *Lancet* 1:534–535, 1961.

Costoff A, Mahesh VB: Primordial follicles with normal oocytes in the ovaries of postmenopausal women. *J Am Geriatr Soc* 23:193–196, 1975.

Cotzias GC, Miller ST, Nicholson AR, et al: Prolongation of the life-span in mice adapted to large amount of L-dopa. *Proc Natl Acad Sci USA* 71:2466–2469, 1974.

Cotzias GC, Miller ST, Tang LC, et al: Levodopa, fertility, and longevity. *Science* 196:541–549, 1977.

Cox RH, Perchuch JS: A sensitive, rapid and simple method for simultaneous spectrophotofluorimetric determination of noradrenaline, dopamine,

5-hydroxytryptamine and 5-hydroxyindolacetic acid in discrete areas of brain. *J Neurochem* 20:1777–1780, 1973.

Crane MG: Hypertension in the aged, in Greenblatt RB (ed): *Geriatric Endocrinology,* vol 5. *Aging*. New York, Raven Press, 1978, pp 115–132.

Crockford PM, Salmon PA: Hormones and obesity: changes in insulin and growth hormone secretion following surgically-induced weight loss. *Can Med Assoc J* 103:147–150, 1970.

Cryer PE, Coran AG, Kelnan BS, et al: Cessation of growth hormone secretion associated with acute elevation of the serum free fatty acids concentration. *Metabolism* 21:867–873, 1972.

Curtis HJ: *Biological Mechanisms of Aging.* Springfield, Ill., Charles C Thomas, 1966.

Curtiss LK, Edgington TS: Identification of a lymphocyte surface receptor for low density lipoprotein inhibitor, an immunoregulatory species of normal human serum LDL. *J Clin Invest* 61:1298–1308, 1978.

Curzon G: Tryptophan pyrrolase—a biochemical factor in depressive illness? *Br J Psychiatry* 115:1367–1374, 1969.

Dafny N, Phillips MI, Taylor A, et al: Dose effects of cortisol on single-unit activity in hypothalamus, reticular formation and hippocampus of freely-behaving rats correlated with plasma steroid levels. *Brain Res* 59:257–272, 1973.

Dairman W, Horst WD, Marchelle ME, et al: The proportionate loss of L-5-hydroxytryptophan decarboxylating activity in rat central nervous system following intracisternal administration of 5,6-dihydroxytryptamine or 6-hydroxydopamine. *J Neurochem* 24:619–623, 1975.

Daniele HW: Smoking, obesity and the menopause. *Lancet* 2:372, 1978.

Danowski TS, Tsai CT, Morgan CR, et al: Serum growth hormone and insulin in females without glucose intolerance. *Metabolism* 18:811–820, 1969.

Danowski TS, Nolan S, Stephan T, et al: Prolonged progestin therapy of menopausal diabetic women. *Behav Neuropsychiatry* 6:1–12, 1975.

Dao TL, Sinha D: Effect of carcinogen on pituitary prolactin synthesis and release. *Proc Am Assoc Cancer Res* 16:28, 1975, abst.

Das Gupta TK, Terz J: Influence of pineal gland on the growth and spread of melanoma in the hamster. *Cancer Res.* 27:1306–1311, 1967.

Daughaday WH, Kipnis DM: The growth promoting and anti-insulin action of somatotropin. *Recent Prog Horm Res* 22:49–99, 1966.

Daughaday WH, Phillips LS, Herington AC: Regulation of somatomedin generation, in Pecile A, Müller EE (eds): *Growth Hormone and Related Peptides.* Amsterdam, Excerpta Medica, 1976, pp 169–177.

Davey FR, Huntington S: Age-related variation in lymphocyte subpopulations. *Gerontology* 23:381–389, 1977.

Davidson PC, Albrink MJ: Insulin resistance in hypertriglyceridemia. *Metabolism* 14:1059–1070, 1965.

Debons AF, Krimsky I, From A, et al: Rapid effect of insulin on the hypothalamic satiety center. *Am J Physiol* 217:1114–1118, 1969.

De Caro LG, Fattorini A, Gorini M: Plasma NEFA response to a glucose load in patients with diabetes, arteriosclerosis and obesity. *Metabolism* 15:65–69, 1966.

Defares JG: Is cancer preventable? *Lancet* 1:135–136, 1971.

De Fronzo RA, Diebert D, Hendler R, et al: Direct evidence of insulin resistance in maturity onset diabetes. *Diabetes* 27(suppl):431, 1978, abst.

Delbridge L, Everitt AV: The effect of hypophysectomy and age on the stabilization of labile cross-links in collagen. *Exp Gerontol* 7:413–441, 1972.

Delespesse G, Duchateau J, Kennes B, et al: Cell-mediated immunity in diabetes mellitus. *Excerpta Medica* (ICS) 316:83-88, 1974.

De Meyts P, Roth J, Neville DM, et al: Insulin interactions with its receptors: experimental evidence for negative cooperativity. *Biochem Biophys Res Commun* 55:154-161, 1973.

Denckla WD: Systems analysis of possible mechanism of mammalian aging. *Mech Ageing Dev* 6:143-152, 1977.

De Waard F: Hormonal factors in the epidemiology of breast cancer. *Excerpta Medica* (ICS) 273:1222-1226, 1973.

De Waard F, Thyssen JHH, Veeman W, et al: Steroid hormone excretion pattern in women with endometrial carcinoma. *Cancer* 22:988-993, 1969.

Dianzani MU, Torrelli MV, Canuto RA, et al: The influence of enrichment with cholesterol on the phagocytic activity of rat macrophages. *J Pathol* 118:193-199, 1976.

Diebel ND, Yamamoto M, Bogdanove EH: Discrepancies between radioimmunoassays and bioassay for rat FSH: Evidence that androgen treatment and withdrawal can alter bioassay-immunoassay ratio. *Endocrinology* 92:1065-1078, 1973.

Dietschy JM, Wilson JD: Regulation of cholesterol metabolism. *N Engl J Med* 282:1128-1138, 1970.

Dietze G, Wicklmayr M, Mehhert H, et al: Effect of phenformin on hepatic balance of gluconeogenic substrates in man. *Diabetologia* 14:243-248, 1978.

Di Girolano M, Owens JL: Glucose metabolism in isolated fat cells. *Horm Metab Res* 8:445-454, 1976.

Dilman VM: On the age-associated elevation of activity of certain hypothalamic centers. *Trans Inst Physiol Acad Sci USSR*. Leningrad, Nauka, 1958, pp 326-336.

Dilman VM: Pituitary inhibitors. Effect of sigetin on the uterine development in immature mice. *Biull Eksp Biol Med* 8:104-106, 1959.

Dilman VM: Age-associated hypercholesterolemia as a sign of elevation of hypothalamic center activity. *Ter Arkh* 32:72-77, 1960.

Dilman VM: *Application of Sex Hormones and their Analogs in Clinical Practice.* Leidykla Mintus, Vilnius, 1961.

Dilman VM; Anahormones. I. The preservation of immunologic properties of the chorionic and pituitary gonadotropins in spite of the gonadotropic effect elimination. *Vopr Onkol* 8:112-113, 1962.

Dilman VM: Anahormones of growth hormone, exophthalmic factor, melanophore-stimulating hormone, adrenocorticotropin and gonadotropin in experimental and clinical endocrinology. *Int J Cancer* 1:239-247, 1966.

Dilman VM: Development of concepts on role of neuroendocrine system in pathogenesis of cancer. *Vopr Onkol* 13:39-59, 1967.

Dilman VM: *Aging, Climacteric and Cancer.* Leningrad, Meditsina, 1968.

Dilman VM: Elevating mechanism of aging and cancer. Need for prophylactic normalization of disturbances in energetic and reproductive homeostasis caused by age increase of resistance of the hypothalamus to inhibition. *Vopr Onkol* 16:45-53, 1970a.

Dilman VM: Malignant growth in the light of elevating mechanism of development and aging, in *Transcript of 141st Session of Scientific Society of Oncologists,* 2:120-122, 1970b.

Dilman VM: Age-associated elevation of hypothalamic threshold to feedback control and its role in development, aging and disease. *Lancet* 1:1211-1219, 1971.

Dilman VM: *Why Do We Die?* Leningrad, Meditsina, 1972.

Dilman VM: *Endocrinologic Oncology.* Leningrad, Meditsina, 1974a.

Dilman VM: Changes in hypothalamic sensitivity in aging and cancer, in Stoll BA (ed): *Mammary Cancer and Neuroendocrine Therapy*. London, Butterworth & Co., 1974b, pp 197–228.

Dilman VM: Aging and growth hormone. *J Clin Endocrinol* 39:183, 1974c.

Dilman VM: Elevating mechanism of development, aging and age-associated pathology. III. Acceleration of the development and age norm. *Hum Physiol* 1:352–359, 1975.

Dilman VM: Improvement of indices of cellular immunity after epithalamin treatment. *Vopr Onkol* 23:7–9, 1977.

Dilman VM: Ageing, metabolic immunodepression and carcinogenesis. *Mech Ageing Dev* 8:153–173, 1978a.

Dilman VM: Transformation of the developmental program into the mechanism of age-associated pathology. Elevation model of human specific age pathology and natural death. *Hum Physiol* 4:579–595, 1978b.

Dilman VM, Blok LP: Anahormones. 2. The influence of the hormonally inactive hypophyseal gonadotropins on the frequency of occurrence of hyperplasia of the ovary transplanted into the spleen. *Vopr Onkol* 8:115–116, 1962.

Dilman VM, Pavlova MV: The secretion of gonadotropins, estrogens and 17-ketosteroids in some pretumourous and tumourous diseases. 2. Breast carcinoma, dysfunctional uterine bleeding. *Vopr Onkol* 9:74–82, 1963.

Dilman VM, Kovaleva IG: Competition of anasomatotropin with active human growth hormone. *Vopr Onkol* 12:30–41, 1964.

Dilman VM, Bobrov YF: Hypercholesterolemia and cancer, in Rakov AI (ed): *Modern Problems of Oncology* (in Russian). Leningrad, Medicine, 1966, pp 76–80.

Dilman, VM, Vasiljeva IA: Inhibition of lipolysis and potentiation of the hypoglycemic effect of insulin by nonhypoglycemic insulin derivatives. *J Endocrinol* 50:373–381, 1971.

Dilman, VM, Anisimov, VN: Increase of hypothalamus sensitivity to inhibitory action of estrogens, caused by L-dopa, Dilantin, epithalamin and phenformin in old rats. *Biull Eksp Biol Med* 79:96–98, 1975.

Dilman VM, Anisimov VN: Potentiation of antitumor effect of clophosphamide and hydrazine sulfate by treatment with the antidiabetic agent, 1-phenylethylbiguanide (phenformin). *Cancer Lett* 7:357–361, 1979.

Dilman VM, Berstein LM, Bobrov YF, et al: Hypothalamopituitary hyperactivity and endometrial carcinoma. *Am J Obstet Gynecol* 102:880–889, 1968.

Dilman VM, Elubajeva GO, Vishnevsky AS, et al: Arguments for Dilantin administration in cancer patients. *Vopr Onkol* 17:70–72, 1971.

Dilman VM, Ostroumova MN, Berstein LM, et al: Recherche de produits faisant baiser senil hypothalamique de freinage homeostatique. II. Etude de l'action des produits Agr. 310 et Agr. 614 et d'extrait dépiphyse. *Agressologie* 14:243–250, 1973.

Dilman VM, Ostroumova MN, Krylova NV, et al: New data on three types of anahormones of LH, GH, ACTH, lipotropin, calcitonin, and parathyroid hormone. *Endocrinol Exp* 8:245–260, 1974.

Dilman VM, Berstein LM, Tsyrlina EV, et al: On the correction of endocrine-metabolic disturbances in oncological patients. The effect of phenformin, buformin, clofibrate and Dilantin. *Vopr Onkol* 11:33–39, 1975.

Dilman VM, Ostroumova MN, Nemirovsky VS, et al: A correlation between immune reactivity and fat-carbohydrate metabolism. The effect of phenformin. *Vopr Onkol* 2:13–17, 1976.

Dilman VM, Ostroumova MN, Blagosklonnaya JV, et al: Metabolic immunodepression. Normalizing effect of phenformin. *Hum Physiol* 3:579–586, 1977a.

Dilman VM, Sofronov BN, Anisimov VN, et al: Elimination of immunodepression induced by 1,2-dimethylhydrazine in the rat, with the aid of phenformin. *Vopr Onkol* 23:50–54, 1977b.

Dilman VM, Berstein LM, Zabezhinski MA, et al: Inhibition of DMBA-induced carcinogenesis by phenformin in the mammary gland of rats. *Arch Geschwulstforsch* 48:1–8, 1978.

Dilman VM, Ostroumova MN, Tsyrlina EV: Hypothalamic mechanisms of ageing and of specific age pathology. II. On the sensitivity threshold of hypothalamic-pituitary complex to homeostatic stimuli in adaptive homeostasis. *Exp Gerontol* 14:175–181, 1979.

Dilman VM, Anisimov VN, Ostroumova MN, et al: Study of the anti-tumor effect of polypeptide pineal extract. *Oncology* 36:274–280, 1979a.

Dilman VM, Lapin JF, Oxenkrug GF: Serotonin and aging, in Essman WB (ed): *Serotonin in Health and Disease.* New York, SP Medical & Scientific Books, 1979b, vol V, pp 111–212.

Dilman VM, Ostroumova MN, Tsyrlina EV: Hypothalamic mechanisms of ageing and of specific age pathology. II. On the sensitivity threshold of hypothalamo-pituitary complex to homeostatic stimuli in adaptive homeostatis. *Exp Gerontol* 14: 175–181, 1979c.

Di Lusio NR, Wooles WR: Depression of phagocytic activity and immune response by methyl palmate. *Am J Physiol* 206:939–943, 1975.

Di Perri T: Iperlipoproteinemia et immunita. *Minerva Med* 66:3397–3405, 1975.

Ditschuneit H: Definition and criteria of prediabetes, in Östman J (ed): *Diabetes.* Amsterdam, Excerpta Medica, 1964, pp 479–485.

Ditschuneit H: Obesity and diabetes mellitus, in Rodriguez RR, Vallance-Owen J (eds): *Diabetes.* Amsterdam, Excerpta Medica, 1971, pp 526–543.

Diszfalusy E, Lauritzen C: *Oestrogens beim Menschen.* Berlin, Springer Verlag, 1961.

Döcke F, Dörner G: The mechanism of the induction of ovulation by estrogens. *J Endocrinol* 33:491–499, 1965.

Dockerty MB, Lovelady SB, Foust GT: Carcinoma of the corpus uteri in young women. *Am J Obstet Gynecol* 61:966–978, 1951.

Doll R: The age factor in the susceptibility of man and animals to radiation. II. Age differences in susceptibility to carcinogensis in man. *Br J Radiol* 35:31–36, 1962.

Doll R: Age in host-environment interaction in the etiology of cancer in man. *IARC Sci Publ* 7:39–48, 1973.

Doll R, Peto R: Mortality in relation to smoking: 20 years' observations on male British doctors. *Br Med J* 2:1525–1536, 1976.

Donegan WL, Hurtz AJ, Rimm AA: The association of body weight with recurrent cancer of the breast. *Cancer* 41:1590–1594, 1978.

Donovan BT: The role of the hypothalamus in puberty, in Schwabe DF, Schade JP (eds): *Progress in Brain Research.* vol 41. Amsterdam, Elsevier, 1974, pp 281–288.

Donovan BT, Van der Werff ten Bosch JJ: The hypothalamus and sexual maturation in the rat. *J Physiol (Lond)* 147:79–92, 1959.

Dragar, NM: Height of diabetic children at onset of symptoms. *Arch Dis Child* 49:616–620, 1974.

Duckworth WC, Kitabchi AE, Heinemann M: Direct measurement of plasma proinsulin in normal and diabetic subjects. *Am J Med* 53:418–422, 1972.

Dudl RJ, Ensinck JW: The role of insulin, glucagon and growth hormone in carbohydrate homeostasis during aging. *Diabetes* 21(suppl):357, 1972, abst.

Dudl RJ, Ensinck JW: Insulin and glucagon relationships during aging in man. *Metabolism* 26:33–41, 1977.

Dudl RJ, Ensinck JW, Palmer HE, et al: Effect of age on growth hormone secretion in man *J Clin Endocrinol Metab* 37:11–16, 1973.

Dyer AR, Stamler J, Berkson DM, et al: High blood-pressure: A risk factor for cancer mortality? *Lancet* 1:1051–1056, 1975.

Eisenberg S, Levy RI: Lipoprotein metabolism. *Adv Lipid Res* 13:1–90, 1975.

Eldridge JC, McPherson JC, Mahesh VB: Maturation of the negative feedback control gonadotropin secretion in the female. *Endocrinology* 14:1536–1540, 1974.

Ellis S, Grindeland RE: Dichotomy between bio- and immuno-assayable growth hormone, in Raiti (ed): *Advances in Human Growth Hormone Research.* Baltimore, HEW Publication, 1973, pp 409–424.

Elubajeva GO, Santcharova AV, Vishnevsky AS, et al: Decreasing of total gonadotropin excretion caused by elipten treatment in breast cancer patients. *Vopr Onkol* 18:92–93, 1972.

Emmanuel NM, Obukhova LK: Types of experimental delay in aging patterns. *Exp Gerontol* 13:25–29, 1978.

Escueta AV, Appel SH: Diphenylhydantoin and potassium transport in isolated nerve terminals. *J Clin Invest* 50:1977–1984, 1971.

Evans DW, Turner SM, Ghosh P: Feasibility of long-term plasma cholesterol reduction by diet. *Lancet* 1:173–174, 1972.

Everitt AV: The thyroid gland in relation to aging and longevity. *Indian J Gerontol* 4, 182:1–10, 1972.

Everitt AV: The hypothalamus-pituitary control of aging and age-related pathology. *Exp Gerontol* 8:265–277, 1973.

Everitt AV, Burgess JA (eds): *Hypothalamus Pituitary and Aging.* Springfield, Ill., Charles C Thomas, 1976.

Exton JH: Gluconeogenesis. *Metabolism* 21:945–990, 1972.

Fabris N, Piantanelli L: Thymus, homeostatic regulation and aging. Presented at *XI International Congress of Gerontology,* Tokyo, 1978, p 17, abst.

Fabris N, Pierpaoli W, Sorkin E: Lymphocytes, hormones and aging. *Nature* 240:557–559, 1972.

Fajans SS, Conn JW: Prediabetes, subclinical diabetes, latent diabetes, in Leibel BS, Wrenshall GA (eds): *On Nature and Treatment of Diabetes.* Amsterdam, Excerpta Medica, 1965, pp 641–656.

Fajans SS, Cloutier MC, Crowther RL: Clinical and etiologic heterogeneity of idiopathic diabetes mellitus. *Diabetes* 27:1112–1125, 1978.

Fassati P, Fassati M, Sonka J, et al: Dehydroepiandrosterone sulphate. A new approach to some cases of angina pectoris therapy. *Agressologie* 11:445–448, 1970.

Felber JP, Magnenat G, Casthelaz M, et al: Carbohydrate and lipid oxidation in normal and diabetic subjects. *Diabetes* 26:693–699, 1977.

Feldman JM, Durchen NG: Inhibition of pancreatic islet monoamine oxidase (MAO) by adrenergic antagonists. *Diabetes* 24(suppl):432, 1975, abst.

Feldman JM, Plonk JW, Bivens CH: Inhibitory effect of serotonin antagonist on growth hormone release in acromegalic patients. *Clin Endocrinol* 5:71–78, 1976.

Felig P: Body fuel metabolism and diabetes mellitus in pregnancy. *Med Clin N Am* 61:43–66, 1977.

Ferguson T, Crichton DN, Price WH: Lymphocyte-counts in relation to age. *Lancet* 2:35, 1977.

Fernandes G, Yunis EJ, Good RA: Suppression of adenocarcinoma by the immunological consequences of caloric restriction. *Nature* 263:504–507, 1976.

Fernandes G, Yunis EJ, Miranda M, et al: Nutritional inhibition of genetically determined renal disease and autoimmunity with prolongation of life in kdkd mice. *Proc Natl Acad Sci USA* 75:2888-2892, 1978.

Fernstrom JD: Modification of brain serotonin by the diet. *Annu Rev Med* 25:1–8, 1974.

Fernstrom JD, Wurtman BJ: Brain serotonin content: physiological dependence on plasma tryptophan levels. *Science* 173:149-151, 1971.

Field EJ, Shenton BK: Inhibition of lymphocyte response to stimulants by unsaturated fatty acids and prostaglandins. *Lancet* 2:725–728, 1974.

Filipp G, Szentivenyi A: Anaphylaxis and the nervous system. Part III. *Ann Allergy* 16:306–311, 1958.

Finch CE: Catecholamine metabolism in the brains of aging male mice. *Brain Res* 52:261–276, 1973.

Finch CE: The regulation of physiological changes during mammalian aging. *Q Rev Biol* 51:49–83, 1976.

Finch CE, Foster JR, Mirsky AE: Ageing and the regulation of cell activities during exposure to cold. *J Gen Physiol* 54:690–712, 1969.

Fineberg SE, Schneider SH: Does hyperinsulinism cause insulin insensitivity? *Diabetes* 24(suppl):432, 1975, abst.

Finkelstein JW, Roffwarg HP, Boyar RM, et al: Age-related change in the twenty-four hour spontaneous secretion of growth hormone. *J Clin Endocrinol Metab* 35:665–670, 1972.

Fishman J, Norton B: Catechol estrogen formation in the central nervous system of the rat. *Endocrinology* 96:1054–1059, 1975.

Fishman LM, Liddle GW, Island DP, et al: Effect of aminoglutethimide on adrenal function in man. *J Clin Endocrinol Metab* 27:481–490, 1967.

Fitzgerald MG, Malins JM, O'Sullivan DJ: Prevalence of diabetes in women thirteen years after bearing a big baby. *Lancet* 1:1950, 1961.

Flerko B: The importance of estrogen-sensitive neurones in the control of cyclic secretion of gonadotropins, in *Proceedings of the First All-Union Conference on Neuroendocrinology*. Leningrad, Hauka, 1974, pp 180–181 (abst).

Flerko B, Mess B: Reduced estradiol-binding capacity of androgen sterilized rats. *Acta Physiol Acad Sci Hung* 33:111–113, 1968.

Florentin RA, Choi BH, Lee KT, et al: Stimulation of DNA-synthesis and cell division in vitro by serum from cholesterol-fed swine. *J Cell Biol* 41:641–645, 1969.

Fluhman CF: Hyperplasia of endometrium and hormones of anterior hypophysis and ovaries. *Surg Gynecol Obstet* 52:1051–1068, 1931.

Fluhman CF: *The Management of Menstrual Disorders.* Philadelphia, WB Saunders, 1956.

Fogelman AM, Edmond J, Seager J, et al: Abnormal induction of 3-hydroxy-3-methylglutaryl coenzyme A reductase in leukocytes from subjects with heterozygous familial hypercholesterolemia. *J Biol Chem* 250:2045—2055, 1975.

Fogelman AM, Seager J, Edwards PA, et al: Mechanism of induction of 3-hydroxy-3-methylglutaryl coenzyme A reductase in human leukocytes. *J Biol Chem* 252:644–645, 1977.

Foglia V, Basabe JC, Chieri RA: Evolution of diabetes after early testosterone treatment in rats. *Diabetologia* 5:258–259, 1969.

Forest MG: Androgènes plasmatiques et maturation de l'axe hypothalamo-hypophyso-gonadique chez le nourrison et l'enfant. *Paediatr Paedol* 5(suppl):13–28, 1977.

Forest MG, De Peretti E, Bertrand J: Hypothalamic-pituitary-gonadal relationships in man from birth to puberty. *Clin Endocrol* 5:551–569, 1976.

Fowler PBS, Swale J: Premyxoedema and coronary-artery disease. *Lancet* 1:1077–1079, 1967.

Franchimont P, Legros JJ, Schaub JC: Exploration de l'axe hypothalamo-hypophyso-somatotrope. *Revue Française d'Endocrinologie Clinique et Metabolisme* 11:105–119, 1970.

Franchimont P, Legros JJ, Maurice J: Effect of several estrogens on serum gonadotropin levels in postmenopausal women. *Horm Metab Res* 4:288–292, 1972.

Francis MG, Peaslee MH: Effects of social stress on pituitary melanocyte-stimulating hormone activity in mice. *Neuroendocrinology* 16:1–7, 1974.

Franks LM, Wilson PD, Whelan RD: The effects of age on total DNA and cell number in the mouse brain. *Gerontologia,* Basel, 20:21–26, 1974.

Frantz AG, Rabkin MT: Effects of estrogen and sex difference on secretion of human growth hormone. *J Clin Endocrinol* 25:1470–1480, 1965.

Frantz AG, Raben MS: Induction of antibodies to human growth hormone in patients with acromegaly. *Excerpta Medica (ICS)* 142:97, 1967, abst.

Fredrickson DS, Levy PJ, Lees RS: Fat transport in lipoproteins—an integrated approach to mechanisms and disorders. *N Engl J Med* 276:34–44, 94–104, 148–155, 273–281, 1967.

Freeman C, Karoly K, Adelman RC: Impairments in availability of insulin to liver in vivo and in binding of insulin to purified hepatic plasma membrane during aging. *Biochem Biophys Res Commun* 54:1573–1580, 1973.

Freychet P: Interactions of polypeptide hormones with cell membrane specific receptors: Studies with insulin and glucagon. *Diabetologia* 19:83–100, 1976.

Friedman M, Green MF, Sharland DE: Assessment of hypothalamic-pituitary-adrenal function in the geriatric age group. *J Geront* 24:292–297, 1969.

Friedman M, Byers S, Rosenman RH, et al: Coronary-prone individuals. *JAMA* 212:1030–1037, 1970.

Friedman M, Byers S, Rosenman RH: Plasma ACTH and cortisol concentration of coronary-prone subjects. *Proc Soc Exp Biol Med* 140:681–684, 1972a.

Friedman M, Byers S, Rosenman RH, et al: Hypocholesterolemic effect of human growth hormone in coronary-prone (type A) hypercholesterolemic subjects. *Proc Soc Exp Biol Med* 141:76–80, 1972b.

Frisch RE: Influences on age of menarche. *Lancet* 1:1007, 1973.

Frisch RE, Revelle R: Height and weight at menarche and a hypothesis of critical body weights and adolescent events. *Science* 169:397–398, 1970.

Frisch RE, McArthur JW: Menstrual cycles. Fatness as a determinant of minimum weight for height necessary for their maintenance or onset. *Science* 185:949–951, 1974.

Frisch RE, Hegsted MD, Joshinaga K: Body weight and food intake at early estrus of rats on a high-fat diet. *Proc Natl Acad Sci USA* 72:4172–4176, 1975.

Fritz JB: Insulin actions in carbohydrates and lipid metabolism, in Litwack G (ed): *Biochemical Actions of Hormones.* New York, Academic Press, 1972, pp 166–214.

Fuxe K, Hökfelt T, Nilsson O: Effect of constant light and androgen-sterilization on the amine turnover of the tuberoinfundibular dopamine neurons: blockade of cyclic activity and induction of a persistent high dopamine turnover in the median eminence. *Acta Endocrinol* 69:625–639, 1972.

Gala RR, Subromanion MG, Peters JA, et al: The effect of serotoninergic and adrenergic receptor antagonists on prolactin release in the monkey. *Life Sci* 20:631–638, 1977.

Ganis FM, Lowe RH, Morris MH, et al: The conversion of [4-^{14}C] -cortisol to [^{14}C] -11p-hydroxyestradiol in a patient with metastatic breast carcinoma: cortisol metabolism and breast cancer. *J Steroid Biochem* 5:543-549, 1974.

Ganong WF: The role of catecholamines and acetylcholine in the regulation of endocrine function. *Life Sci* 15:1401-1414, 1974.

Garrison RJ, Kannel WG, Feinlei M, et al: Cigarette smoking and HDL cholesterol. *Atherosclerosis* 30:17-25, 1978.

Gavin GR, Roth J, Neville DM, et al: Insulin-dependent regulation of insulin receptor concentrations; a direct demonstration in cell culture. *Proc Natl Acad Sci USA* 71:84-88, 1974.

Gerich JE, Lorenzi M, Bier DM, et al: Effect of physiological levels of glucagon and growth hormone on human carbohydrate and lipid metabolism. *J Clin Invest* 57:875-884, 1976.

Gerretsen GJ, Kremer E, Bleumink JO, et al: Dinitrochlorobenzene sensitization test in woman on hormonal contraceptives. *Lancet* 2:347-349, 1975.

Ginsberg H, Olefsky JM, Reaven GM: Further evidence that insulin resistance exists in patients with chemical diabetes. *Diabetes* 23:674-678, 1974.

Glass DN, Russell AS, Davies R: Human growth hormone and lung carcinoma. *Lancet* 1:683-684, 1972.

Glick SM, Roth J, Yalow RS, et al: The regulation of growth hormone secretion. *Recent Prog Horm Res* 21:241-283, 1965.

Glicksman AS, Rawson RW: Diabetes and altered carbohydrate metabolism in patients with cancer. *Cancer* 9:1127-1134, 1956.

Glueck CJ, Garstide PS, Steiner PM, et al: Hyperalpha- and hypobetalipoproteinemia in octogenarian kindreds. *Atherosclerosis* 27:387-406, 1977.

Gofman J, Jones H, Lindgren H, et al: Blood lipids and human atherosclerosis. *Circulation* 5:119-134, 1952.

Gold J: Enhancement by hydrazine sulfate of antitumor effectiveness of cytoxan, mitomycin C, methotrexate and bleomycin in Walker 256 carcinosarcoma in rats. *Oncology* 31:44-53, 1970.

Gold J: Inhibition by hydrazine sulfate and various hydrazides, of in vivo growth of Walker 256 intramuscular carcinoma, B-16 melanoma, Murphy-sturm lymphosarcoma and L-1210 solid leukemia. *Oncology* 27:69-80, 1973.

Gold PW, Goodwin FK: Neuroendocrine responses to levodopa in affective illness. *Lancet* 1:1007, 1977.

Goldstein JL, Brown MS: Lipoprotein receptors, cholesterol metabolism and atherosclerosis. *Arch Pathol Lab Med* 99:181-184, 1975.

Gommers A, de Gasparo M: Variation de l'insulinémie en function de l'âge chez le rat mâle non traité. *Gerontologia* 18:176-184, 1972.

Gonzalez R, Dempsey ME: Sterol synthesis in cultured human renal cell cancer. *J Urol* 117:708-711, 1977.

Good RA: Relationship between immunity and malignancy. *Proc Natl Acad Sci USA* 69:1026-1032, 1972.

Goodman MA, McMaster JH, Allon L, et al: Metabolic and endocrine alterations in osteosarcoma patients. *Cancer* 42:603 – 610, 1978.

Gordon EE, de Hartog M: Gluconeogenesis in renal-cortical tubules: effect of phenformin. *Diabetes* 22:50-57, 1973.

Gordon P, Tobin SS, Doty B, et al: Drug effects on behavior in aged animals and man: diphenylhydantoin and procainamide. *J Gerontol* 23:434-444, 1968.

Gosden RG, Bancroft L: Pituitary function in reproductively senescent female rats. *Exp Gerontol* 11:157-160, 1976.

Goth M, Gönczi J: Effect of insulin-induced hypoglycemia on the plasma cortisol and growth-hormone levels in obese and diabetic persons. *Endocrinologie* 60:8-16, 1972.

Grad B, Kral VA, Fayne RC, et al: Plasma and urinary corticoids in young and old persons. *J Gerontol* 22:66–71, 1967.

Grant DB: Fasting serum insulin levels in childhood. *Arch Dis Child* 42:375–378, 1967.

Greenberg JL, Yunis EJ: Histocompatibility determinants, immune responsiveness and aging in man. *Fed Proc* 37:1258–1267, 1978.

Greenblatt DJ, Shader RI: Benzodiazepines. *N Engl J Med* 291:1011–1015, 1974.

Gregerman RL: The age-related alteration of thyroid hormone function and thyroid hormone metabolism in men, in Gitman L (ed): *Endocrines and Aging*. Springfield, Ill., Charles C Thomas, 1967, pp 161–173.

Gregerman RL, Bierman EL: Hormones and aging. in Williams RH (ed): *Textbook of Endocrinology*. Philadelphia, WB Saunders, 1974, pp 1059–1070.

Griffiths CT, Hall TC, Saba L, et al: Preliminary trial of aminoglutethimide in breast cancer. *Cancer* 32:31–37, 1973.

Grimm Y, Reichlin S: Thyrotropin-releasing hormone (TRH): neurotransmitter regulation of secretion by mouse hypothalamic tissue in vitro. *Endocrinology* 93:626–631, 1973.

Grodin JM, Silteri PK, MacDonald PC: Source of estrogen production in postmenopausal women. *J Clin Endocrinol* 36:207–214, 1973.

Grodsky GM, Karam JH, Pavlatos FC, et al: Reduction by phenformin of excessive insulin levels after glucose loading in obese and diabetic subjects. *Metabolism* 12:278–286, 1963.

Gruen PH: Endocrine changes in psychiatric diseases. *Med Clin North Am* 62:285–296, 1978.

Guillemin R: Physiological and clinical significance of hypothalamic and extrahypothalamic brain peptides. *Triangle* 15:1–7, 1976.

Hadfield HG: Uptake and binding of catecholamines: effect of diphenylhydantoin and a new mechanism of action. *Arch Neurol* 26:78–84, 1972.

Hales CW, Greenwood FC, Mitchell FL, et al: Blood-glucose, plasma-insulin and growth hormone concentration of individuals with minor abnormalities of glucose tolerance. *Diabetologia* 4:73–82, 1968.

Hallgren HM, Wood NE: Phytohemagglutinin response and antibodies in aging humans. *Fed Proc* 31:649, 1972, abst.

Hallgren HM, Buckley CE, Gilbertsen VA, et al: Lymphocyte phytohemagglutinin responsiveness, immunoglobulins and autoantibodies in aging humans. *J Immunol* 111:1101–1107, 1973.

Hamlin CR, Kohn RK, Luschin JH: Apparent accelerated aging of human collagen in diabetes mellitus. *Diabetes* 24:902–904, 1975.

Hancock RW, Mosely R, Coup AJ: Height and Hodgkin's disease. *Lancet* 2:1364, 1976.

Hann S, Kaye R, Folkner B: Subpopulations of peripheral lymphocytes in juvenile diabetes. *Diabetes* 25:101–103, 1976.

Hansen AP: Abnormal serum growth hormone response to exercise in juvenile diabetics. *J Clin Invest* 49:1467–1478, 1970.

Hansen AP: Normalization of growth hormone hyperresponse to excercise in juvenile diabetics after "normalization" of blood sugar. *J Clin Invest* 50:1806–1811, 1971.

Hansen AP: Serum growth hormone patterns in female juvenile diabetics. *J Clin Endocrinol* 36:638–647, 1973a.

Hansen AP: Abnormal serum growth hormone response to exercise in maturity-onset diabetes. *Diabetes* 22:619–628, 1973b.

Hansen AP: Immunoreactive growth hormone in plasma and urine in juvenile diabetics before and during initial treatment. *Acta Endocrinol* 75:50–64, 1974.

Harman D, Hendricks S, Eddy DE, et al: Free radical theory of aging: effect of dietary fat on central nervous system function. *J Am Geriatr Soc* 24:301–307, 1976.

Harrison LC, Martin FIR, Melick RA: Correlation between insulin receptor binding in isolated fat cells and insulin sensitivity in obese human subjects. *J Clin Invest* 58:1435–1441, 1976.

Hart RW, D'Ambrosio SM, Kwokei J, et al: Longevity, stability, and DNA repair. *Mech Ageing Dev* 9:203–223, 1979.

Haubrich DR, Denzer JS: Simultaneous extraction and fluorimetric measurement of brain serotonin, catecholamine, 5-hydroxyindoleacetic acid and homovanillic acid. *Anal Biochem* 55:306–312, 1973.

Haven FL, Bloor WR, Randall C: Lipids of the carcass, blood plasma, and adrenals of the rat in cancer. *Cancer Res* 9:511–514, 1949.

Hayflick L: The limited in vitro lifetime of human diploid cell strains. *Exp Cell Res* 37:614–636, 1965.

Hayflick L: Current theories of biological aging. *Fed Proc* 34:9–13, 1975.

Hayflick L: The cell biology of human aging. *N Engl J Med* 295:1302–1308, 1976.

Heald FP, Arnold G, Seabold W, et al: Plasma levels of free fatty acids in adolescents. *Am J Clin Nutr* 20:1010–1014, 1967.

Heiniger HJ, Chen HW, Applegate OL, et al: Elevated synthesis of cholesterol in human leukemic cells. *J Mol Medicine* 1:109–116, 1976.

Helderman JH, Strom TB: Emergence of insulin receptors upon alloimmune T cells in the rat. *J Clin Invest* 59:338–344, 1977.

Hems G: Epidemiological characteristics of breast cancer in middle and late age. *Br J Cancer* 14:226–235, 1970.

Hemsell DL, Grodin JM, Brenner PF, et al: Plasma precursors of estrogen. II. Correlation of the extent of conversion of plasma androstenedione to estrone with age. *J Clin Endocrinol* 38:476–479, 1974.

Henderson WR, Rowlands IW: Gonadotropic activity of anterior pituitary gland in relation to increased intracranial pressure. *Br Med J* 1:1094–1097, 1938.

Hendricks SE: Influence of neonatally administered hormone and early gonadectomy on rat's sexual behavior. *J Comp Physiol Psychol* 69:408–413, 1969.

Henneman DH: Effect of estrogen and growth hormone on collagen. *Excerpta Medica* (ICS) 273:1109–1114, 1973.

Hertenlendy F, Kipnis DM: Studies on growth hormone secretion. V. Influence of plasma free fatty acid levels. *Endocrinology* 92:410–420, 1973.

Hess GD, Riegle GD: Effects of chronic ACTH stimulation on adrenocortical function in young and aged rats. *Am J Physiol* 222:1458–1461, 1972.

Heuson JC, Legros N: Influence of insulin deprivation on growth of the 7,12-dimethylbenz(a)anthracene-induced mammary carcinoma in rats subjected to alloxan diabetes and food restriction. *Cancer Res* 32:226–232, 1972.

Hilf R, Goldenberg H, Michel L, et al: Enzymes, nucleic acids and lipids in human breast cancer and normal breast tissues. *Cancer Res* 30:1874–1882, 1970.

Himsworth HP, Kerr RB: Age and insulin sensitivity. *Clin Sci Mol Med* 4:153–157, 1939.

Hjermann I, Helgeland A, Holme I, et al: The intercorrelation of serum cholesterol, cigarette smoking and body weight. *Acta Med Scand* 200:479–487, 1976.

Ho YK, Brown MS, Bilhaimer DW, et al: Regulation of low density lipoprotein receptor activity in freshly isolated human lymphocytes. *J Clin Invest* 58:1465–1474, 1976a.

Ho YK, Brown MS, Keyden HJ, et al: Binding, internalization and hydrolysis of low density lipoprotein in long-term lymphoid cell lines from a normal subject and a patient with homozygous familial hypercholesterolemia. *J Exp Med* 144:444–455, 1976b.

Ho JR, Faust JR, Bilheimer DW, et al: Regulation of cholesterol biosynthesis by low density lipoproteins in isolated human lymphocytes. *J Exp Med* 145:1531–1549, 1977.

Hoffmann JC: Light and feedback control of gonadotropin secretion. *Excerpta Medica* (ICS) 273:886–890, 1973.

Hofman D, Soergel T: Untersuchungen über das Menarchen und Menopausenalter. *Geburtshilfe Frauenheilkd* 32:969–997, 1972.

Hofstatter L, Sonnenberg A, Kountz WB: The glucose tolerance in elderly patients, in Moore RA (ed): *Biological Symposium.* vol 11. Lancaster, Penn, The Jaques Cattell Press, 1945, pp 87–95.

Hohlweg W, Döhrn M: Beziehungen zwischen Hypophysenvorderlappen und Keimdrusen. *Wien Arch Inn Med* 21:337–350, 1931.

Holland OB, Gomez-Sanchez CE: Prolactin in hypertension. *Lancet* 2:1033, 1977.

Holley RW: A unifying hypothesis concerning the nature of malignant growth. *Proc Natl Acad Sci USA* 69:2840–2841, 1972.

Holley RW, Baldwin JH, Kiernan JA: Control of growth of a tumor cell by lipollic acid. *Proc Natl Acad Sci USA* 71:3976–3978, 1974.

Hollingsworth JW, Hashizume A, Jablon S: Correlation between tests of aging in Hiroshima subjects—an attempt to define "physiologic" age. *Yale J Biol Med* 38:11–26, 1965.

Hollinshead AC, McWright CG, Alfrod TC, et al: Separation of skin-reactive intestinal cancer antigen from the carcinoembryonic antigen of Gold. *Science* 177:887–889, 1972.

Horowitz SD, Borchording W, Bargman GJ: Suppressor T-cell function in diabetes mellitus. *Lancet* 2:1291, 1977.

Howard BV, Kritchevsky D: The lipids of human diploid (WI-38) and SV40-transformed human cells. *Int J Cancer* 4:393–402, 1969.

Hradec J: The role of cholesteryl 14-methylhexadecanoate in gene expression and its significance for cancer, in Carroll KK (ed): *Progress in Biochemical Pharmacology, Lipids and Tumors.* Basel, S Karger, 1975, pp 197–227.

Huang HH, Meites J: Reproductive capacity of aging female rats. *Neuroendocrinology* 17:289–295, 1975.

Humphries GMK, McConnell HM: Potent immunosuppression by oxidized cholesterol. *J Immunol* 122:121–126, 1979.

Hunter WM, Clarke BF, Duncan LJP: Plasma growth hormone after an overnight fast and following glucose loading in healthy and diabetic subjects. *Metabolism* 15:596–607, 1966.

Illei-Donhoffer A, Flerko B, Mess B: Reduction of estradiol-binding capacity of neural target tissues in light-sterilized rats. *Neuroendocrinology* 14:187–194, 1974.

Irvine, WJ, Clarke BF, Scarth L, et al: Thyroid and gastric autoimmunity in patients with diabetes mellitus. *Lancet* 2:163–168, 1970.

Isaacs AF, Havard CWH: Effect of piperazine oestrone sulphate on serum oestrogen and gonadotropin levels in postmenopausal women. *Clin Endocrinol* 9:297–302, 1978.

Jackson WPU: Present status of prediabetes. *Diabetes* 9:373-378, 1960.

Jackson WPU, Mieghen W, Keller P: Insulin excess as the initial lesion in diabetes. *Lancet* 1:1040-1041, 1972.

Jacobsson B, Holm V, Björntorp P, et al: Influence of cell size on the effects of insulin and noradrenaline on human adipose tissue. *Diabetologia* 12:69-72, 1976.

Jafarey NA, Yunns Khan M, Jafarey SN: Role of artificial lighting in decreasing the age of menarche. *Lancet* 2:471, 1970.

Jahnke K, Cries F, Engelhardt A, et al: Adaptive and genetically determined regulations of metabolism in obesity, in Rodriguez RR, Vallance-Owen J (eds): *Diabetes.* Amsterdam, Excerpta Medica, 1971, pp 507-516.

Jankovic BD, Janczic A, Popeskovic: Effect of neonatal epipectomy on humoral and cellular immune reactions in the rat. *Immunology* 28:597-609, 1975.

Jenner MR, Kelch RP, Kaplan SL, et al: Hormonal changes in puberty. IV. Plasma estradiol, LH and FSH in prepubertal children, pubertal females, and in precocious puberty, premature thelarche, hypogonadism, and in a child with a feminizing ovarian tumor. *J Clin Endocrinol* 34:521-530, 1972.

Jezkova Z, Pokorny J: The appearance of a wide variety of antibodies in atherosclerosis. *Angiologia,* 4:359-368, 1967.

Joffe BI, Vinik AI, Jackson WPU: Insulin reserve in elderly subjects. *Lancet* 1:1292-1293, 1969.

Johansen K: A new principle for the comparison of insulin secretory responses. *Acta Endocrinol* 74:511-523, 1973a.

Johansen K: A new principle for the comparison of insulin secretory responses. The effect of obesity on insulin secretion. *Acta Endocrin* 74:524-541, 1973b.

Johnson WM: Different weight response to the same provocation. *JAMA* 133:1238, 1947.

Jones EC, Krohn PL: The effect of hypophysectomy on age changes in the ovaries of mice. *J Endocrinol* 21:497-509, 1961.

Jones RJ: The hyperlipoproteinemias. *Med Clin North Am* 57:47-61, 1973.

Jose DG, Good RA: Immune resistance and malnutrition. *Lancet* 1:314, 1972.

Jose DG, Stutman O, Good RA: Long term effects of immune function of early nutritional deprivation. *Nature* 241:57-58, 1972.

Jouvet M: Biogenic amines and the states of sleep. *Science* 163:32-41, 1969.

Judd HL, Judd GE, Lucas WE, et al: Endocrine function of the postmenopausal ovary: concentration of androgens and estrogens in ovarian and peripheral vein blood. *J Clin Endocrinol Metab* 39:1020-1028, 1974.

Jung V, Khurana RC, Corredor DG, et al: Reactive hypoglycemia in women: results of a health survey. *Diabetes* 20:428-434, 1971.

Juret P, Couette, JE, Mandard AM, et al: Age of menarche as a prognostic factor in human breast cancer. *Eur J Cancer* 12:701-704, 1976.

Kahn CR: Membrane receptor for hormones and neurotransmitters. *J Cell Biol* 70:261-286, 1976.

Kalk WJ, Vinik AJ, Pimatone BL, et al: Growth hormone response to insulin hypoglycemia in the elderly. *J Gerontol* 28:431-433, 1973.

Kamberi IA: Biogenic amines and neurohumoral control of gonadotropin and prolactin secretion. *Excerpta Medica* (ICS) 273:112-119, 1973.

Kamberi IA, Mical RS, Porter JC: Effect of anterior pituitary perfusion and intraventricular injection of catecholamines and indolamines on LH release. *Endocrinology* 87:1-12, 1970.

Kamberi IA, Mical RS, Porter JC: Effect of anterior perfusion and intraventricular injection of catecholamines on FSH release. *Endocrinology* 88:1003–1011, 1971a.

Kamberi IA, Mical RS, Porter JC: Effect of anterior pituitary perfusion and intraventricular injection of catecholamines on prolactin release. *Endocrinology* 88:1012–1020, 1971b.

Kandutsch AA, Chen HW: Consequences of blocked sterol synthesis in cultured cells. *J Biol Chem* 252:409–415, 1977.

Kandutsch AA, Chen HW, Heiniger HJ: Biological activity of some oxygenated sterols. *Science* 201:498–501, 1978.

Kansal PC, Boshell BR, Bure J, et al: Hyperinsulinemic hypoglycemic effect of epinephrine suppression. *Horm Metab Res* 9:510–512, 1977.

Karess RE, Hayward WS, Hanafusa H: Cellular information in the genome of recovered avian sarcoma virus directs the synthesis of transforming protein. *Proc Natl Acad Sci USA* 76:3154–3158, 1979.

Kärki NT: The urinary excretion of noradrenaline and adrenaline in different age groups, its diurnal variation and the effect of muscular work on it. *Acta Physiol Scand* 39(suppl):7–96, 1956.

Kastin A, Schally AV: Autoregulation of release of melanocyte stimulating hormone from the rat pituitary. *Nature* 213:1238–1240, 1967.

Kavetsky RE: *Tumor and Organism.* Kiev, Meditsina, 1962.

Kelch RP, Kaplan SL, Grumbach MM: Suppression of urinary and plasma follicle-stimulation hormone by exogenous extrogens in prepubertal and pubertal children. *J Clin Invest* 52:1122–1128, 1973.

Kennedy GC, Mitra J: Body weight and food intake as initiating factors for puberty in the rat. *J Physiol* 166:408–418, 1963.

Kent S: Is diabetes a form of accelerated aging? *Geriatrics* 3:140–151, 1976.

Kent S: Can normal aging be explained by the immunological theory? *Geriatrics* 32:111–116, 1977.

Kershbaum A, Khorsandian R, Caplan RF, et al: The role of catecholamines in the free fatty acid response to cigarette smoking. *Circulation* 28:52–57, 1963.

Keys A, Brozek J: Body fat in adult man. *Physiol Rev* 33:245–325, 1953.

Keys A, Taylor HL, Crande F: Basal metabolism and age of adult man. *Metabolism* 22:579–587, 1973.

Kigoshi S, Ito R.: High levels of FFA in lymphoid cells with special reference to their cytotoxicity. *Experientia* 29:1408–1410, 1973.

Kigoshi S, Akiyama M: Change in levels of cholesterol and FFA of lymphoid cells during tumor growth. *Experientia* 31:1225–1227, 1975.

Kitay JI, Altschule MD: *The Pineal Gland: A Review of the Physiologic Literature.* Cambridge, Mass, Harvard University Press, 1954.

Kitay JI, Holub DA, Jailer JW: Inhibition of pituitary ACTH release: an extra-adrenal action of exogenous ACTH. *Endocrinology* 64:475–482, 1959.

Kledzik GS, Meites J: Reinitiation of estrous cycles in light-induced constant estrous female rats by drugs. *Proc Soc Exp Biol Med* 146:989–992, 1974.

Kleinberg DL, Noel GL, Frantz AG: Chlorpromazine stimulation and L-dopa suppression of plasma prolactin in man. *J Clin Endocrinol Metab* 33:873–876, 1971.

Klimek R: Obserwacje i wyniki leczenia galaktorhei za pocoma cyklopeptydowych hormonow. *Ginekol Pol* 39:1009–1014, 1968.

Klimek R: Enzyme determination of biological age of fetus. *Symposium of Criteria for Determination of Biological Age in Man* Leningrad, Nauka, 1974, p. 103, abst.

Klimov AN: Immunobiological mechanisms of atherosclerosis. *Summaries of Reports to the 34th Session of the General Meeting of the USSR AMS,* 1973.

Klotz HP, Jayle MF: L'hyperoestrogénurie post-ménopausique (ménopause naturelle et chirurgicale). *Ann Endocrinol* 12:931-937, 1951.

Knab DR: Estrogen and endometrial carcinoma. *Obstet Gynecol Surv* 32:267-281, 1977.

Knatterud GL, Meiner CL, Klimt ChR: Effects of hypoglycemic agents on vascular complications in patients with adult-onset diabetes. *JAMA* 217:777-784, 1971.

Knopp RH, Sondek CB, Arky RA, et al: Two phases of adipose tissue metabolism in pregnancy: maternal adaptations for fetal growth. *Endocrinology* 99:984-988, 1973.

Knudson AG: Mutation and cancer in man. *Cancer* 39:1882-1886, 1977.

Kondrashova MN, Evtodienko YV, Mironova GD, et al: The norm and pathology in the light of mitochondrial energy processes. *Biophysics of Complex Systems and Radiation Disorders.* Moscow, Nauka, 1977.

Korneva EA, Klimenko VM, Shinek EK: *Neuro-Humoral Provision of Immune Homeostasis.* Leningrad, Nauka, 1978.

Kovaleva IG, Vishnevsky AS, Dilman VM: Estrogens as inhibitors of the effect produced by the growth hormone on the free fatty acids mobilization. *Biull Eksp Biol Med* 10:53-55, 1964.

Kovaleva IG, Rischka IF, Dilman VM: Inhibition of lipolytic activity of human growth hormone with sheep prolactin derivative (anaprolactin). *Acta Endocrinol* 69:209-218, 1972.

Krieger DT: The central nervous system and Cushing's disease. *Med Clin North Am* 62:261-268, 1978.

Krieger DT, Allen WA, Rizzo F, et al: Characterization of the normal temporal pattern of plasma corticosteroid levels. *J Clin Endocrinol Metab* 32:266-284, 1971.

Krieger HP, Krieger DT: Chemical stimulation of the brain: effect on adrenal corticoid release. *Am J Physiol* 218:1632-1641, 1970.

Kritchevsky D: Diet and atherosclerosis. *Am J Pathol* 84:615-632, 1976.

Kroes R, Weiss JW, Weisburger JH: Immune suppression and chemical carcinogenesis, in Grundmann E, Gross R (eds): *The Ambivalence of Cytostatic Therapy.* Berlin, Springer-Verlag, 1975, pp 65-75.

Krug U, Krug F, Cuatrecasas P: Emergence of insulin receptors on human lymphocytes during in vitro transformation. *Proc Natl Acad Sci USA* 69:2604-2608, 1972.

Kruger GRF, Harris D: Is phenytoin carcinogenetic? *Lancet* 1:323, 1972.

Kulin HE, Reiter EO: Gonadotropin suppression by low dose estrogen in men: evidence for differential effects upon FSH and LH. *J Clin Endocrinol Metab* 35:836-839, 1972.

Kulin HE, Grumbach MM, Kaplan SL: Gonadal-hypothalamic interaction in prepubertal and pubertal man: effect of clomiphene citrate on urinary follicle-stimulating hormone and luteinizing hormone in plasma. *Pediatr Res* 6:162-171, 1972.

Kuo PT: Metabolic basis of human atherosclerosis. *Metabolism* 18:631-634, 1969.

Kushima K, Kamio K, Okuda V: Climacterium, climacteric disturbances on rejuvenation of sex center. *Tohoku J Exp Med* 74:113-129, 1961.

Laborit H: *Les Regulations Metaboliques.* Paris, Masson et cie, 1965.

Laborit H: Correlations between protein and serotonin synthesis during various activities of the central nervous system. *Res Commun Chem Pathol Pharmacol* 3:51-81, 1972.

Lamberts SWF, Temmermans HAT, De Jong FH, et al: The role of dopaminergic depletion in the pathogenesis of Cushing's disease: on the possible consequences for medical therapy. *Clin Endocrinol* 7:185–193, 1977.

Lancet: Aging and cancer, editorial. 1:131–132, 1976.

Lang VF: Arterial hypertension. Leningrad, Meditsina, 1950.

Lapin IP, Oxenkrug VF: Intensification of the central serotoninergic processes as a possible determinant of the thymoleptic effect. *Lancet* 1:132–136, 1969.

Lapin V: The pineal and neoplasia. *Lancet* 1:341, 1975.

Lapin V, Ebels F: Effects of some low molecular weight sheep pineal fractions and melatonin on different tumors in rats and mice. *Oncology* 33:101–148, 1976.

Laporte M, Astrue M, Tabacik C, et al: 3-hydroxy-3-methylglutaryl coenzyme A reductase of human lymphocytes: kinetic properties. *FEBS Lett* 86:225–229, 1978.

Larson LL, Spilman CH, Foote RH: Uterine uptake of progesterone and estradiol in young and aged rabbits. *Proc Soc Exp Biol Med* 141:463–466, 1972.

Lau AF, Krzyzek RA, Brugge JS, et al: Morphological revertants of an avian sarcoma virus-transformed mammalian cell line exhibit tumorigenicity and contain $pp60^{src}$. *Proc Natl Acad Sci USA* 76:3904–3908, 1979.

Laurell S: Turnover rate of unesterified fatty acids in human plasma. *Acta Physiol Scand* 41:158–167, 1972.

Lawrence AM, Goldfine ID, Kirsteins I: Growth hormone dynamics in acromegaly. *J Clin Endocrinol Metab* 31:239–247, 1970.

Lazarev AF, Izotov VK: Effect of antiserum to growth hormone on Croker's sarcoma. *Biull Eksp Biol Med* 9:99–101, 1965.

Lee PA, Juffe RB, Midyley AR: Serum gonadotropin, testosterone and prolactin concentrations through puberty in boys: a longitudinal study. *J Clin Endocrinol Metab* 39:664–672, 1974.

Ledet T: Growth hormone antiserum suppresses the growth effect of diabetic serum. *Diabetes* 26:798–803, 1977.

Lehman FP, McArthur DA, Hendrics SE: Pharmacological induction of ovulation in old and neonatally androgenized rats. *Exp Gerontol* 13:107–114, 1978.

Lémarchand-Béraud T, Scazziya BR, Vannotti A: Plasma thyrotropin levels in thyroid disease and effect of treatment. *Acta Endocrinol* 62:593–600, 1969.

Lender M, Lawrence AM, Paloyan J: Diabetes, autoimmune thyroid disease, and breast cancer. *Lancet* 1:1110, 1977.

Lentle BC, Thomas JP: Adrenal function and the complications of diabetes mellitus. *Lancet* 2:544–549, 1964.

Lewis BK, Wexler BC: Serum insulin changes in male rats associated with age and reproductive activity. *J Gerontol* 29:139–144, 1974.

Lewis BK, Wexler BC: Changes in LH and prolactin in arteriosclerotic female breeder rats. *Atherosclerosis* 21:301–314, 1975.

Liddle GW: Tests of pituitary-adrenal suppressibility in the diagnosis of Cushing's syndrome. *J Clin Endocrinol Metab* 20:1539–1560, 1960.

Lindholm F, Kenlet H, Blichert-Toft M, et al: Discrepancy between ACTH and cortisol responses to insulin induced hypoglycaemia. *Clin Endocrinol* 9:371–374, 1978.

Lints FA: Life span in *Drosophila. Gerontologia* 17:33–51, 1971.

Lints FA: Growth components, ageing and longevity. Presented at *XI International Congress of Gerontology,* vol 2. Tokyo, 1978, p 10, abst.

Lipschutz A: *Steroid Homeostasis, Hypophysis and Tumorigenesis.* Cambridge, England, Heffer & Sons Ltd, 1957.

Lipsett MB: Prospects in endocrinology for chemotherapy. *Cancer Res* 29:2408–2411, 1969.

Lipton A, Santen RJ: Medical adrenalectomy using aminoglutethimide and dexamethasone in advanced breast cancer. *Cancer* 33:503–512, 1974.

Llanos JME: Circadian rhythms in DNA, cell reproductions and growth hormone. Amsterdam, *Excerpta Medica* (ICS) 273:244–250, 1973.

Loeb H: Variations in glucose tolerance during infancy and childhood. *J Pediatr* 68:237–242, 1966.

Loffer FD: Decreased carbohydrate tolerance in pregnant patients with an early menarche. *Am J Obstet Gynecol* 123:180–184, 1975.

Londono H, Gallaher TF, Bray GA: Effect of weight reduction, triiodothyronine and diethylstilbestrol on growth hormone in obesity. *Metabolism* 18:986–992, 1969.

Louis LH, Conn JW: Diabetogenic polypeptide from animal pituitaries similar to that excreted by proteinuria of diabetic patients. *Metabolism* 21:1–9, 1972.

Lu KH, Meites J: Effect of serotonin precursors and melatonin on serum prolactin release in rats. *Endocrinology* 93:152–155, 1973.

Lu KH, Huang HH, Chen HT, et al: Positive feedback by estrogen and progesterone on LH release in old and young rats. *Proc Soc Exp Biol Med* 154:82–85, 1977.

Lucas WE: Causal relationships between endocrine-metabolic variables in patients with endometrial carcinoma. *Obstet Gynecol Surv* 29:507–528, 1974.

Lucke C, Glick SM: Effect of medroxyprogesterone acetate on the sleep induced peak of growth hormone secretion. *J Clin Endocrinol Metab* 33:851–853, 1971.

Lucke C, Glick SM: Experimental modification of the sleep-induced peak of growth hormone secretion. *J Clin Endocrinol Metab* 35:413–416, 1972.

Lucke C, Adelman N, Glick SM: The effect of elevated free fatty acids on the sleep-induced human growth hormone peak. *J Clin Endocrinol Metab* 35:407–412, 1972.

Luft R, Cerasi E: Human growth hormone in blood glucose homeostasis. Amsterdam, *Excerpta Medica* (ICS) 158:373–381, 1968.

Luft R, Guillemin R: Growth hormone and diabetes. *Diabetes* 23:783–787, 1974.

Luft R, Efendic S, Hökfelt T: Somatostatin—both hormone and neurotransmitter? *Diabetologia* 14:1–13, 1978a.

Luft R, Schmulling RM, Eggstein M: Lactic acidosis in biguanide-treated diabetics. *Diabetologia* 14:75–87, 1978b.

Lundbaek K: Abnormal growth hormone secretion as a causal factor in the development of basal membrane abnormalities. Amsterdam, *Excerpta Medica* (ICS) 273:1137–1143, 1973.

Lundbaek K, Johansen K, Orskov H, et al: Anxiety, growth hormone and glucose tolerance in normal children. *Acta Med Scand* 192:539–542, 1972.

Lupparello TJ, Stein M, Park CD: Effect of hypothalamic lesions on rat anaphylaxis. *Am J Physiol* 207:911–914, 1964.

MacCuish AC, Urbaniak SI, Campbell CJ, et al: Phytohemagglutinin transformation and circulating lymphocyte subpopulations in insulin-dependent diabetes. *Diabetes* 23:708–712, 1974.

MacDonald PC, Rombaut RP, Silteri PK: Plasma precursor of estrogen. I. Extent of conversion of plasma delta-4-androstenedione to estrone in normal males and nonpregnant, normal, castrate and adrenalectomized females. *J Clin Endocrinol Metab* 27:1103–1111, 1967.

Machlin LJ, Takahashi Y, Horino M, et al: Regulation of growth hormone secretion in non-primate species. *Excerpta Medica* (ICS) 158:245-305, 1968.

MacKay WD, Edwards MH, Bulbrook RD, et al: Relation between plasma-cortisol, plasma-androgen-sulphates and immune response in women with breast cancer. *Lancet* 2:1001-1002, 1971.

MacKay IR, Whittingham SF, Mathews JD: The immunoepidemiology of aging, in Makinodan T, Yunis E (eds): *Immunology and Aging*. New York, Plenum Publishing Corporation, 1977, pp 35-50.

Makinodan T: Immunity and aging, in Birren JE (ed): *Handbook of the Biology of Aging*. New York, Van Nostrand Reinhold Company, 1977.

Makinodan T: Mechanism of senescence of immune response. *Fed Proc* 37:1239-1241, 1978.

Marble A: Definition and criteria of the prediabetic state, in Ostman J (ed). *Diabetes,* Ambsterdam, Excerpta Medica, 1964, pp 473-475.

Marmorston J, Weiner JM, Hopkins L, et al: Abnormalities in urinary hormone patterns in lung cancer and emphysema. *Cancer* 19:985-995, 1966.

Marquie G, Agid R, Amiel S: Evolution of the activity of several endocrine glands in cholesterol fed rabbits. *Ann Endocrinol* 34:271 – 282, 1973.

Martin JB: Neural regulation of growth hormone secretion. *N Engl J Med* 288:1384-1393, 1973.

Mass JW: Biogenic amines and depression. *Arch Gen Psychiatry* 32:1357-1365, 1965.

Mathews JD, Freery RJ: Cholesterol and immune response to influence of antigens. *Lancet* 2:1212-1213, 1978.

Mayer J: Metabolism of adipose tissue in experimental obesity, in Renold AE, Cahill GF (eds): *Handbook of Physiology, Sec. 5, Adipose Tissue.* Washington, American Physiological Society, 1965, pp 645-651.

Mayer J, Arees EA: Ventromedial hypothalamic region concerned with food intake. *Excerpta Medica* (ICS) 213:210-213, 1970.

McCann SM, Kalra PS, Kalra SP, et al: Control of adenohypophyseal secretion by hypothalamic releasing and inhibiting neurohormones. *Excerpta Medica* (ICS) 273:107-111, 1973.

McClain DA, Maness PF, Edelman GM: Assay for early cytoplasmic effects of the src gene product of Rous sarcoma virus. *Proc Natl Acad Sci USA* 75:2750-2754, 1978.

McMahon B, Cole P, Brown J: Etiology of human breast cancer: a review. *JNCI* 50:21-42, 1973.

McPherson JC, Costoff A, Mahesh VB: Effect of aging on the hypothalamic-hypophyseal-gonadal axis in female rats. *Fertil Steril* 28:1365-1370, 1977.

Meade CJ, Mertin J: Fatty acids and immunity. *Adv Lipid Res* 16:127-166, 1978.

Medawar PB: *An Unsolved Problem of Biology*. London, HK Lewis, 1952.

Meier-Ruge W: Experimental pathology and pharmacology in brain research and aging. *Life Sci* 17:1617-1636, 1975.

Meites F: Control of prolactin secretion in animals, in Pasteels JL, Robyn C (eds): *International Symposium on Human Prolactin*. Amsterdam, *Excerpta Medica,* 1973, pp 105-118.

Meites F, Lu KH, Wuttke W, et al: Recent studies on functions and control of prolactin secretion in rats. *Recent Prog Horm Res* 28:471-526, 1972.

Meites F, Huang HH, Simpkins FW: Recent studies on neuroendocrine control of reproductive senescence in rats, in Schneider EL (ed): *The Aging Reproductive System*. New York, Raven Press, 1978, pp 213-235.

Mendelson WD, Sitaram N, Wyatt RJ, et al: Methscopolamine inhibition of sleep-related growth hormone secretion: evidence for a cholinergic secretory mechanism. *J Clin Invest* 61:1683–1690, 1978.

Menon S, Smith PA, White RWR, et al: Diurnal variations of fibrinolytic activity and plasma 11-hydroxycorticosteroid levels. *Lancet* 2:531–532, 1967.

Merimee TJ, Fineberg SE: Dietary regulation of human growth hormone secretion. *Metabolism* 22:1491–1497, 1973.

Merimee TJ, Fineberg SE: Growth hormone secretion in starvation: a reassessment. *J Clin Endocrinol* 39:385–386, 1974.

Merimee TJ, Felig Ph, Marliss E, et al: Glucose and lipid homeostasis in the absence of human growth hormone. *J Clin Invest* 50:574–582, 1971.

Merimee TJ, Hollander W, Fineberg SE: Studies of hyperlipidemia in the HGH-deficient state. *Metabolism* 21:1053–1061, 1972.

Merimee TJ, Fineberg SE, Hollander W: Vascular disease in the chronic human growth hormone-deficient states. *Diabetes* 22:813–819, 1973.

Mertin J, Hughes D: Specific inhibitory action of polyunsaturated fatty acids on lymphocyte transformation induced by PHA and PPD. *Int Arch Allergy Appl Immunol* 48:203–210, 1975.

Mertin J, Hunt R: Influence of polyunsaturated fatty acids on survival skin allografts and tumor incidence in mice. *Proc Natl Acad Sci USA* 73:928–931, 1976.

Mertin J, Meade CJ: Relevance of fatty acids in multiple sclerosis. *Br Med Bull* 33:67–71, 1977.

Mertin J, Stackpoole A: Suppression by essential fatty acids of experimental allergic encephalomyelitis is abolished by indomethacin. *Prostaglandins Med* 1:283–292, 1978.

Metz R, Surmaczynska B, Berger S, et al: Glucose tolerance, plasma insulin, and free fatty acids in elderly subjects. *Ann Intern Med* 64:1042–1048, 1966.

Miettinen TA: Cholesterol production in obesity. *Circulation* 44:842–850, 1971.

Miettinen TA: Mechanism of hyperlipidemias in different clinical conditions. *Adv Card,* vol 8. Basel: Karger, 1973, pp. 85–99.

Mikhall MN, Guiggis FK, Abdel-Hai MM, et al: Lipid metabolism in prediabetics. *Atherosclerosis* 16:51–60, 1972.

Milcu SM, Pavel S, Neascu C: Biological and chromatographic characterization of a polypeptide with pressor and oxytocic activity isolated from the bovine pineal gland. *Endocrinology* 72:563–566, 1963.

Miller DL, Hanson W, Schede HP, et al: Proliferation rate and transport time of mucosal cells in small intestine of the diabetic rat. *Gastroenterology* 73:1326–1332, 1977a.

Miller NE, Weistein DE, Carew T, et al: Interaction between high density and low density lipoproteins during uptake and degradation of cultured human fibroblasts. *J Clin Invest* 60:78–88, 1977b.

Mills TM, Mahesh VB: Pituitary function in aging men and women, in Greenblatt RB (ed): *Geriatric Endocrinology,* vol 5. New York, Raven Press, 1978, pp 1–12.

Mitchell FL, Pearson J, Strauss WT: Plasma lipids and glucose in normal health, diabetes and cardiovascular disease. *Diabetologia* 4:105–108, 1968.

Mitchell ML, Raben MS, Ernesti M: Use of growth hormone as a diabetic stimulus in man. *Diabetes* 19:196–199, 1970.

Mitra J, Hayward JL: Hypothalamic-pituitary-thyroid axis in breast cancer. *Lancet* 1:885–888, 1974.

Mitra J, Perrin J, Kumaoka S: Thyroid and other autoantibodies in British and Japanese women: an epidemiological study of breast cancer. *Br Med J* 1:257–260, 1976.

Mjøs OD, Thelle DS, Førde OH, et al: Family study of high density lipoprotein cholesterol and the relation to age and sex. *Acta Med Scand* 201:323–329, 1977.

Mølsted-Pedersen L: Aspects of carbohydrate metabolism in newborn infants of diabetic mothers. *Acta Endocrinol* 79:174–188, 1972.

Monroe SE, Jaffe RE, Midgley AR: Regulation of human gonadotropins. III. Increase in serum gonadotropins in response to estradiol. *J Clin Endocrinol Metab* 31:342–347, 1972.

Morell B, Froesch ER: Fibroblasts as an experimental tool in metabolic and hormone studies. II. Effects of insulin and nonsuppressible insulin-like activity (NSILA-S) on fibroblasts in culture. *Eur J Clin Invest* 3:119–123, 1973.

Morgan WW, Rudden PK, Pfeil KA: Effect of immobilization stress on serotonin content and turnover in regions of the rat brain. *Life Sci* 17:143–150, 1975.

Moroz BB, Kendych IN: *Radiobiological Factors and Endocrine System.* Moscow, Atomizdat, 1975.

Morozov VG, Khavinson VH: Effect of hypothalamic and pineal extracts on certain functions of the organism. *Proc Scient Conf Cadets SM Kirov Millitary Medical Academy,* Leningrad, 1971, p 127, abst.

Mougdal NR, Jagannadha RA, Maneckjee R, et al: Gonadotropins and their antibodies. *Recent Prog Horm Res* 30:47–77, 1974.

Mueller PS, Watkin DM: Plasma unesterified fatty acid concentrations in neoplastic diseases. *J Lab Clin Med* 57:95–108, 1961.

Muggeo M, Fedele D, Tiengo A, et al: Human growth hormone and cortisol response to insulin stimulation in aging. *J Gerontol* 30:546–555, 1975.

Müller EE: Nervous control of growth hormone secretion. *Neuroendocrinology* 11:338–369, 1973.

Müller EE, Cocchi D, Villa A: Involvement of brain catecholamines in the gonadotropins-releasing mechanism(s) before puberty. *Endocrinology* 90:1267–1276, 1972.

Müller EE, Nistricò G, Scapagnini U: *Neurotransmitters and Anterior Pituitary Function.* New York, Academic Press, 1977.

Munkres KD, Minssen M: Aging of *Neurospora crassa.* 1. Evidence for the free radical theory of aging from studies of a natural-death mutant. *Mech Ageing Dev* 5:79–98, 1976.

Muntoni S: Inhibition of fatty acid oxidation by biguanides: implication for metabolic physiopathology. *Adv Lipid Res* 12:311–377, 1974.

Nakagawa K, Mashimo K: Suppressibility of plasma growth hormone levels in acromegaly with dexamethasone and phentolamine. *J Clin Endocrinol Metab* 37:238–246, 1973.

Naor D, Bonovida B, Walford RL: Autoimmunity and aging: the age-related response to mice of a long-lived strain to trinitrophenylated synergic mouse red blood cells. *J Immunol* 117:2204–2208, 1976.

Napalkov NP: Blastogenic action of thyreostatic substances, in Kholdin SA (ed): *Modern Problems of Oncology.* Leningrad, Meditsina, 1965, pp 34–43.

Napalkov NP, Alexandrov VA: The study of antenatal and postnatal carcinogen and its role in cancer prevention. *Environment Aspects of Tumor Prevention,* All-union symposium, Leningrad, 1978, pp 44–50.

Neckers L, Sze PJ: Regulation of 5-hydroxytryptamine metabolism in mouse brain by adrenal glucocorticoids. *Brain Res* 93:123–132, 1975.

Nelson JF, Latham KR, Finch CE: Plasma testosterone levels in C57Bl/67 male mice: effect of age and disease. *Acta Endocrinol* 80:744–752, 1975.

Nemirovsky VB, Ostroumova MN, Blagosklonnaya JV, et al: Improvement of functional-morphological parameters of mononuclear blood cells produced by clofibrate treatment. *Vopr Onkol* 24:65–68, 1978.

Nervi FD, Dietschy JM: The mechanisms of and the interrelationships between bile acids and chylomicron-mediated regulation of hepatic cholesterol synthesis in the liver of the rat. *J Clin Invest* 61:895–909, 1978.

Nestel PJ, Whyte HM: Plasma free fatty acid and triglyceride turnover in obesity. *Metabolism* 17:1122–1128, 1968.

Netter A, Lambert A: Étude hormonale preliminare de la premenopause, in Bernard I, Kollenc M, Audebert A (eds): *La Menopause—Colloque Internationale de Biarritz de College de Gynecologie de Bordeaux et du Sud Quest.* Paris, Imprimerie E Drouillard, 1975, pp 28–37.

Newsholme EA: Mechanism for starvation suppression and refeeding activation of infection. *Lancet* 1:654, 1977.

Ng KY, Chase TN, Golburn RW, et al: L-dopa induced release of cerebral monoamines. *Science* 170:76–77, 1970.

Niehans CE, Nicocle A, Wootton R, et al: Influence of lipid concentrations and age on transfer of plasma lipoprotein into human arterial intima. *Lancet* 2:469–470, 1977.

Nigro ND, Campbell RL, Gantt TS, et al: A comparison of the effects of the hypocholesterolemic agents, cholestyramine and candicidin, on the induction of intestinal tumors in rats by azoxymethane. *Cancer Res* 37:3198–3203, 1977.

Nikkilä EA, Kastl M, Ehnholma Ch, et al: Increase of serum high-density lipoproteins in phenytoin users. *Br Med J* 2:99–100, 1978.

Nisticò G, Scapagnini U, Preziosi P: Metabolic changes in depression. *Lancet* 2:159, 1969.

Noel GL, Suh HK, Stone JG, et al: Human prolactin and growth hormone release during surgery and other conditions of stress. *J Clin Endocrinol Metab* 35:840–851, 1972.

Novak LP: Aging, total body potassium, fat-free mass, and cell mass in males and females between ages 18 and 85 years. *J Gerontol* 27:438–443, 1972.

O'Brien JR, Etherington M, Jamieson S: Acute platelet changes after large meals of saturated and unsaturated fats. *Lancet* 1:878–880, 1976.

O'Conner PJ, Skinner LG: The effect of chronic diethylstilbestrol administration and subsequent withdrawal on pituitary gonadotropin excretion in patients with mamary carcinoma. *Acta Endocrol* 45:623–630, 1964.

O'Hanlon JTJ, Campusano HC, Horvath SM: A fluorimetric assay for subnanogram concentrations of adrenaline (A) and noradrenaline (Na) in plasma. *Anal Biochem* 34:568–581, 1970.

Okada F, Saito Y, Fujieda T, et al: Monoamine changes in the brain of rats injected with L-5-hydroxytryptophan. *Nature* 238:355–356, 1972.

Okuno A, Niskimura Y, Kawarazaky T: Changes in plasma 11-hydroxycorticosteroids after ACTH, insulin and dexamethasone in neonatal infants. *J Clin Endocrinol Metab* 34:516–520, 1972.

Olefsky JM: Mechanism of decreased insulin responsiveness of large adipocytes. *Endocrinology* 100:1169–1177, 1977.

Olefsky JM, Reaven VM: Insulin binding to monocytes and total mononuclear leukocytes from normal and diabetic patients. *J Clin Endocrinol Metab* 43:226–228, 1976.

Olefsky JM, Bacon VC, Baur S: Insulin receptors of skeletal muscle: specific insulin binding sites and demonstration of decreased numbers of sites in obese rats. *Metabolism* 25:179–191, 1976.

Oliver MF: Reduction of serum lipid and uric acid levels by an orally active androsterone. *Lancet* 1:1321–1323, 1962.

Oliver MF, Boyd GS: The influence of sex hormones on the circulating lipids and lipoproteins in coronary sclerosis. *Circulation* 13:82–91, 1956.

Olpe, HP, McEwen BS: Glucocorticoid binding to receptor-like proteins in rat brain and pituitary: ontogenetic and experimentally induced changes. *Brain Res* 105:121–128, 1976.

O'Reilly MV, MacDonald RT: Efficacy of phenytoin in the management of ventricular arrhythmias induced by hypokalemia. *Br Heart J* 55:631–634, 1973.

Orgel LE: The maintenance of the accuracy of protein synthesis and its relevance to aging. *Proc Natl Acad Sci USA* 49:517–521, 1963.

Orts RJ, Benson B, Cook BF: LH inhibitory properties of aqueous extracts of rat pineal glands. *Life Sci* 14:1501–1510, 1974.

Östman J, Backman L, Hallbery D: Cell size and lipolysis by human subcutaneous adipose tissue. *Acta Med Scand* 193:469–475, 1973.

Ostroumova MN: The peculiarities of chemical content of gonadotropin residue in cancer of body uteri. *Vopr Onkol* 16:76–80, 1970.

Ostroumova MN: Decrease of excretion of antigonadotropic factor in endometrial and breast cancer patients. *Vopr Onkol* 18:38–41, 1972.

Ostroumova MN: Age-associated decrease in hypothalamic-pituitary complex sensitivity to dexamethasone suppression test. The effect of stress, epithalamin and phenformin. *Probl Endokrinol* 24:59–64, 1978.

Ostroumova MN, Dilman VM: The influence of the pineal extract on the threshold of hypothalamic sensitivity to prednisolone suppression. *Vopr Onkol* 18:53–55, 1972.

Ostroumova MN, Vasiljeva IA: Effect of polypeptide pineal extract on fat-carbohydrate metabolism. *Probl Endokrinol* 22:66–69, 1976.

Ostroumova MN, Tsyrlina EV, Nuller JL, et al: Age-associated shift of homeostatic regulation in adaptive homeostat and age-associated pathology. *Hum Physiol* 4:629–635, 1978.

O'Sullivan JB, Mahan CM, Freelender AE, et al: Effect of age on carbohydrate metabolism. *J Clin Endocrinol Metab* 33:619–623, 1971.

Panksepp J, Reilly P: Medial and lateral hypothalamic oxygen consumption as a function of age, starvation and glucose administration in rats. *Brain Res* 94:133–140, 1975.

Parker DC, Rossman LG: Human growth hormone release in sleep, nonsuppression by acute hyperglycemia. *J Clin Endocrinol Metab* 32:65–69, 1971.

Parsons WB: Reduction of hepatic synthesis of cholesterol from ^{14}C-acetate in hypercholesterolemic patients by nicotinic acid. *Circulation* 24:1099–1100, 1961.

Passa P, Gauville C, Caniver J: Influence of muscular exercise on plasma level of growth hormone in diabetics with and without retinopathy. *Lancet* 2:72–74, 1974.

Peckham WD, Yamaji T, Dierschke DJ, et al: Gonadal function and the biological and physiochemical properties of follicle-stimulating hormone. *Endocrinology* 92:1660–1666, 1973.

Pedersen J, Mølsted-Pedersen L: The hyperglycemia-hypersulinism theory and the weight of the newborn baby, in Rodriquez RR, Vallance-Owen J (eds): *Diabetes.* Amsterdam, Excerpta Medica, 1971, pp 678–685.

Pelham RW, Vaughan GM, Sandock KL, et al: Twenty-four hour cycle of a melantonin-like substance in the plasma of human males. *J Clin Endocrinol Metab* 37:341–344, 1973.

Peng Ming-Tsung, Peng Ya-Mei: Changes in the uptake of tritiated estradiol in the hypothalamus and adenohypophysis of old female rats. *Fertil Steril* 24:534–539, 1973.

Peracchi M, Reschini E, Cantalamessa L, et al: Effect of somatostatin on blood glucose, plasma GH, insulin, and FFA in normal subjects and acromegalic patients. *Metabolism* 23:1099–1115, 1974.

Peto R, Roe FJC, Lee PN, et al: Cancer and ageing in mice and men. *Br J Cancer* 32:411–426, 1975.

Petrusz P, Nagy E: On the mechanism of sexual differentiation of the hypothalamus: decreased hypothalamic estrogen sensitivity in androgen-sterilized female rats. *Acta Biol Acad Sci Hung* 18:21–26, 1967.

Pfeiffer EF: Recognized diabetogenic hormones and diabetes in man, in Neibel BS, Wrenshall GA (eds): *On the Nature and Treatment of Diabetes.* Amsterdam, Excerpta Medica, 1965, pp 368–386.

Pfeiffer EF: Does diabetes begin with insulin resistance? in Camerini-Dávolos RA, Cole HS (eds): *Early Diabetes.* New York, Academic Press, 1970, pp 146–153.

Philipott JR, Cooper AG, Wallach DFH: Regulation of cholesterol biosynthesis by normal and leukemic (L_2C) guinea pig lymphocytes. *Proc Natl Acad Sci USA* 74:956–960, 1977.

Piacsek BE, Streur JJ: Effect of exposure to continuous light on estrogen-induced precocious sexual maturation in female rats. *Neuroendocrinology* 18:86–91, 1975.

Pick R, Stamler K, Rodbard S, et al: The inhibition of coronary atherosclerosis by estrogens in cholesterol-fed chicks. *Circulation* 6:276–280, 1952.

Pierpaoli W: Changes of hormonal status in young mice by restricted caloric diet. Relation to life span extension: preliminary results. *Experientia* 33:1612–1613, 1977.

Pierpaoli W, Sorkin E: Immunological blockade of adenohypophysis and its possible application in prophylaxis and therapy of neoplasia. *Experientia* 28:336–339, 1972.

Pierpaoli W, Besedovsky HO: Role of the thymus in programming of neuroendocrine function. *Clin Exp Immunol* 20:323–338, 1975.

Pierpaoli W, Fabris N, Sorkin E: Developmental hormones and immunological maturation. *Ciba Found Symp* 36:126–143, 1970.

Pierpaoli W, Kopp HG, Bianchi E: Interdependence of thymic and neuroendocrine functions in ontogeny. *Clin Exp Immunol* 24:501–506, 1976.

Pisciotta AV, Westring DW, DePrey C, et al: Mitogenic effect of PHA at different ages. *Nature* 215:193–194, 1967.

Pitis M, Milea E, Simionescu L, et al: Growth hormone secretion after insulin-induced hypoglycemia in the aged. *Rev Roum d'Endocr* 10:59–61, 1973.

Pitot HC: Carcinogenesis and aging—two related phenomena. (Review article) *Am J Pathol* 87:444–472, 1977.

Poortman J, Thijssen JHH, Schwarz F: Androgen production and conversion to estrogens in normal postmenopausal women and in selected breast cancer patients. *J Clin Endocrinol Metab* 37:101–109, 1973.

Postnov, YV: On some problems of pathogenesis of chronic arterial hypertony. *Arkh Patol* 7:3–9, 1973.

Post RH, Arbor A: Early menarchial age of diabetic women. *Diabetes* 11:287–290, 1962.

Pozefsky T, Colker JL, Langs MM, et al: The cortisone-glucose tolerance test: the influence of age on performance. *Ann Intern Med* 63:989–997, 1965.

Premachandra BN: Biochemical and pathophysiological observations in active thyroid immunity, in *Recent Advances in Endocrinology.* Amsterdam, Excerpta Medica, 1971, pp 102–120.

Presl J, Herzmann J, Röhling S, et al: Developmental changes in regional distribution of estrogenic metabolites in the female rat hypothalamus. *Endocrinol Exper* 7:189–192, 1973.

Procopè BJ: Studies on the urinary excretion, biological effects and origin of estrogens in postmenopausal women. *Acta Endocrinol* 60(suppl):1–110, 1969.

Pyke DA: Parting and the incidence of diabetes. *Lancet* 1:818–820, 1956.

Pyoräla K, Pyoräla T: Glucose tolerance, plasma insulin and lipids in postmenopausal women during oestradiol-valerate treatment. *Diabetologia* 7:402–403, 1971, abst.

Quabbe HJ, Ramek W, Luyckx AS: Growth hormone, glucagon and insulin response to depression of plasma FFA and the effect of glucose infusion. *J Clin Endocrinol Metab* 44:383–391, 1977.

Quadri SK, Kledzik GS, Meites J: Reinitiation of estrous cycles in old constant-estrous rats by central-acting drugs. *Neuroendocrinology* 11:248–255, 1973.

Quay WB: Pineal homeostatic regulation of shifts in the circadian activity rhythm during maturation and aging. *Ann NY Acad Sci* 34:239–254, 1972.

Rabinowitz D: Some endocrine and metabolic aspects of obesity. *Annu Rev Med* 21:241–258, 1970.

Rabinowitz D, Merimee T, Nelson JK, et al: Insulin release in states of growth hormone excess and deficiency. *Excerpta Medica* (ICS) 140:122, 1967, abst.

Rakoff AE, Nowroozi K: The female climacteric, in Greenblatt RB (ed): *Geriatric Endocrinology,* vol 5. New York, Raven Press, 1978, pp 165–190.

Rakoff JS, Rigg LA, Yen, SSC: The impairment of progesterone-induced pituitary release of prolactin and gonadotropin in patients with hypothalamic chronic anovulation. *Am J Obstet Gynecol* 130:807–812, 1978.

Ramaley IA: Effects of dexamethasone before and after puberty on the daily corticosterone rhythm. *Neuroendocrinology* 17:203–210, 1975.

Ramirez VD, McCann SM: Comparison of the regulation of luteinizing hormone secretion in immature and adult rats. *Endocrinology* 72:452–464, 1963.

Randle PJ: The glucose fatty acid cycle, in Leibel BS, Wrenshall GA (eds): *On the Nature and Treatment of Diabetes.* Amsterdam, Excerpta Medica, 1965, pp 361–367.

Rao LGS: Lung cancer as an endocrine disease. *Nature* 235:220–222, 1972.

Rasmussen H: Organization and control of endocrine system, in Williams RH (ed): *Textbook of Endocrinology.* Philadelphia, WB Saunders Co, 1968, pp 2–30.

Ratzmann KP: In vitro untersuchungen zur Mobilisation frier fettsäuren aus dem Fettwebs. *Z Gesamte Inn Med* 28:677–680, 1973.

Ray PD, Hanson RL, Lardy HA: Inhibition by hydrazine of gluconeogenesis in the rat. *J Biol Chem* 245:690–696, 1970.

Reaven GM, Olefsky JM: The role of insulin resistance in the pathogenesis of diabetes mellitus, in Levine R, Luft R (eds): *Advances in Metabolic Disorders,* vol 9, no. 4. New York, Academic Press, 1978, pp 313–331.

Reaven GM, Lerner RL, Stern MO, et al: Role of insulin in endogenous hypertriglyceridemia. *J Clin Invest* 46:1756–1767, 1967.

Reaven GM, Olefsky J, Farquhar JW: Does hyperglycemia or hyperinsulinemia characterize the patients with chemical diabetes? *Lancet* 1:1247–1249, 1972.

Rechless JPD, Weinstein DB, Steinberg D: Lipoproteins and cholesterol metabolism in rabbit arterial endothelial cells in culture. *Biochim Biophys Acta* 529:475–487, 1978.

Reddy BS, Mastromarino A, Wynder E: Diet and metabolism: large bowel cancer. *Cancer* 39:1815–1819, 1977.

Reichlin S, Siperstein R, Jackson IM, et al: Hypothalamic hormones. *Annu Rev Physiol* 38:389–424, 1976.

Riegle GD: Chronic stress effects on adrenocortical responsiveness in young and aged rats. *Neuroendocrinology* 11:1–10, 1973.

Riegle GD: Aging and adrenocortical function, in Everitt AV, Burgers JA (eds): *Hypothalamus Pituitary and Aging.* Springfield, Ill, Charles C Thomas, 1976, pp 547–552.

Riley V, Spackman D, McClanahan, et al: The role of stress in malignancy. *Third International Symposium on Detection and Prevention of Cancer,* Seattle, 1976, p 39 (abst).

Robertson OH, Wexler BC: Histological changes in the organs and tissues of senile castrated Kokance salmon *(Oncorhynchus nerka Rennerlyi). Gen Comp Endocrinol* 2:458–472, 1962.

Robertson RP, Smith PH: Inhibition of triglyceride secretion by stress in *Psammomys obesus. Diabetes* 24(suppl):441, 1975, abst.

Robertson OH, Krupp MA, Thomas SF, et al: Hyperadrenocorticism in spawning migratory and non-migratory Rainbow trout *(Salmo gairdnerii);* comparison with Pacific salmon *(genus Oncorhynchus). Gen Comp Endocrinol* 1:473–484, 1961a.

Robertson OH, Wexler BC, Miller BF: Degenerative changes in the cardiovascular system of the spawning Pacific salmon. *Circulat Res* 9:826–834, 1961b.

Robinson DS: Changes in monoamine oxidase and monoamines with human development and aging. *Fed Proc* 34:103–107, 1975.

Robinson DS, Nies A, Davis JN, et al: Aging, monoamines and monoamine oxidase levels. *Lancet* 1:290–291, 1972.

Robinson DS, Sourkes TL, Nies A, et al: Monoamine metabolism in human brain. *Arch Gen Psychiatry* 34:89–92, 1977.

Rodin AE: The growth and spread of Walker 256 carcinoma in pinealectomized rats. *Cancer Res* 23:1545–1548, 1963.

Rodriguez JL, Ghiselli GC, Torreggiani D, et al: Very low density lipoproteins in normal and cholesterol-fed rabbits: lipid and protein composition and metabolism. Part 1. Chemical composition of very low density lipoprotein in rabbits. *Atherosclerosis* 23:73–83, 1976.

Rönnemaa T, Lentonen A, Tammi M, et al: Running, HDL-cholesterol, and atherosclerosis. *Lancet* 2:1261–1262, 1978.

Root AW, Oski FA: Effects of human growth hormone in elderly males. *J Gerontol* 24:97–104, 1969.

Ross GT, Cargille C, Lipsett M, et al: Pituitary and gonadal hormones in women during spontaneous and induced ovulatory cycles. *Recent Prog Horm Res* 26:1–26, 1970.

Roth GS, Livingston JN: Reduction in glucocorticoid inhibition of glucose oxidation and presumptive glucocorticoid receptor content in rat adipocytes during aging. *Endocrinology* 99:831–839, 1976.

Roth GS, Chang WC, Gesell MS: Hormone receptor and responsiveness changes during aging. *Eleventh International Congress of Gerontology.* Tokyo, 1978a, vol 2, p 18–19, abst.

Roth GS, Schocken DD, Spurgeon HA, et al: The cell membrane and control of hormone action during senescence. *Eleventh International Congress of Gerontology.* Tokyo, 1978b, vol 2, p 15–16, abst.

Roth J, Kahn CR, Lesniak MA, et al: Receptors for insulin, NSILA-S, and growth hormone: applications to disease states in man. *Recent Prog Horm Res* 31:95–139, 1975.

Rothfeld B, Pare WP, Margolis S, et al: Effect of glucagon and stress on cholesterol metabolism and deposition in tissues. *Biochem Med* 11:189–193, 1974.

Ruderman NB, Toews CJ, Shafrir E: Role of free fatty acids in glucose homeostasis. *Arch Intern Med* 123:299–313, 1969.

Rust CC, Meyer RK: Effect of pituitary autografts on hair color in the short tailed weasel. *Gen Comp Endocrinol* 51:548–551, 1968.

Rutherford RB, Ross R: Platelet factors stimulate fibroblasts and smooth muscle cells quiescent in plasma serum to proliferate. *J Cell Biol* 69:196–203, 1976.

Ryan KJ, Naftolin F, Reddy V, et al: Estrogen formation in the brain. *Am J Obstet Gynecol* 114:454–459, 1972.

Sachar EJ: Hormonal changes in stress and mental illness. *Hosp Pract* 10:49–55, 1975.

Sachar EJ, Finkelstein J, Hellman L: Growth hormone responses in depressive illness. *Arch Gen Psychiatry* 25:263–269, 1971.

Saez S: Corticotropin secretion in relation to breast cancer, in Stoll BA (ed): *Mammary Cancer and Neuroendocrine Therapy.* London, Butterworth & Co, 1974, pp 101–122.

Saez S, Martin PM, Chouvet CD: Estradiol and progesterone receptor levels in human breast adenocarcinoma in relation to plasma estrogen and progesterone levels. *Cancer Res* 38:3468–3473, 1978.

Sakuma M, Knobil E: Inhibition of endogenous growth hormone secretion by exogeneus growth hormone infusion in the Rhesus monkey. *Endocrinology* 86:890–894, 1970.

Saller CF, Stricker EM: Hyperphagia and increased growth in rats after intraventricular injection of 5,7-dihydroxytryptamine. *Science* 192:385–387, 1976.

Samaan N, Pearson OH, Gonzalez D, et al: Paradoxical secretion of growth hormone in patients with breast cancer. *J Lab Clin Med* 68:1011 (abst), 1966.

Samorajski T: Central neurotransmitter substances and aging: a review. *J Am Geriatr Soc* 25:337–348, 1977.

Sandberg H, Yoshimine N, Maeda S, et al: Effects of an oral glucose load on serum immunoreactive insulin, free fatty acid, growth hormone and blood sugar levels in young and elderly subjects. *J Am Geriatr Soc* 21:433–439, 1973.

Sassin JF, Parker DC, Mace JW, et al: Human growth hormone release: relation to slow-wave sleep and sleep-walking cycles. *Science* 165:513–515, 1969.

Scapagnini U, Annuziato L, Preziosi P: Role of brain norepinephrine in stress regulation, in Nemeth S (ed): *Hormones, Metabolism and Stress.* Bratislava, Slovak Academy of Science, 1973, pp 25–41.

Schafer EJ, Eisenberg SH, Levy RI: Lipoprotein apoprotein metabolism. *J Lipid Res* 19:667–687, 1978a.

Schafer EJ, Levy RI, Anderson DW, et al: Plasma triglycerides in regulation to HDL-cholesterol levels. *Lancet* 2:391–393, 1978b.

Schally AV, Arimura A, Bowers CJ, et al: Hypothalamic neurohormones regulating anterior pituitary function. *Recent Prog Horm Res* 24:497–588, 1968.

Schally AV, Kastin AJ, Arimura A: The hypothalamus and reproduction. *Am J Obstet Gynecol.* 114:423–442, 1972.

Schildkraut JJ: The catecholamine hypothesis of affective disorders: a review of supporting evidence. *Am J Psychiatry* 122:509–522, 1965.

Schilling FJ, Christokis GJ, Bennett J, et al: Studies of serum cholesterol in 4244 men and women. *Am J Public Health* 54:461–474, 1964.

Schindler WJ, Hutchins NO, Septimus EJ: Growth hormone secretion and control in the mouse. *Endocrinology* 91:483–490, 1972.

Schinitzky M, Inbar M: Microviscosity parameters and protein mobility in biological membrane. *Biochim Biophys Acta* 433:133–144, 1976.

Schlierf G, Dorow E: Diurnal patterns of triglycerides, free fatty acids, blood sugar, and insulin during carbohydrate-induction in man and their modification by nocturnal suppression of lipolysis. *J Clin Invest* 52:732–740, 1973.

Schwartz BH, Bianco AR, Handwerger BS, et al: Demonstration that monocytes rather than lymphocytes are the insulin-binding cells in preparations of human peripheral blood mononuclear leukocytes: implications for studies of insulin-resistant states in man. *Proc Natl Acad Sci USA* 72:474–478, 1975.

Schwartz E, Echemendia E, Schiffer M, et al: Mechanism of estrogenic action in acromegaly. *J Clin Invest* 48:260–270, 1969.

Schwarz EJ, Kovaleva IG, Rosenberg OA: Cholesterol content in lymphocytes in patients with Down's syndrome. Presented at the Third All-union Symposium: *Structure, Biosynthesis and Metabolism of Lipids in the Organisms of Animals and Human Beings*. Leningrad, Nauka, 1978, pp 146–147.

Segall PE, Timiras PC: Patho-physiologic finding after chronic tryptophan deficiency in rats: a model for delayed growth and aging. *Mech Ageing Dev* 5:109–124, 1976.

Seifter E, Rettura G, Demetrion AA, et al: Inhibition of murine sarcoma development by deoxycorticosterone acetate. *JNCI* 53:1809–1812, 1974.

Selye H, *The Story of the Adaptation Syndrome*. Montreal, Medical Publishers, 1952.

Selye H, Tuchweber B: Stress in relation to aging and disease, in Everitt AV, Burgess JA (eds): *Hypothalamus Pituitary and Aging*. Springfield, Ill, Charles C Thomas, 1976, pp 553–569.

Sever PS, Birch M, Osikowska B, et al: Plasma-noradrenaline in essential hypertension. *Lancet* 2:1078–1081, 1977.

Shafrir E, Gutman A: Patterns of decrease of free fatty acids during glucose tolerance tests. *Diabetes* 14:77–83, 1965.

Shagan BP: The diabetes: a model for aging. *Med Clin North Am* 60:1209–1211, 1976.

Shapiro AP: Essential hypertension—why idiopathic. *Am J Med* 54:1–6, 1973.

Shapot VS: Some biochemical aspects of relationship between tumor and the host. *Adv Cancer Res* 15:253–286, 1972.

Shapot VS: Isoenzymes and cancer *Mendeleev Chemistry Journal, USSR* 35:7–13, 1973.

Sharpe RM, Shahamanes HM: Influence of age and duration of treatment of the effects of testosterone on serum and pituitary follicle-stimulating hormone levels in male rats. *J Endocrinol* 63:571–578, 1974.

Sheehan HL: Neurohypophysis and hypothalamus, in Bloodworth JMB (ed): *Endocrine Pathology*. Baltimore, Williams and Wilkins, 1968, pp 12–74.

Sherman RM, West JH, Korenman SG: The menopause transition: analysis of LH, FSH, estradiol and progesterone concentration during menstrual cycles of older women. *J Clin Endocrinol Metab* 42:629–636, 1976.

Sherwin RS, Insel PA, Tobin JD, et al: Computer modeling: an aid to understanding insulin action. *Diabetes* 21(suppl):347, 1972, abst.

Shin SH, Howitt, CJ, Milligan JV: A paradoxical castration effect on LH-RH levels in male rat hypothalamus and serum. *Life Sci* 14:2491–2496, 1974.

Shock NW: Ageing of homeostatic mechanisms, in Lansing AI (ed):

Cowdry's Problems of Aging. Baltimore, Williams and Wilkins, 1952, pp 415–446.

Shock NW: System integration, in Finch CE, Hayflick L (eds): *Handbook of the Biology of Aging*. New York, Van Nostrand Reinhold Company, 1977, pp 639–665.

Sims EAH, Horton ES: Endocrine and metabolic adaptation to obesity and starvation. *Am J Clin Nutr* 2:1455–1470, 1968.

Singhal SK, Roder JC, Duwl AK: Suppressor cells in immunosenescence. *Fed Proc* 37:1245–1252, 1978.

Sinha AK, Shattil SJ, Colmân RW: Cyclic AMP metabolism in cholesterol rich patients. *J Biol Chem* 252:3310–3314, 1977.

Siperstein MD: Feedback control of cholesterol synthesis in normal, malignant and premalignant tissues. *Canadian Cancer Conf* 7:152–162, 1967.

Siperstein MD, Fagan VM, Morris HP: Further studies on the depletion of the cholesterol feedback system in hepatomas. *Cancer Res* 26:1–7, 1966.

Sirtori CR, Catapano A, Ghiselli GC, et al: Metformin: an antiatherosclerotic agent modifying very low density lipoproteins in rabbits. *Atherosclerosis* 26:79–89, 1977a.

Sirtori CR, Tremoli E, Sirtori M, et al: Treatment of hypertriglyceridemia with metformin. *Atherosclerosis* 26:583–592, 1977b.

Sizonenko PC, Pannicz L: Hormonal changes in puberty. III. Correlation of plasma dehydroepiandrosterone, testosterone, FSH, and LH with stages of puberty and bone age in normal boys and girls and in patients with Addison's disease or hypogonadism or with premature or late adrenarche. *J Clin Endocrinol Metab* 41:894–904, 1975.

Sjöström L: Adult human adipose tissue cellularity and metabolism. *Acta Med Scand* 544:1–52, 1972.

Sjöström L: Carbohydrate-stimulated fatty acid synthesis de novo in human adipose tissue of different cellular types. *Acta Med Scand* 194:387–404, 1973.

Smelik E, Papoikonamon E: Steroid feedback mechanisms in pituitary-adrenal function. *Prog Brain Res* 39:99–109, 1973.

Smith ER, Slater RS: Relationship between low-density lipoprotein in aortic intima and serum levels. *Lancet* 1:463–469, 1972.

Smith IE, Fitzharris BM, McKinna JA, et al: Aminoglutethimide in treatment of metastatic breast cancer. *Cancer* 2:646–649, 1978.

Smith II, Stuart AE: Effect of simple lipids on macrophages in vitro. *J Pathol* 115: 13–16, 1975.

Smith MA, Evans T, Steel CH: Age-related variation in proportion of circulating T-cells. *Lancet* 2:922–924, 1974.

Smith MJ, Hall MRP: Carbohydrate tolerance in the very aged. *Diabetologia* 9:387–390, 1973.

Smith OW, Emerson K: Urinary estrogens and related compounds in postmenopausal women with mammary cancer: effect of cortisone treatment. *Proc Soc Exp Biol Med* 85:264–267, 1954.

Smythe GA: The role of serotonin and dopamine in hypothalamo-pituitary function. *Clin Endocrol* 7:325–342, 1977.

Smythe GA, Lazarus L: Suppression of human growth hormone secretion by melatonin and cyproheptadine. *J Clin Invest* 54:116–121, 1974.

Smythe GA, Stuart MC, Lazarus L: Stimulation and suppression of somatomedin activity by serotonin and melatonin. *Experientia* 30:1356–1358, 1974.

Sobine JR: Metabolic control in precancerous liver. Time course of loss of dietary feedback control of cholesterol synthesis during carcinogen treatment. *Eur J Cancer* 12:299–304, 1976.

Sodhi HS, Kudchodkar BJ: Synthesis of cholesterol in hypercholesterolemia and its relationship to plasma triglycerides. *Metabolism* 22:895-912, 1973.

Solomon GF, Amkraut AA, Kasper Ph: Immunity, emotions and stress, with special reference to the mechanisms of stress effects on the immune system. *Psychother Psychosom* 23:209-228, 1974.

Sommers SC, Teloh HA: Ovarian stromal hyperplasia in breast cancer. *Arch Pathol* 53:160-166, 1952.

Sonenberg M, Money WL: Inhibition of pituitary hormone activity with derivatives of pituitary preparations. *Endocrinology* 61:12-29, 1957.

Sonenberg M, Dellacha JM, Free CA, et al: Growth hormone activity in man of chymotryptic digests of bovine growth hormone. *J Endocrinol* 44:255-265, 1969.

Sönksen PH, Srivastava MC, Tompkins CV, et al: Growth hormone and cortisol response to insulin infusion in patients with diabetes mellitus. *Lancet* 2:155-159, 1972.

Sönksen PH, Soeldner JS, Gleasson PE, et al: Abnormal serum growth hormone response in genetically potential male patients with normal oral glucose tolerance: evidence for insulin-like action of growth hormone in vivo. *Diabetologia* 9:426-437, 1973.

Spector A: Fatty acid metabolism in tumors, in Carrol KK (ed): *Progress in Biochemical Pharmacology. Lipids and Tumors.* Basel, S Karger, 1975, pp 43-75.

Spellacy WN, Buhi WC, Birk SA: The effect of estrogens on carbohydrate metabolism. *Am J Obstet Gynecol* 114:378-392, 1972.

Stamler J, Berkson DM, Lindberg HA, et al: Does hypercholesterolemia increase the risk of lung cancer in cigarette smokers? *Circulation* 38(suppl):188, 1968, abst.

Steelman SL, Pohley FM: Assay of follicle-stimulating hormone based on augmentation with human chorionic gonadotropin. *Endocrinology* 53:604-616, 1953.

Stein V, Stein O: Cholesterol removal in isolated cells and in tissue culture. *Triangle* 15:63-69, 1976.

Stephan T, Khurana RC, Nolan S, et al: Growth hormone levels in chemical diabetes. *J Am Geriatr Soc* 21:481-485, 1973.

Stoll BA: Breast cancer and hypothyroidism. *Cancer* 18:1431-1436, 1965.

Stoll BA: Brain catecholamines and breast cancer: a hypothesis. *Lancet* 1:431, 1972.

Stoll BA: Psychoendocrine factors and breast cancer growth, in Stoll BA (ed): *Mammary Cancer and Neuroendocrine Therapy.* London, Butterworth and Co, 1974, pp 401-412.

Stoll BA: Psychosomatic factors and tumor growth, in Stoll BA (ed): *Risk Factors in Breast Cancer,* vol 2. Chicago, William Heinemann Medical Books, 1976, pp 193-203.

Stout RW: Insulin-stimulated lipogenesis in arterial tissues in relation to diabetes and atheroma. *Lancet* 2:702-703, 1968.

Stout RW: The relationship of abnormal circulating insulin levels to atherosclerosis. *Atherosclerosis* 27:1-13, 1977.

Stout RW, Brunzell, JD, Porte D, et al: Effect of phenformin on lipid transport in hypertrigylceridemia. *Metabolism* 23:815-828, 1974.

Streeten DHP, Gerstein MM, Marmor BM, et al: Reduced glucose tolerance in elderly human subjects. *Diabetes* 14:579-583, 1965.

Strelkauskas AJ, Davies IJ, Drag S: Longitudinal studies showing alternations in the levels and functional response of T and B lymphocytes in human pregnancy. *Clin Exp Immunol* 32:531-539, 1978.

Strom TB, Bear RA: Insulin-induced augmentation of lymphocyte-mediated cytotoxity. *Science* 187:1206–1208, 1975.

Stumpe KD, Kolloch R, Higuch M, et al: Hyperprolactinaemia and antihypertensive effect of bromcriptine in essential hypertension. Identification of abnormal central dopamine control. *Lancet* 2:211–214, 1977.

Stutman O: Lymphocyte subpopulations in NZB mice: deficit of thymus-dependent lymphocytes. *J Immunol* 109:602–611, 1972.

Sukkar MJ, Hunter WM, Passmore R: Changes in plasma levels of insulin and growth hormone levels after a protein meal. *Lancet* 2:1020–1022, 1967.

Sutherland HW: On the biological role of cyclic AMP. *JAMA* 214:1281–1288, 1970.

Sutherland HW, Fisher PM, Stowers JM: Evaluation in the maternal carbohydrate metabolism by the venous glucose tolerance test in early life, in Camerini-Davolos RA, Cole HS (eds): *Early Diabetes*. New York, Academic Press, 1975, pp 365–371.

Synder F, Blank ML, Morris HP: Occurrence and nature of O-alkyl and O-alk-1-enyl moieties of glycerol in lipids of Morris transplanted hepatomas and normal rat liver. *Biochim Biophys Acta* 176:502–510, 1969.

Szepsenwol J: Carcinogenic effect of cholesterol in mice. *Proc Soc Exp Biol Med* 121:168–171, 1966.

Szilard L: On the nature of the aging process. *Proc Natl Acad Sci USA* 45:30–45, 1959.

Taggart NR, Holliday RM, Billiwicz WZ, et al: Changes in skinfolds during pregnancy. *Br J Nutr* 21:439–451, 1967.

Tajic M, Longhino N: Urinary gonadotropin values in healthy individuals. *Gynecol Invest* 165:333–337, 1968.

Takahashi S, Kondo H, Yoshimura M, et al: Growth hormone responses to administration of L-5-hydroxytryptophan in manic-depressive psychoses. *Folia Psychiatr Neurol Jpn* 27:197–206, 1973.

Takenchi N, Jamamura J, Katayama Y, et al: Impairment of feedback control and induction of cholesterol synthesis in rats by aging. *Exp Gerontol* 11:121–126, 1976.

Taleisnik S, Celis ME: Control of melanocyte-stimulating hormone secretion. *Excerpta Medica* (ICS) 273:100–105, 1973.

Talwar GP, Sharma NC, Dubey SK, et al: Isoimmunization against HCG with conjugates of processed β-subunit of the hormone and tetanus toxoid. *Proc Natl Acad Sci USA* 73:218–222, 1976.

Tannenbaum A: Nutrition and cancer, in Homburger F (ed): *The Physiopathology of Cancer*. New York, Hoeber-Harper, 1959, pp 519–562.

Tanner JM: *Foetus into Man. Physical Growth from Conception to Maturity*, Cambridge, Harvard University Press, 1978.

Tanner JM: Events in the interaction between the environment and the genetic potential during the growth of the child are critical to the health of the adult. *Sci Am* 229:35–43, 1973.

Tapp E, Blumfield M: The weight of the pineal gland in maliganancy. *Br J Cancer* 24:67–70, 1970.

Tasca C, Damian E, Stefaneanu L: Disappearance of aortic lesions in the rabbits with experimental atheromatosis after pineal extraction administration. *Rev Roum d'Endocr* 11:209–13, 1974.

Tavadia HB, Fleming KA, Hume PD, et al: Circadian rhythmicity of human plasma cortisol and PHA-induced lymphocyte transformation. *Clin Exp Immunol* 22:190–193, 1975.

Tchobroutsky G: Plasma growth hormone after lunch in diabetics and nondiabetics. *Acta Endocrol* 74:67–68, 1973.

Teasdale C, Thatcher J, Whitehead RH, et al: Age dependence of T-lymphocytes. *Lancet* 1:1410, 1976.

Telegdy G, Vermes I: Effect of adrenocortical hormones on activity of the serotoninergic system in limbic structures in rats. *Neuroendocrinology* 18:16–26, 1975.

Temin HM: Control of cell multiplication in uninfected chicken cells and chicken cells converted by avian sarcoma viruses. *J Cell Physiol* 74:9–16, 1969.

Timiras PS: Aging of homeostatic control systems. *Fed Proc* 34:81–82, 1975.

Tomatis L, Turusov V, Day N, et al: The effect of long-term exposure to DDT on CF-1 mice. *Int J Cancer* 10:489–506, 1972.

Toyoshima S, Osawa T: Lectins from *Wistaria floribunda* seeds and their effect on membrane fluidity of human peripheral lymphocytes. *J Biol Chem* 250:1655–1660, 1975.

Toyoshima S, Osawa T: Cholesterol inhibition of the temporary increase of membrane fluidity of lymphocytes induced by mitogenic lectins. *Exp Cell Res* 102:438–441, 1976.

Truswell AS: Diet and plasma lipids: a reappraisal. *Am J Clin Nutr* 31:977–989, 1978.

Trygstad O: A purified human LMF with hyperglycemic activity. *Acta Endocrinol* 58:277–294, 1968.

Turnell RW, Clarke LH, Burton AF: Studies on the mechanism of corticosteroid-induced lymphocytolysis. *Cancer Res* 33:203–212, 1973.

Tzagournis M, Seidensticker JF, Hamwi GJ: Metabolic abnormalities in premature coronary disease: effect of therapy. *Ann NY Acad Sci* 148:945–957, 1968.

Tzagournis M, Chiles R, Herrold Y, et al: The role of endogenous insulin in different hyperlipemic states. *Diabetologia* 8:215–220, 1972.

Tzagournis M, George J, Herrold J: Increased growth hormone in partial and total lipoatrophy. *Diabetes* 22:388–396, 1973.

Ullenbrock JTJ: Effect of ovariectomy and subsequent estrogen treatment on serum luteinizing hormone in androgen sterilized rats. *J Endocrinol* 57, 1973, abst.

Unger RH, Orci L: The essential role of glucagon in the pathogenesis of diabetes mellitus. *Lancet* 1:14–16, 1975.

Vanhaelst L, Golstenin J, Smets Ph, et al: Asymptomatic autoimmune thyroiditis and coronary heart disease. *Lancet* 2:155–158, 1977.

Vanha-Pertulla TP, Hapsu VK: High incidence of malignancies in persistent-estrous rats. *Acta Pathol Microbiol Scand* 64:286–288, 1965.

van Look FH, Lothian H, Hunter WM, et al: Hypothalamic-pituitary-ovarian function in perimenopausal women. *Clin Endocrinol* 7:13–32, 1977.

Vasiljeva IA, Dilman VM: Insulin sensitivity in patients with cancer of colon, lung, and body uteri. *Vopr Onkol* 19:35–38, 1973.

Vekemans M, Robyn C: Influence of age on serum prolactin levels in women and men. *Br Med J* 4:738–739, 1975.

Vermes JJ, Telegdy K, Lissak K: Correlation between hypothalamic serotonin content and adrenal function during acute stress. Effect of adrenal corticosteroids on hypothalamic serotonin content. *Acta Physiol Acad Sci Hung* 43:33–42, 1973.

Vermeulen A, Verdonck L: Sex hormone concentrations in post-menopausal woman. Relation to obesity, fat mass, age and years postmenopause. *Clin Endocrol* 9:59–66, 1978.

Vermeulen A, Rulens R, Verdonck L: Testosterone secretion and metabolism in male senescence. *J Clin Endocrinol Metab* 34:730–735, 1972.

Verzár F: *Lectures on Experimental Gerontology*. Springfield, Ill, Charles C Thomas, 1953.

Verzár F: Aging of connective tissue. *Gerontology* 1:363–370, 1957.

Vigneri R, Squatrio S, Motta L, et al: Regulation of growth hormone: attempt at a comprehensive interpretation. *Acta Diabetol Lat* 10:91–108, 1973.

Vilenchik, MM: *Specific Molecular Genetic Effect of Chemical Carcinogens*. Moscow, Nauka, 1977.

Vinik AI, Jackson WPU: Diabetes in the elderly. Is it a disease? *Excerpta Medica* (ICS) 140:195, 1967, abst.

Vishnevsky AS, Dilman VM: Varying influence of estrogens and preparations suppressing ovulation on the carbohydrate tolerance. *Akush Ginekol* 7:59–61, 1972.

Vishnevsky AS, Dilman VM, Krylova NV, et al: Effect of elipten on gonadotropins and phenolsteroids excretion. *Vopr Onkol* 15:94–95, 1969.

Vogelberg KH: Die Kombination von Clofibrate und Phenformin in der Behandlung endogener Hypertriglyceridaemien. *Dtsch Med Wochenschr* 101:1868–1871, 1976.

Vorontsov IM, Zinevich LM, Andresen VP, et al: Some peculiar processes of acceleration and hematological shifts. *Pediatria* 12:40–44, 1973.

Waddell CC, Taunton OD, Twomly JJ: Inhibition of lymphoproliferation by hyperlipoproteinemic plasma. *J Clin Invest* 58:950–954, 1976.

Wahlberg F: The intravenous glucose tolerance test in atherosclerotic disease with special reference to obesity, hypertension, diabetic heredity and cholesterol values. *Acta Med Scand* 171:1–8, 1962.

Wahlqvist ML, Kaijser L, Lassers VW, et al: Fatty acid as a determinant of myocardial substrate and oxygen metabolism in men. *Acta Med Scand* 113:89–96, 1973.

Waldorf DS, Willkens RF, Decker JL: Impaired delayed hypersensitivity in an aging population. *JAMA* 203:831–834, 1968.

Walford RL: *The Immunologic Theory of Aging*. Copenhagen, Munksgaard, 1969.

Walford RL: An immunologic theory of aging: current status. *Fed Proc* 33:2020–2027, 1974.

Walker RF, McMahon KM, Pivorun EB: Pineal gland structure and respiration as affected by age and hypocaloric diet. *Exp Gerontol* 13:91–99, 1978.

Walker WJ: Success story: the program against major cardiovascular risk factors. *Geriatrics* 1:97–109, 1976.

Way S: *Malignant Disease of the Female Genital Tract*. London, Churchill, 1951.

Weber G, Convery HJH, Lea MA, et al: Feedback inhibition of key glycolytic enzymes in liver: action of free fatty acids. *Science* 154:1357–1360, 1966.

Weil R: Pituitary growth hormone and intermediary metabolism. *Acta Endocrinol* 98(49 suppl):1–92, 1965.

Weiss G, Schmidt C, Kleinbery DL, et al: Positive feedback of oestrogen or LH secretion in women on neuroleptic drugs. *Clin Endocrinol* 6:423–427, 1977.

Weiss NS: Relationship of menopause to serum cholesterol and arterial blood pressure. *Am J Epidemiol* 46:237–241, 1972.

Welborn TA, Brockenridge A, Rubinstein AH, et al: Serum-insulin in essential hypertension and in peripheral vascular disease. *Lancet* 1:1336–1337, 1966.

Welborn TA, Stenhouse NS, Johnstone CG: Factors determining serum-insulin response in a population sample. *Diabetologia* 5:263–266, 1969.

Werner W: Diabetes mellitus und carcinom. Statistische untersuchungen anhand von 25147 Sektionsfällen. *Z Krebsforsch* 60:399–407, 1955.

Wertelecki W, Mantel N: Increased birth weight in leukemia. *Pediatr Res* 7:132–138, 1973.

Westerman MP: Hypocholesterolaemia and anaemia. *Br J Haematol* 31:87–99, 1975.

Wexler BC: Spontaneous arteriosclerosis in repeatedly bred male and female rats. *Atherosclerosis* 4:57–80, 1964.

Wexler BC: Comparative aspects of hyperadrenocorticism and arteriosclerosis. *Hum Pathol* 2:180–181, 1971.

Wexler BC: Comparative aspects of hyperadrenocorticism and aging, in Everitt AV, Burgess JA (eds): *Hypothalamus Pituitary and Aging*. Springfield, Ill, Charles C Thomas, 1976, pp 333–361.

Wexler BC, Kittinger GW: Adrenocortical function in arteriosclerotic female breeder rats. *Atherosclerosis* 5:317–329, 1965.

Wexler BC, Lutmer RF: ACTH content of pituitary glands of arteriosclerotic breeder vs non-arteriosclerotic virgin rats. *Atherosclerosis* 22:199–214, 1975.

Whittingham S, Pitt DB, Sharma DLB, et al: Stress deficiency of the T-lymphocyte system exemplified by Down syndrome. *Lancet* 1:163–166, 1977.

Whyte A: Human chorionic gonadotropin and trophoblast antigenicity. *Lancet* 2:1003, 1978.

Wiedemann E, Schwartz E: Suppression of growth hormone-dependent human serum sulfation factor by estrogen. *J Clin Endocrinol Metab* 34:51–58, 1972.

Wilansky DL, Hahn I: Modification of latent diabetes by short term phenformin administration. *Metabolism* 16:199–203, 1967.

Wilkins L, Bongiovanni AM, Clayton GW, et al: Virilising adrenal hyperplasia: its treatment with cortisone and the nature of the steroid abnormalities, in Wolstenholme GEW, Cameron MP (eds): *Ciba Foundation Colloquia on Endocrinology,* vol 8. London, Churchill Ltd, 1955, pp 460–481.

Williams P, Robinson D, Bailey A: High-density lipoprotein and coronary risk factors in normal men. *Lancet* 1:72–75, 1979.

Williams RH: *Diabetes.* New York, Paul B Hoeber Inc, 1960.

Wilson RA: The roles of estrogen and progesterone in breast and genital cancer. *JAMA* 182:327-331, 1962.

Wilson RG, Singhal VK, Perry-Robb I, et al: Response of plasma prolactin and growth hormone to insulin hypoglycemia. *Lancet* 2:1283–1285, 1972.

Wirz-Justice A, Hackmann E, Lichtsteiner M: The effect of oestradiol dipropionate and progesterone on monoamine uptake in rat brain. *J Neurochem* 22:187–189, 1974.

Wise AJ, Gross MA, Schalch DS: Quantitative relationship of the pituitary gonadal axis in postmenopausal women. *J Lab Clin Med* 81:28–36, 1973.

Wood PD, Haskell W, Klin H, et al: The distribution of plasma lipoproteins in middle-aged male runners. *Metabolism* 25:1249–1257, 1976.

Woods SC, Porte D: The central nervous system, pancreatic hormones, feeding and obesity, in Levine R, Luft R (eds): *Advances in Metabolic Disorders,* vol 4. New York, Academic Press, 1978, pp 283–312.

World Health Statistics Annual, vol 1. Vital statistics and cause of death. Geneva, World Health Organization, 1967.

Wurtman RJ: The pineal gland: endocrine interrelationships. *Adv Intern Med* 16:155–169, 1970.

Wurtman RJ: The effect of light on the human body. *Sci Am* 233:68–79, 1975.

Wurtman RJ, Fernstrom JD: Control of brain neurotransmitter synthesis by precursor availability and nutritional state. *Biochem Pharmacol* 25:1961–1966, 1976.

Wybran J, Fudenberg HH: Human thymus-derived rosette-forming cells: their role in immunocompetence and immunosurveillance, in Williams RC (ed): *Lymphocytes and their Interactions.* New York, Raven Press, 1975, pp 113–132.

Wyle FA, Kent JR: Immunosuppression by sex steroids hormones. I. The effect upon PHA and PPD stimulated lymphocytes. *Clin Exp Immunol* 27:407–415, 1977.

Wynder EL: Nutrition and cancer. *Proc Soc Exp Biol Med* 35:1309–1315, 1976.

Wynn V, Doar WH: Some effects of oral contraceptives on carbohydrate metabolism. *Lancet* 2:761–768, 1969.

Yadley RA, Rodbard D, Chrambach A: Isohormones of human growth hormone. III. Isolation by preparative polyacrylamide gel electrophoresis and characterization. *Endocrinology* 94:866–873, 1973.

Yalow RS, Berson SA: Secretory responses of human growth hormone and ACTH in diabetic and non-diabetic subjects. *Diabetes* ICS No. 231:741–756, 1971.

Yalow RS, Goldsmith SJ, Berson SA: Influence of physiologic fluctuations in plasma growth hormone on glucose tolerance. *Diabetes* 18:402–408, 1969.

Yamamoto WS: Homeostasis continuity and feedback, in Yamamoto WS, Brobeck JR (eds): *Physiological Control and Regulations.* Philadelphia, WB Saunders, 1965, pp 14–31.

Yamamoto WS, Yamamura J: Changes of cholesterol metabolism in the aging rat. *Atherosclerosis* 13:365–374, 1971.

Yen SSC, Tsai, CC: The biphasic pattern in the feedback action of ethinyl estradiol on the release of pituitary FSH and LH. *J Clin Endocrinol* 33:882–887, 1971.

Yevtushenko TP, Bobrov YF: Age-dependent hypothalamo-pituitary complex sensitivity to the inhibitory action of triiodothyronine. *Hum Physiol* 4:650–653, 1978.

Young FG: Insulin and the action of growth hormone. *Excerpta Medica* (ICS) No. 158, 1968, abst.

Zimmerman E, Critchlow V: Negative feedback and pituitary-adrenal function in female rats. *Am J Physiol* 216:148–155, 1969.

Zondek B: *Hormone des Ovariums und des Hypophysenvorderlappens.* Vienna, Springer-Verlag, 1935.

Zondek H, Leszynsky H, Wolfsohn G: Blutcholesterin bei Hypophysar-Diencephalen Erkrankungen. *Schweiz Med Wochenschr* 30:746–747, 1948.

Zor U, Lamprecht SA, Misulovin Z, et al: Refractoriness of ovarian adenylate cyclase to continued hormonal stimulation. *Biochim Biophys Acta* 428:761–765, 1976.

INDEX